Pediatric Urology

Warren T. Snodgrass
Editor

Pediatric Urology

Evidence for Optimal Patient Management

Springer

Editor
Warren T. Snodgrass
Department of Pediatric Urology
University of Texas Southwestern Medical Center
and Children's Medical Center Dallas
Dallas, TX, USA

ISBN 978-1-4614-6909-4 ISBN 978-1-4614-6910-0 (eBook)
DOI 10.1007/978-1-4614-6910-0
Springer New York Heidelberg Dordrecht London

Library of Congress Control Number: 2013934223

Printed on acid-free paper

Springer is part of Springer Science+Business Media (www.springer.com)

Preface

The primary aim of this book is to assemble data needed by clinicians in their daily decision making.

The format differs from usual textbooks in that it assumes a basic knowledge of pediatric urology and so is focused on pivotal clinical questions. Each chapter begins with a statement of the primary and secondary aims for the diagnosis and treatment of the condition, followed by a synopsis of the evidence we found for those aims. Information from the primary sources is summarized so that readers know how studies were done and reported.

To write the book an outline for each chapter was made including questions frequently encountered in diagnosis and management, and then broad-based computer searches were done to identify articles potentially answering them. We followed the general methodology of a guidelines panel to review materials and results for pertinent information to extract.

We gave greater emphasis to meta-analyses, such as Cochrane Reviews, RCTs, and prospective studies, as well as to well-done retrospective analyses with clearly defined objectives and well-described results. In the absence of these, useful information still could be obtained from primary sources that otherwise would not rate high in current evidence-based standards.

Why do this?

Numerous studies report wide variations in practice among pediatric urologists, despite the obvious truth that recommendations a patient receives should not be an accident of geography. One step towards greater consistency is summarizing the expected findings and outcomes from diagnostic and management options. Rather than base decisions on surgeon opinion and preference, this book facilitates rapid review of published data to guide treatment.

Study of the available evidence for most topics in this book also highlights need for multicenter cooperation to enroll sufficient patients in trials to answer important clinical questions. Most urologic conditions in children simply do not affect sufficient numbers of patients for single centers to perform high-quality studies. For example, no RCT proves benefit of antibiotic prophylaxis in children with either prenatally detected hydronephrosis or VUR, and several centers would need to pool their patients to power such a trial.

Management of various conditions by pediatric urologists has been challenged by outside specialties for focusing too much on surgical outcomes rather than benefits to the child. We are experts in correcting reflux, or predicting when it will spontaneously resolve, but pediatricians are asking which children need this expertise. A common theme throughout this book is that there is less evidence on health benefits from therapy than on surgical success rates. To that end, the book may also stimulate new avenues of research.

Writing this book has changed our own practice in many ways. When questions arise, for example, in preoperative conferences, we no longer ask each surgeon what he or she would do, but instead review available published information to narrow the options. Although we each trained in different centers and bring different perspectives to discussions, this process has reduced variations in our individual practice, with the additional benefits of simplifying on-call coverage, instructions to nurses, and fellow training. Studying the sometimes weak evidence on which clinical decision making is based has stimulated us to design better prospective trials, some in collaboration with other centers.

Here are three specific examples of changes made in our practices prompted by this book. We operate much less often on an "undescended" testis in boys older than 1 year, especially when records from the hospital and initial primary care provider indicate it was descended at birth, given the evidence cited in Chap. 5 that even specialists are sometimes fooled by retractile testes and most of those testes not in the scrotum after a normal newborn exam return to the scrotum during puberty. We no longer consider baseline renal function or diuretic washout times indications for pyeloplasty, since repair most often does not improve differential function and "obstructive" drainage curves do not predict future function loss. We now use results of semen analysis at age 17 to recommend varicocelectomy, since testicular size discrepancy does not appear to correlate with fertility potential.

Our work inevitably has similar shortcomings as textbooks. It is not possible to include every published study in a review, and while we tried to cast a broad net to identify articles and then extract the best data from them, we still could have overlooked a pertinent report. To minimize intrusion of our own opinions we emphasized summaries from the original sources, but it is difficult to be completely objective.

Nevertheless, we believe this book will be useful to pediatric urologists in training and at all stages of practice, and hope it helps to improve care for the children entrusted to us all.

The book is designed for use as a manual, and so studies are sometimes mentioned in several sections within a chapter. It was written over a 1.5-year period beginning in March 2011, with final editing completed in October 2012. An outline with specific clinical questions was used as a guide by authors, who then performed computer searches to identify articles containing information to answer those questions. After drafts were completed and edited, we met as a committee, repeating selected computer searches and reviewing and critiquing each chapter to finalize the manuscript.

Two authors have advanced degrees of relevance, one a Master's in Public Health and Epidemiology and the other a Master's in Clinical Studies. Nevertheless, the Editor bears final responsibility for the reporting in this book.

Dallas, TX, USA

Warren T. Snodgrass
Linda A. Baker
Nicol C. Bush
Patricio C. Gargollo
Micah A. Jacobs

Contents

Contributors

Linda A. Baker Department of Pediatric Urology, University of Texas Southwestern Medical Center and Children's Medical Center Dallas, Dallas, TX, USA

Nicol C. Bush Department of Pediatric Urology, University of Texas Southwestern Medical Center and Children's Medical Center Dallas, Dallas, TX, USA

Patricio C. Gargollo Department of Pediatric Urology, University of Texas Southwestern Medical Center and Children's Medical Center Dallas, Dallas, TX, USA

Micah A. Jacobs Department of Pediatric Urology, University of Texas Southwestern Medical Center and Children's Medical Center Dallas, Dallas, TX, USA

Warren T. Snodgrass Department of Pediatric Urology, University of Texas Southwestern Medical Center and Children's Medical Center Dallas, Dallas, TX, USA

Urinary Tract Infection

1

Warren T. Snodgrass and Nicol C. Bush

Primary goals in the diagnosis of urinary tract infection (UTI) and the subsequent evaluation of underlying factors predisposing to UTI:

1. **Reduce recurrent UTI.**
2. **Prevent acquired renal damage.**

Summary of evidence for these goals:

- **After first febrile UTI (fUTI), less than one-third of patients will develop a second fUTI within 1–2 years.**
- **Approximately 15 % of children will develop renal scarring after fUTI.**
- **Vesicoureteral reflux (VUR) increases risk for renal scarring by approximately 2.5 times, but no evidence demonstrates management reduces future acquired renal damage.**
- **Patients with negative DMSA after UTI have ≤5 % risk for future abnormal DMSA with recurrent UTI.**
- **Potential interventions to reduce risk for recurrent UTI include circumcision and therapy for voiding dysfunction and/or constipation. However, no RCT demonstrates circumcision after infection is more effective than the natural history of diminishing UTI occurrence in males. No RCTs have been reported concerning efficacy of therapy for voiding dysfunction or constipation to reduce UTI.**
- **Observations that renal scars occur in a minority of patients after fUTI, and that those without scarring on DMSA scan have <5 % risk for developing scars with recurrent UTI suggest there are two general populations of children—those with a greater versus a lesser risk for scarring.**

UTI occurs in approximately 8 % of children. While most have no discernible underlying etiology, and so their infections are presumed to reflect disturbed bacterial–host interaction, infection can indicate structural anomalies of the urinary tract, as well as functional bladder disturbances, or constipation. In the past, children with UTI, especially febrile infection, routinely underwent radiologic investigations, and those found to have anomalies, most often VUR, routinely had treatment. Several recent RCTs have called into question this paradigm, as reviewed below.

Diagnosis

The standard for diagnosis of UTI is greater than 10^5 cfu/mL of a pure bacterial growth on urine culture from a symptomatic patient.

2011 AAP guidelines recommend diagnosis based on ≥50,000 cfu/mL and a urinalysis that demonstrates pyuria and/or bacilluria.

Suprapubic aspiration is considered the gold standard to obtain urine samples with the

W.T. Snodgrass, M.D. (✉) • N.C. Bush, M.D., M.S.C.S.
Department of Pediatric Urology,
University of Texas Southwestern Medical Center
and Children's Medical Center Dallas,
1935 Medical District Drive, MS F4.04,
Dallas, TX 75235, USA
e-mail: warren.snodgrass@childrens.com

W.T. Snodgrass (ed.), *Pediatric Urology: Evidence for Optimal Patient Management*,
DOI 10.1007/978-1-4614-6910-0_1,

least risk for contamination in infants and non-toilet-trained children, but is not often performed. One study found catheterized specimens more accurate than voided samples in girls, but not in uncircumcised boys.

One retrospective analysis reported likelihood for true UTI was greatest in uncircumcised males with >10^5, and in females with >10^4 growth on catheterized specimens, with indeterminate probability at lower colony counts.

Urine gram stain, urine dipstick for leukocyte esterase (LE) and/or nitrite, and urine microscopy may be useful to increase or decrease suspicion for UTI during the 24- to 48-h delay needed for urine culture results.

Gram stain showing any bacteria in uncentrifuged urine best predicts UTI.

Nearly as reliable as gram stain is urine dipstick. UTI is very likely when both LE and nitrite are positive and very unlikely when both are negative, with intermediate reliability if only one of the tests is positive. Negative dipstick results are less reliable to exclude UTI in children <2 years of age.

Standard microscopy showing ≥5 WBCs per high power field is less reliable than gram stain or dipstick, except in children <2 years of age in which microscopy results are the same as dipstick.

Microscopy showing both pyuria and bacteria has similar accuracy to dipstick positive for LE and nitrite to rule in UTI.

Catheterized Versus Voided Specimens

Pure growth of 10^3 colony-forming units has been considered diagnostic for catheterized specimens, versus 10^5 for voided urine specimens (AAP guidelines 1999). The 2011 AAP guidelines recommend a minimum 50,000 cfu/mL in a specimen obtained by catheterization or suprapubic aspiration.

A prospective study compared clean catch versus catheterized urine specimens in 98 asymptomatic children <2 years (mean 6 months, SD 4.3) undergoing a voiding cystourethrogram (VCUG) after prior UTI ($n=71$) or in evaluation of prenatal HN ($n=27$). There were 82 males, all uncircumcised, and 16 females. All were receiving prophylactic antibiotics, and all obtained specimens were negative for WBCs and nitrite. Colony counts were greater in voided specimens in both boys and girls. However, if mixed bacterial colonies were considered evidence of contamination, catheterized and clean catch specimens showed similar false-positive rates regardless of a threshold of 10^3, 10^4, or 10^5. There was moderate agreement between clean catch versus catheterized specimens when comparing any bacterial growth to no growth in uncircumcised boys (Kappa 0.42) but poor agreement in girls (Kappa 0.18). In other words, a catheterized specimen in girls was more accurate than a voided specimen, but the same was not true in boys, implying catheterized specimens in uncircumcised boys are prone to contamination (Lau et al. 2007).

Colony Counts

A retrospective study compared results of urine obtained by catheterization in children 1- to 18-months old (median age 6 months). There were 952 samples, 492 (52 %) collected from uncircumcised boys and the remainder from girls. Of these, 435 (46 %) had bacterial growth that was pure in 352 (81 %) and mixed in 83. Patients were considered to have fUTI on the basis of positive LE and nitrite and WBCs by microscopy, and response to antibiotics. There were 212 patients diagnosed with fUTI, with 198 (93 %) having pure colony growth and 14 (7 %) with mixed growth. Another 740 patients did not have UTI, with 223 (30 %) having positive growth that was pure in 154 (69 %) and mixed in 69 (31 %). In uncircumcised boys, only colony counts >10^5 indicated high likelihood for UTI (LR20.2 [95 % CI 12.01–34.02]). In females, 10^4 to 10^5 colony counts had a likelihood ratio (LR) 8.95 (95 % CI 3.08–25.98). Lesser cfu/cc yielded indeterminate probability for true UTI, leading to the conclusion that catheter urine cultures have to be interpreted within the clinical context (Cheng and Wong 2005).

Gram Stain, Dipstick, and Microscopy

Meta-analysis was done on 26 articles published between 1966 and 1998 regarding rapid diagnostic testing for UTI in children:

- Gram stain demonstrating any bacteria in uncentrifuged urine was most accurate to predict UTI, with a positive LR of 18.5 and negative LR of 0.07.
- Dipstick had a positive LR of 12.6 when both LE and nitrites were positive, and a negative LR of 0.13 when both LE and nitrites were negative.
- Microscopy (>5 WBC/hpf in centrifuged urine) offered no advantage over dipstick with lower sensitivity and specificity.

Most of the tests were found to have significant heterogeneity among the included studies, depending, for example, on how stringent was the diagnosis of UTI and what age patients were evaluated (Gorelick and Shaw 1999).

Another meta-analysis reviewed search databases from their inception until 2004, finding 70 for inclusion concerning rapid testing to diagnose UTI in children under 5 years of age.

- UTI was likely when dipstick was LE and nitrite positive (pooled LR 28.2 [95 % CI 17.3–46.0]) or microscopy was positive for both WBC and bacteria (pooled LR 37.0 [95 % CI 11.0–125.9]).
- UTI was ruled out when dipstick was negative for both LE and nitrite (pooled LR 0.20 [95 % CI 0.16–0.26])
- Microscopy was negative for both WBC and bacteria (pooled LR 0.11 [95 % CI 0.05–0.23]). Definition of pyuria and bacteriuria on microscopy was not stated (Whiting et al. 2005).

A third meta-analysis reviewed published articles from 1966 to 2009 for studies comparing dipstick to microscopy in infants versus older children. A total of six met inclusion criteria, finding the following:

- Dipstick was useful to rule in bacteriuria when both LE and nitrites were positive (LR 38.54 [95 % CI 22.49–65.31]), and useful to rule out bacteriuria when both were negative (LR 0.13 [95 % CI 0.07–0.25]). Reliability of dipstick to predict likelihood for UTI was reduced when dipstick was only LE- or nitrite-positive.
- Dipstick was significantly less reliable in children <2 years versus older children
- Dipstick was more reliable to make a rapid diagnosis of UTI than standard microscopy (>5 WBC/hpf in centrifuged urine) in children >2 years of age and the tests were nearly equivalent in patients <2 years.

Given the small number of studies, the authors stated results should be interpreted with caution, and it was not clear why tests had variable results by age (Mori et al. 2009).

Pyelonephritis Versus Febrile UTI

Febrile UTI refers to urinary infection associated with fever ≥38 °C, whereas pyelonephritis specifically refers to renal inflammation.

Acute DMSA scintigraphy demonstrates that only approximately 50 % of fUTIs show radiologic evidence of renal parenchymal inflammation.

Follow-up (late) DMSA scintigraphy indicates renal scars do not develop in patients with negative acute scans, and are found in 15–38 % of children with positive acute scans in the region of prior inflammation.

The minimum time after acute infection needed for inflammation to resolve so that late DMSA scintigraphy demonstrates permanent renal damage is unknown.

As part of a prospective trial, 309 children 1–24 months of age with first known fUTI had acute DMSA scintigraphy within 48 h of diagnosis. Of these, 190 (61 %) were positive, demonstrating renal inflammation that involved a mean of 31 % of renal parenchyma. Repeat DMSA scintigraphy was obtained in 275 (89 %) patients 6 months later. All those with negative acute scans had negative follow-up scans, while 26 (15 %) of 173 whose initial scan was positive had apparent scar formation that involved a mean of 8 % of renal parenchyma (Hoberman et al. 2003).

Another prospective study of first symptomatic UTI in term neonates ≤28 days of age also performed acute DMSA scintigraphy (≤72 h of diagnosis) and late DMSA scintigraphy at 6 months. Results in 72 patients were reported per renal unit: 27 (19 %) of 144 kidneys demonstrated apparent parenchymal inflammation, of which 10 had presumed renal scar on the 6 months follow-up scan. No patient with an initially normal scan had an abnormal late scan, while 10 (37 %) of those with positive acute scans had presumed scar on the 6-month scan (Siomou et al. 2009).

A third prospective study of DMSA scintigraphy after first fUTI in 105 children a mean of 5.9±4.7 years of age found 37 (35 %) patients had acute parenchyma lesions. Follow-up DMSA scans were then done at 6 and 12 months in those with positive acute studies. Of the 37 children, 3 were excluded for recurrent infection, leaving 34 undergoing repeat DMSA at 6 months, of which 13 (38 %) continued to show renal defects. These 13 children then had a final DMSA scan at 12 months, with only 6 (18 %) still having a defect (Agras et al. 2007).

Fifty children with positive DMSA scintigraphy 6 months after first fUTI responded to a letter 3 years later inviting study participation for a second DMSA evaluation. There were 30 females, and patient age was 0–18 years, with 24 (48 %) less than 2 years of age at time of first DMSA study. Comparison of the two DMSA scans was done by three blinded observers, reporting that of the 88 initial defects, there was no change in lesion in 24 (27 %), partial resolution in 56 (63 %), and complete resolution in 8 (9 %) (Parvex et al. 2008).

Incidence

Approximately 2 % of males and 8 % of females will develop UTI.

Most UTIs in males occur at ≤3 months of age. Prevalence is 10 times less in circumcised versus uncircumcised males at this age, and the likelihood for infection decreases rapidly thereafter in both circumcised and uncircumcised infants.

First UTIs occur most often during infancy, comprising 75 % of UTIs in males and 50 % in females. After 1 year of age, most UTIs occur in females.

Meta-analysis of articles published from 1950 to 2009 reporting prevalence data for UTI in symptomatic children (fever and/or urinary tract symptoms) 0–19 years of age indicated the following:

- Prevalence of UTI in febrile infants <2 years old was 7 % (CI 5.5–8.4). Most boys were less than 3 months of age with declining likelihood of UTI thereafter, while most UTIs in females occurred within the first year of life.
- Prevalence in febrile circumcised boys less than 3 months was 2.4 % (95 % CI 1.4–3.5) versus 20.1 % (95 % CI 16.8–23.4) in uncircumcised boys. Only one study reported prevalence of fUTI in circumcised versus uncircumcised boys 6–12 months, finding 0.3 % versus 7.3 %, respectively. No data regarding prevalence after 12 months were found.
- Prevalence in children 2–19 years was 7.8 % (95 % CI 6.6–8.9), which combined both febrile and afebrile infections (Shaikh et al. 2010).

A prospective study of first symptomatic infections in 304 consecutive children (169 boys) less than 5 years of age presenting to the emergency department of a pediatric hospital found 64 % were <1 year old, comprising 75 % of infections in males and 50 % in females (Craig et al. 1998).

Similarly, another prospective report of 209 consecutive children (77 boys) with first known symptomatic UTI presenting to the emergency department found 58 % occurred at age <1 year, and 75 % by age 2 years (Ismaili et al. 2011).

Retrospective review was done of consecutive infants born in 1996 in 12 facilities of the Kaiser Permanente Medical Care Program of Northern California, comprising 28,812 infants (52 % males). Diagnosis of UTI over the following 12 months of life was determined from computerized databases using ICD-9 codes, reporting the following:

- 446 (1.5 %) had UTI; 2 % uncircumcised males, 0.2 % in circumcised males, 2 % in females.

- Mean age at hospitalization for UTI was 2.5 months in uncircumcised males.
- Mean age at hospitalization for UTI was 6.5 months in females (Schoen et al. 2000).

Recurrent UTI After Initial Infection

Less than one-third of patients with or without VUR evaluated after a first fUTI will have a second fUTI within 1–2 years.

Of those with recurrent infection, most will have a single recurrence with less than 10 % of patients with or without VUR having three or more recurrences within 1–2 years.

Recurrence rates are not significantly different in males versus females.

Even though need and efficacy of antibiotic prophylaxis relate to risk for recurrent infection, likelihood for recurrent UTI after first known infection has not been widely reported.

A retrospective analysis of 262 children admitted to hospital for therapy of their first known UTI and then followed with monthly surveillance urine cultures for 2 years found a subsequent positive culture in 33 %, evenly distributed by gender (all boys were uncircumcised). Of these, 71 % were symptomatic infections, while the remainder were diagnosed by scheduled urine culture in asymptomatic children; 61 % recurred within 3 months, and 92 % by 1 year, of the initial infection. During 3 years' follow-up in the 88 children with recurrent UTI, 48 (54 %) had only one recurrence, and another 25 (28 %) had only two. Patients with obstructive or neuropathic uropathies were excluded from the study. VCUG was performed in 121 (46 %) patients after first UTI, and analysis excluded the seven patients prescribed antibiotic prophylaxis. VUR grades 3–5 were found a risk factor for recurrence versus grades 1–2 and no VUR (Nuutinen and Uhari 2001).

A review of electronic medical records from 27 primary care pediatricians within a common network also evaluated recurrent infection after first known UTI. A cohort of 611 children was assembled, of which 83 (14 %) had subsequent infection (0.12 per person-year after first UTI), a rate the authors noted was lower than in studies including asymptomatic bacilluria detected by surveillance cultures, which were not done in these patients. Risk factors for recurrence included white race (multivariable HR 1.97 [95 % CI 1.22–3.16]), age 2–6 years (HR 2.01 [95 % CI 1.20–3.37]), and VUR grades 4–5 (HR 4.38 [95 % CI 1.26–15.29]), but not gender, no VCUG, or grades 1–3 reflux. VCUG was not performed in 400 (65.5 %) after initial UTI (Conway et al. 2007).

A study of 290 children less than 5 years of age presenting with first UTI included imaging with renal ultrasonography and VCUG, with antibiotic prophylaxis prescribed to the 29 % with VUR and the 1 % with obstructive uropathy. Recurrent UTI developed in 34 (12 %) children within 12 months. These recurrences were associated with age <6 months at initial diagnosis (OR 2.9 [95 % CI 1.4–6.2]) and VUR grades 3–5 (OR 3.6 [95 % CI 1.5–8.3]), but not with gender (OR 1.5 [95 % CI 1–2.2]) (Panaretto et al. 1999).

Data regarding recurrent UTI can also be extracted from several prospective RCTs comparing antibiotic prophylaxis to no antibiotic therapy in patients with and without reflux (Table 1.1). In those studies in which all patients had VUR, at least one recurrent fUTI occurred in from 16 to 37 % of patients followed for 18–24 months (Pennesi et al. 2009; Roussey-Kesler et al. 2008; Brandstrom et al. 2010). Lower rates of recurrent fUTI ranging from 2.5 to 13 % were noted in three other studies, in which approximately half the patients had reflux and there was shorter follow-up of 1 year (Garin et al. 2006; Montini et al. 2009; Craig et al., 2009). Most patients with recurrent UTI had only a single episode, with only 6 % having three or more recurrent fUTIs (Pennesi et al. 2009; Craig et al. 2009).

Data collected in 740 consecutive patients with VUR between 1970 and 2008, who were all prescribed antibiotic prophylaxis with either trimethroprim or nitrofurantoin, found recurrent UTI during 58,856 person-months in 278 (38 %) children. This equated to 8.4 episodes of UTI per 1,000 person-months (95 % CI 7.7–9.2). Of patients with recurrent UTI, 21 % had a single recurrence, 10 % had two, and 7 %

Table 1.1 Recurrent UTI in patients on no antibiotic prophylaxis after UTI

Author	Study type	Patients		Source patients	Age patients	Duration f/u	Recurrent fUTI	
		VUR⊕ (grade)	VUR–		(mean or median)		VUR ⊕	VUR–
Series of patients ± VUR								
Garin 2006	RCT	58 (1–3)	60	fUTI, Excluded VUR g 4,5	3 month–18 year (2 year)	1 year	1 (1.7 %)	2 (3.3 %)
Montini 2009	RCT	46 (1–3)	81	First fUTI	2 month–7 year (15 month)	1 year	9 (19.6 %)	3 (3.7 %)
Craig 2009	RCT	121 (1–5)	115[a]	≥1 UTI	<18 year (15 month)	1 year	36 (13 %)	
Series of patients all with VUR								
Roussey-Kesler 2008	RCT	122	–	First fUTI, g 1–3 VUR	1 month–3 year (11 month)	18 month	19 (15.5 %)	–
Pennesi 2008	RCT	50	–	First fUTI, g 2–4 VUR	<30 month (8 month)	2 year	15 (30 %)	–
Brandstrom 2010	RCT	68	–	First fUTI, g 3–4 VUR	1–2 year (1.8)	2 year	25 (37 %)	–

[a]VUR status unknown in another 52 patients

had three or more. The likelihood for recurrence diminished with time, from 16.8 episodes per 1,000 person-months in the first 24 months, to 7.8 between 24 and 48 months and was <5 episodes per 1,000 person-months thereafter to 10 years follow-up (Dias et al. 2010).

Associated Conditions

Anatomic Anomalies

Obstructive uropathies and various renal anomalies occur in <10 %.

VUR is diagnosed in ≤33 % of children imaged after fUTI. Most VUR is grades 1–3.

One prospective study using the 1999 AAP imaging guidelines (renal US and VCUG in children <24 months after fUTI) in 309 children (33 boys) ages 1–24 months presenting with first known fUTI reported renal US was normal in 88 %, with another 5 % having findings likely to be insignificant (extrarenal pelvis, pelvic dilation, ureteral duplication); 4.5 % had "hydronephrosis or pelvicaliectasis." VCUG was normal in 61 % of patients, demonstrating reflux in the remaining 39 %. In these 115 children with reflux, 96 % had grades 1–3, 5 had grade 4, and none had grade 5 (Hoberman et al. 2003)

Another prospective study of 297 consecutive children under age 5 years with first symptomatic UTI were imaged according to 1999 AAP recommendations. Renal US demonstrated "obstructive uropathy" in three, a megaureter in seven, a horseshoe kidney in two, and duplex ureters in five. Accordingly, potentially significant findings (obstructive conditions and megaureters) were noted in 3 %. VUR was diagnosed in 28 % (95 % CI 23.3–33.6); grades were not reported (Craig et al. 1998).

A prospective study analyzed 72 term neonates 0–28 days of age with symptomatic UTI (fever, vomiting, poor feeding, failure to thrive). Renal US findings were not reported, except to note that one patient had ureteropelvic junction obstruction (UPJO) and another with VUR had congenital hypodysplasia of the ipsilateral kidney. VUR was reported by renal units, occurring in 22 %, and was noted equally in males and females. However, grades 4–5 reflux, which accounted for 25 % of detected VUR, was found only in boys. The authors noted other studies with similar findings that together suggest VUR is less commonly found after UTI in neonates versus in older children (Siomou et al. 2009).

Analysis of prospective data on 209 children presenting at median age 10 months (0.2–204) with first known UTI reported on antenatal US had been done in 198 (95 %), finding UPJO in 2.5 %, posterior urethral valve (PUV) in 0.5 %, and primary megaureter in 0.5 %. Renal US was repeated in all patients, finding one new case each of PUV and primary megaureter. VUR was diagnosed in 25 %, with grades 1–3 comprising 85 % (Ismaili et al. 2011).

A retrospective study reviewed renal US findings in 203 consecutive infants, 80 males, 5 days to 6 months of age with fUTI who had normal VCUG. Abnormalities were detected in 32 patients (16 %), but management was altered in only 9 (4 %) for UPJO ($n=1$), ectopic ureter ($n=2$), renal calculus ($n=1$), UVJO ($n=3$), multicystic dysplastic kidney (MCDK) ($n=1$), and renal scar ($n=1$) (Giorgi et al. 2005).

Bladder Dysfunction

Lack of standardized means and criteria to diagnose bladder dysfunction limits reliability of reported studies to determine prevalence of these disorders in children presenting with UTI.

In one retrospective study of 109 consecutive children, 82 % female, referred for urologic evaluation of UTI and/or voiding symptoms, children were systematically queried for history of urinary frequency and urgency, with or without diurnal incontinence, considered indicative of urge syndrome. In females older than 3 years old with infection, 40 % had urge syndrome symptoms. Of all females older than 3 years with urge syndrome symptoms, 66 % had a history of UTI (Snodgrass 1991).

During a 4-year period, 3,500 children were evaluated for urinary incontinence, of which 1,000 underwent invasive urodynamic studies for the following indications: history of UTI, small bladder capacity, repeated dysfunctional uroflow, ultrasonographic abnormalities, and resistance to therapy. Diagnostic categories assigned by UD were urge syndrome (detrusor instability during filling with normal voiding), dysfunctional voiding (sphincteric activity during voiding diminishing or interrupting urine flow), and lazy bladder (greater than predicted bladder capacity without detrusor contraction during voiding). Mean patient age was approximately 10 years, with 524 males and 476 females. UTI was reported in 5 % of males with urge syndrome and 7 % with dysfunctional voiding (no male was diagnosed with lazy bladder), versus 30 % of females with urge syndrome, 36 % with dysfunctional voiding, and 53 % with lazy bladder (Hoebeke et al. 2001).

Another study defined dysfunctional elimination syndrome (DES) as "daytime wetting or soiling," or the presence of at least three of the following: voiding <3 times daily, Vincent's curtsy, thick-walled bladder by ultrasound, trabeculated or spinning top bladder on cystogram, or bladder capacity >30 % predicted value for age. All 2,759 patients referred for these symptoms and/or UTI and reflux over a 14-year period were identified from a database for multivariable logistic regression analysis. DES was diagnosed in 52 % of children having UTI and normal radiologic testing, versus 38.5 % of those with VUR. Girls were more likely than boys to have DES (Chen et al. 2004).

Constipation

Constipation is considered a risk factor for development of UTI, but the lack of standardized means and criteria to establish the diagnosis hinders determination of its prevalence in children with urinary infection.

Rome III criteria, currently recommended to diagnose pediatric functional constipation, are two or more of the following:

- Two or fewer defecations per week.
- At least one episode of fecal incontinence per week.
- Stool-retentive posturing.
- Painful or hard bowel movements.
- Presence of a large fecal mass in the rectum.
- Large-diameter stools that may obstruct the toilet.

Additional criteria include the following:

- Without objective evidence of a pathological condition.
- Without fulfilling irritable bowel syndrome criteria.

Infants up to 4 years of age have to fulfill two or more criteria for at least 1 month. Children >4 years should have two or more criteria from ≥2 months (Tabbers et al. 2011).

A prospective study reported an association between constipation and UTI in patients >5 years old (176 boys) referred to an encopresis clinic for soiling at least once a week for 6 months. Additional diagnostic criteria for functional constipation were not stated, except to note that all had fecal retention on rectal examination and 45 % had a palpable abdominal mass from stool. Diurnal urinary incontinence was reported by 29 % of patients without gender difference, whereas UTI occurred in 3 % of males versus 33 % of females ($p<0.001$). Of the 19 girls with UTI, 8 reported only one infection. The remaining 11 had recurrent infections, 4 also having structural urinary tract anomalies including reflux in 3 and a "large" bladder diverticulum in 1. Successful relief of constipation was said to prevent further UTI. Infections were not categorized as febrile versus nonfebrile, and neither the number of infections nor time interval during which they occurred was stated for those with recurrent UTI. Patients with recurrent UTI received antibiotic prophylaxis for nonspecified intervals, with five continuing therapy at time of last follow-up. This follow-up was performed at a mean of 15 months, most often by a questionnaire mailed to families, or by phone call (Loening-Baucke 1997).

Other studies linking constipation to UTI, mostly from the 1980s or earlier, suffer from small numbers of patients, lack of uniform definition of constipation, and poor study design without controls or multivariable statistical analyses. For example, one evaluation of 131 children with UTI diagnosed constipation in 45 (34 %) based on symptoms including hard stools, infrequent stooling, fecal soiling, chronic laxative use, or rectal fissures. Effective therapy for constipation was reported to prevent UTI recurrence at 1 year, although success was only defined as "regular bowel movements of normal size" (Neumann et al. 1973).

Circumcision Status

Circumcision reduces the risk of UTI, with relative risk (RR) 4.5 (95 % CI 2.4–8.4) in uncircumcised versus circumcised infants <1 month of age, and RR 3.7 (95 % CI 2.8–4.9) during the first year of life.

One retrospective study reported first infection occurred at mean age 4 months in uncircumcised boys, with recurrent UTI in 35 % a mean of 3 months later.

Although circumcision reduces UTI risk, more than 100 circumcisions are needed to prevent one UTI. Calculated number needed to treat to prevent one UTI in boys with grades 3–5 VUR is 4, which supports circumcision for this higher-risk group.

Meta-analysis of four articles concerning UTI and circumcision status reported prevalence of febrile infection in 2.4 % (95 % CI 1.4–3.5) of circumcised boys <3 months of age versus 20.1 % (95 % CI 16.8–23.4) in those uncircumcised. For infants 6–12 months of age, prevalence for fUTI in one study was 0.3 % in circumcised versus 7.3 % in uncircumcised males. No data were found concerning febrile UTI after 1 year age (Shaikh et al. 2008).

A prospective matched cohort study compared 29,217 circumcised to the same number of uncircumcised Canadian newborns to determine relative risk for hospital admission for UTI. There were 1.88 infections per 1,000 person-years of observation in circumcised boys versus 7.02 per 1,000 person-years in uncircumcised boys. RR for infection in uncircumcised boys was 4.5 (95 % CI 2.4–8.4) in the first month of life, and 3.7 (95 % CI 2.8–4.9) during the first year of life. The authors noted this reduction in risk was much less than the 10–20 times higher rate of UTI in uncircumcised boys commonly quoted, and calculated that 195 circumcisions would be needed to prevent a single hospital admission for UTI (To et al. 1998).

A retrospective review concerned recurrence of UTI after initial infection in 128 uncircumcised boys within the first year of life in Finland. Mean age for initial UTI was 0.33 years (SD 0.23), and in the following 3 years 35 % had a second infection occurring at a mean of 85 days (SD 92 days) (Nuutinen and Uhari 2001).

A meta-analysis of published data regarding effect of circumcision on UTI risk obtained information on 402,908 boys in 12 studies. From this, the number to treat to prevent one UTI was calculated to be 111. For boys with grades 3–5 VUR, the number to treat to prevent one UTI is 4 (Singh-Grewal et al. 2005).

Imaging After UTI

Renal Ultrasound and VCUG

The 1999 AAP guidelines recommended renal US and VCUG after first known fUTI in children ages 1–24 months. 2011 AAP guidelines only recommend renal US unless there is "hydronephrosis, scarring, or other findings suggesting high-grade VUR."

Findings reported by prospective studies in consecutive children undergoing these tests are summarized in the section "Anatomic Anomalies."

Diagnostic Accuracy of Cystography

A single-fill (noncycled) cystogram fails to detect VUR in approximately 20 % of cases. Accuracy is increased with cycled cystography.

Approximately 20 % of patients found to have unilateral VUR on initial (non-cycled) VCUG will be found to have contralateral VUR on subsequent cystography.

Cycling during NC also increases diagnostic yield; one study reported 15 % of VUR found during the second cycle.

One study of consecutive children undergoing both VCUG and NC found NC significantly more accurate to detect both VUR overall and high-grade VUR.

A prospective study compared findings after the first cycle to findings after a second cycle of VCUG in 275 children ≤2 years of age, 90 % following UTI. Overall, VUR was detected in 68 (25 %) patients. However, the first cycle only demonstrated reflux in 18 cases, whereas the second in another 50. Of the 257 children with a negative initial cycle, the additional 50 found with VUR during the second cycle represented another 19.5 % that otherwise would have been missed. Grades found on the second cycle ranged from 1 to 5 (Papadopoulou et al. 2002).

Another prospective study analyzed first versus second cycle of cystrography in children after fUTI (n=124, all girls) and in follow up of known VUR (n=135, 127 girls). NC was done in 249 children and VCUG in 10. Patient age ranged from 3 weeks to 17 years. Of 124 studies after fUTI, VUR was found in the first cycle in 40/124 and the second in 7/76, meaning 15 % of VUR was detected in the second cycle. For follow-up patients, VUR was seen during the first cycle in 90/135 and the second in 8/34, indicating 8 % had VUR detected by a second cycle (Gelfand et al. 1999).

To determine relative accuracy of VCUG versus NC, 124 consecutive children 1 month to 9 years of age (mean 2 years) being imaged following UTI, prenatal hydronephrosis, or multicystic dysplastic kidney underwent both studies. VCUG was performed first, with NC then obtained immediately in 73, within 3 days in 21, and a mean of 17 days in 30 patients. VCUG was done twice in children less than 3 years of age. NC was not cycled. Voiding occurred in all studies. Findings were concordant in 84 % of renal units, and 93 % for diagnosis of grades 4–5 VUR, corresponding to "severe" VUR on NC. However, there were 4 refluxing units only detected by VCUG versus 36 seen only with NC (p=0.0001), of which VCUG did not exclusively detect severe VUR while NC did in 17/27 renal units (p=0.004). Considering findings in patients, VCUG failed to detect VUR found on NC in 23, 12 of which had severe VUR on at least one side. NC failed to detect VUR in three patients, grade 1 in two and grade 2 in one (Polito et al. 2000).

A retrospective study considered new contralateral VUR after initial VCUG showed only unilateral reflux. Therefore, all patients had ≥2 VCUGs, ranging to seven. Those found to have new contralateral VUR had a statistically significant greater number of cystograms (3.5±1.4 vs. 2.6±1, p<0.001). Overall, new contralateral VUR was found in 33 (21 %) of 167 patients, comprising grade 1 in 4, grade 2 in 18, grade 3 in 9, and grade 4 in 1, with grade not determined due to nuclear cystography in 1. The methods regarding VCUG cycling were not clearly stated (cycled only if initial imaging was "unsatisfactory"); the interval between studies was not stated, and whether new reflux was seen on a second versus later cystogram was not reported (Barroso et al. 2008).

"Top-Down" Imaging Using DMSA Scintigraphy

"Top-down" imaging limiting VCUG to patients with positive acute or delayed DMSA scintigraphy reduces the number of VCUGs.

One study reported top-down imaging would have reduced VCUG by 50 % while not detecting VUR in 15 % of patients, all but one of which had grades 1–2.

Another study obtained DMSA later, at ≥3 months after fTUI, and found VCUG would have been done in 20 % of patients if limited to those with abnormal findings.

A prospective study using DMSA scintigraphy at ≤7 days of onset of fever or urinary symptoms combined with renal US and VCUG reported an 83 % positive predictive value and a 92 % negative predictive value for "clinically significant VUR" Significant VUR was defined as including ≥ grade 3 reflux, recurrent UTI, and renal scarring. It is noteworthy that 73 % of the 121 children (mean age 3.6 years, median 2.4, range 2 months-11 years) had positive acute DMSA scans, so the potential avoidance of VCUGs would be limited by their protocol to a maximum 27 % of patients (Herz et al. 2010).

Another prospective observational study also evaluated acute DMSA imaging (≤2 weeks of onset of symptoms), in children <1 year old with first known symptomatic UTI. There were 290 children, with positive DMSA scans in 51 % and VUR in 18 %. Abnormal DMSA occurred in 44 % of children without VUR, 72 % with grades 1–2 VUR, and 96 % of those with ≥ grade 3 reflux. Reserving VCUG to those with positive acute DMSA studies would have reduced the number of VCUGs by 50 %, missing VUR in 15 % which was grades 1–2 in all but one patient with grade 3 (Preda et al. 2007).

A single "late" DMSA scan was done ≥3 months after fUTI in another prospective study of 565 consecutive children referred for urologic evaluation. Scintigraphy was obtained at a mean of 7 months (median 4 months) after UTI. Focal cortical defects, whether resolving renal inflammation or scars, were present in only 15.5 %. Another 4 % had presumed congenital nephropathy (<44 % ipsilateral function with no focal cortical defect). If VCUG was only obtained in patients with abnormal DMSA ≥3 months after fUTI, it would have been done in only 19 % of patients (Snodgrass et al. 2012).

Antibiotic Therapy

Intravenous Versus Oral Therapy

Children with fUTI can be treated with oral therapy using third-generation cephalosporins (following gram stain to exclude gram-positive cocci).

Those judged too ill for initial oral therapy can receive initial intravenous antibiotics until clinical symptoms improve sufficiently to complete therapy orally.

There is no difference in duration of fever or renal scarring based on mode of antibiotic administration.

No data are available to guide optimal antibiotic therapy in children with known uropathies, especially obstructive conditions or renal hypodysplasia in which antibiotic penetration into the affected kidney might be reduced and/or the risk of scarring increased.

A Cochrane Database review in 2010 included 23 studies with 3,407 children, finding the following:

- No difference in duration of fever or in renal damage as assessed 6 and 12 months after fUTI based upon oral antibiotic therapy (ceftibuten, cefixime, or amoxicillin/clavulanic acid) for 10–14 days versus initial intravenous therapy (cefotaxime or ceftriaxone) for 3 days followed by 10 days of oral therapy.
- No difference in renal scars between intravenous therapy for 3 days plus 10 days oral therapy versus intravenous therapy for 7–10 days.

Ten of the 23 studies excluded patients with known "severe urinary tract abnormalities" (Hodson et al. 2010).

One RCT compared oral cefixime for 14 days to initial intravenous cefotaxime for 3 days followed by oral cefixime for 11 days in children ≤2 years of age with fUTI. Initial evaluation included urine gram stain, with gram-positive cocci an exclusion criteria. No significant differences were found in duration of fever (oral: 25 h vs. IV plus oral: 24 h), or renal scarring on DMSA performed at entry and at 6 months (oral:11 % vs. IV plus oral: 8 %). Exclusion from the study included known genitourinary anomalies and severe clinical illness defined as systolic blood pressure <60 mmHg or capillary refill >3 min (Hoberman et al. 1999).

Longer Versus Shorter Duration of Antibiotic Therapy

There is no difference in renal scarring based on 3 days initial intravenous antibiotic therapy plus 5 days oral therapy versus 8 days of intravenous therapy in patients without uropathy.

There are no data regarding optimal duration of therapy in those with known uropathies.

The Cochrane Database review mentioned above reported no significant difference in persistent renal damage between initial IV therapy for 3–4 days followed by oral therapy versus IV therapy for 7–14 days (3 studies, 341 children: RR 1.13 [95 % CI 0.86–1.49]) (Hodson et al. 2010).

The shortest duration of therapy (8 days) reported for fUTI was part of a RCT comparing outcomes in 383 children at median age 15 months (3 months-16 years) with first fUTI. All received 3 days intravenous antibiotics (netilmicin for 48 h plus ceftriaxone for 72 h) followed by either 5 additional days of intravenous ceftriaxone or oral antibiotic based on sensitivities. Exclusion criteria were known uropathy, or obstructive uropathy (pelvis dilation >10 mm) or renal hypoplasia (length < 2 SD) on renal US. There was no difference in renal scarring determined by DMSA at median 8 months later (17 % longer intravenous therapy vs. 13 % shorter intravenous therapy) (Bouissou et al. 2008).

Immediate Versus Delayed Therapy

Delay in starting antibiotic therapy was reported to progressively and significantly increase positive acute DMSA findings in one report.

Three prospective studies found renal scar at DMSA 6–12 months after fUTI did not vary according to antibiotic therapy started within 1 day of fever onset versus a delay in treatment.

The prospective study by Bouissou et al. (2008) described in the preceding section analyzed risk for renal scar on DMSA a median of 8 months after first known fUTI for children starting intravenous antibiotic therapy <2 days versus ≥2 days after onset of fever, finding no difference in renal scar (OR 1.34 [95 % CI 0.73–2.45]).

Another prospective study included 287 children 1 month to 7 years of age with first known fUTI and positive acute DMSA scan who had follow-up scintigraphy 12 months later. Risk for renal scar was evaluated according to duration of fever before antibiotic therapy of <1 day to ≥5 days. Overall prevalence of renal scar was 31 %, with no difference in renal damage based on delay in starting therapy (Hewitt et al. 2008).

A third prospective study evaluated 278 infants (153 boys) aged 6–12 months with first known fUTI started on antibiotics at <1 day to ≥ day 4 of fever to determine effect of timing of antibiotic therapy on renal scarring. Second DMSA scans were obtained 5–26 months later (median 6.5 months) in those with initially positive findings. There was a significantly increased number of renal defects observed during acute DMSA scintigraphy with progressive delay in therapy (41 % at <1 day, 59 % at day 2, 68 % at day 3, and 75 % at ≥ day 4 [$p=0.000$]). Of 158 positive acute scans, follow-up scans were obtained in 76 without recurrent fUTI, with no difference in persistently positive scan (overall 51 %) in those treated at <1 day versus those later (Doganis et al. 2007).

Cranberry Supplements

One study found no difference in the number of children who developed UTIs in patients drinking cranberry juice versus placebo, but did report a decrease in the number of UTIs in those with cranberry juice.

Two other trials reported a decrease in the number of patients with UTI taking cranberry juice versus placebo.

In a multicenter Finnish trial, 263 children, 88 % female, mean age 4 years (1–16) were randomized to cranberry juice versus placebo for 6 months and monitored for UTI (fever and/or symptoms) for a 1-year period; 20 (16 %) in the cranberry group and 28 (22 %) in the placebo group had at least one recurrent UTI, $p=0.21$. While the intervention did not reduce the number of children with recurrent UTIs, it did reduce the number of recurrences, with 27 and 47 in the cranberry and placebo groups with a UTI incidence density per person-year at risk of 0.25 versus 0.41 in the cranberry versus placebo group ($p=0.03$, CI −0.31 to −0.01) as well as the total days on antibiotics (11.6 vs. 17.6 days, $p<0.001$) (Salo et al. 2011).

Eighty-four girls mean age 7.5 years (3–14) with normal renal function and no genitourinary anomalies with more than one UTI due to *E. coli* were randomized to cranberry juice (50 mL OD), lactobacillus (100 mL of 4×10^7 cfu lactobacillus

5 days/month), or control for 6 months. The results were that 34/80 (42.5 %) had at least one UTI, with fewest in the cranberry treatment group; 5/17 (18.5 %) cranberry, 11/26 (42 %) lactobacillus, and 18/27 (48 %) controls ($p < 0.05$) (Ferrara et al. 2009).

Thirty-nine girls and one boy mean age 9.5 years who had ≥2 non-febrile UTIs in the year prior to enrollment were randomly assigned to receive daily cranberry juice versus placebo over 1 year. The incidence of non-febrile UTI was 0.4 in the cranberry versus 1.15 in the placebo arm ($p = 0.045$), representing a RR reduction of 65 % (Afshar et al. 2012).

Renal Scar

Renal scars determined by DMSA scintigraphy occur in approximately 15 % of children evaluated following first known fUTI.

Renal scars were also found in 15 % of patients referred to urologic management after fUTI and/or VUR diagnosis.

The meta-analysis by Shaikh et al. described above included 33 studies to determine prevalence of acute phase (≤15 days) and follow-up (>5 months) DMSA scintigraphy in children after first known UTI, finding the following:

- 57 % (95 % CI 50–64) had positive acute-phase DMSA changes.
- 15 % (95 % CI 11–18) had persistently positive follow-up DMSA scans.

The authors found significant heterogeneity between studies, but noted the rate of 15 % renal scar was stable in reports since 2002 (Shaikh et al. 2010).

Prospective evaluation of 565 consecutive children referred for urologic assessment after fUTI and/or VUR diagnosis included DMSA scintigraphy ≥3 months after infection, if present. Twenty-four (4 %) had congenital reflux nephropathy defined as ≤44 % ipsilateral function without cortical defect, while 84/541 (15.5 %) had focal defects on scan done a mean of 7.4 months (median 4 months) after infection (Snodgrass et al. 2012).

Versus Age at UTI

Despite common belief, renal scars are found *less often*, or at the same frequency, in infants as in older children.

A prospective study of first symptomatic UTI in term neonates ≤28 days of age obtained acute DMSA scintigraphy (at ≤72 h of diagnosis) and late DMSA scintigraphy at 6 months. Results in 72 patients were reported per renal unit: 27 (19 %) of 144 kidneys demonstrated apparent parenchymal inflammation, of which 10 (7 %) had renal scar on the follow-up scan (Siomou et al. 2009).

Another prospective analysis of 309 children <2 years of age presenting with first known fUTI included acute-phase (≤48 h) DMSA scan, with follow-up DMSA 6 months later obtained in 275 (89 %). Renal scarring was found on the second scan in 9.5 %, occurring with equal frequency in those <1 year versus >1 year at initial infection (Hoberman et al. 2003).

A third prospective study included 287 children 1 month to 7 years of age after first fUTI who all had acutely (<10 days) positive DMSA scans. This inflammation resulted in a renal scar on DMSA 1 year later in 55/184 (30 %) <1 year of age versus 34/103 (33 %) at greater age during initial infection. Quartiles from age 1 to 24 months and 2 to 7 years showed no differences in renal scarring (Hewitt et al. 2008).

A fourth prospective study enrolled 316 consecutive children ages 1 month to 14 years with first fUTI. Acute-phase (<5 days) DMSA was obtained in all, with late (>6 months) follow-up scan if the initial study was positive. There was no difference in renal scarring in those <1 year versus 1–4 years (OR 1.45 [95 % CI 0.62–3.37]), but greater scarring in those 5–14 years (OR 3.35 [95 % CI 1.04–10.78]) (Pecile et al. 2009).

The prospective study by Snodgrass et al. (2012) described above, with 565 consecutive patients referred for urologic assessment after fUTI and/or VUR, reported focal DMSA defects on scans done a mean of 7 months (median 4 months) in 6 % of patients <1 year of age versus 18 % of those >1 year, with each year of life increasing the odds of abnormal DMSA by 20 % (OR 1.2 [95 % CI 1.1–1.3]).

Table 1.2 Renal scar versus VUR in 452 consecutive urology patients with fUTI and/or VUR

VUR grade	Total patients	No. abnormal DMSA	OR estimate	95 % CI	*p*
0	112	17	1.00	–	–
1	23	4	3.94	1.05–14.85	0.04
2	133	15	3.12	1.35–7.21	0.008
3	130	19	3.93	1.68–9.22	0.002
4	44	21	28.91	10.73–77.88	<0.0001
5	10	6	77.37	16.62–360.20	<0.0001

Versus VUR

VUR increases risk for renal scar by 2.5 times in children following first fUTI.

One study of patients referred for urology assessment reported risk was greater in all grades versus no VUR, with greatest risk in grades 4–5.

A retrospective study of children with VUR similarly reported increased scar in those with grades 4–5 versus 1–3.

The meta-analysis mentioned above by Shaikh et al. (2010) was done specifically to assess risk for renal scarring in children with UTI. Published articles were included if they reported acute-phase (≤15 days) or follow-up (>5 months) DMSA results in patients 0–18 years of age, resulting in 33 studies for review. As stated above, 57 % of children had positive acute-phase scans, of which 15 % demonstrated renal scar on follow-up scan. Those with VUR had increased risk for scarring (RR 2.6 [95 % CI 1.7–3.9]), based on review of four articles. Risk by individual grade was not reported, but those with grades 3–5 were 2.1 times (95 % CI 1.4–3.2) more likely to have renal scar versus those with grades 1–2. However, in these four articles, one included only five patients with grade 4 and none with grade 5 VUR, and the other three lumped grades 3–5 together.

Renal scar risk was analyzed by individual reflux grades in a prospective series of 565 consecutive patients referred after fUTI and/or VUR diagnosis described above (Snodgrass et al. 2012). Among consecutive patients referred for urologic evaluation after UTI and/or VUR diagnosis, multiple regression analysis showed all grades of VUR increased risk for DMSA defects versus no VUR, with similar odds for grades 1–3 and greatly increased odds for grades 4 and 5 (Table 1.2).

A retrospective study included 182 children (32 boys) with VUR and UTI who had DMSA scintigraphy to determine renal scarring 4–6 months after a positive acute-phase scan. Risk for scar for those with grades 1–3 VUR was 30/94 (32 %) versus 37/44 (84 %) with grades 4–5, $p = 0.000$ (Soylu et al. 2008).

Versus Number of fUTIs

Few data are available regarding impact of recurrent UTI on renal scar risk.

Most recent RCTs included patients with first known fUTI, or did not specify number of fUTIs before enrollment.

New DMSA defects after UTI in patients with prior negative DMSA occur in approximately 5 % of patients, as discussed in the next section.

A study based on protocol assessment and management of children with symptomatic UTI from 1970 to 1979 included IVP-based diagnosis of renal scar (calyceal deformity with overlying parenchymal defect). Prevalence of renal scar progressively increased from 5 % in those without history of fUTI to 9 % of those with one, 15 % with two, 35 % with three, and 58 % with four or more episodes of fUTI (Jodal 1987). Logistic regression analysis to control influence of VUR grade was not done.

Cross-sectional analysis of 565 consecutive children with fUTI reported by Snodgrass et al. (2012) as described above analyzed renal scar prevalence versus reported number of fUTIs in 529 patients (Table 1.3). A single fUTI did not

Table 1.3 Renal scar versus number of reported febrile UTIs in consecutive referred patients with UTI and/or VUR

No. febrile UTIs	Total patients	No. abnormal DMSA	OR estimate	95 % CI	*p*
0	81	9	1.00	–	–
1	226	18	0.60	0.25–1.44	0.25
2	85	17	2.65	1.22–5.74	0.01
≥3	137	36	3.97	2.06–7.63	<0.0001

increase renal scars over patients with no history of infection, although 9/81 (11 %) with no infection history had DMSA defects, possibly indicating UTI attributed to other illnesses. Two or more fUTI did increase scarring, although it could not be determined if scarring occurred after the first or a subsequent infection.

Scar Risk After Recurrent UTI When Initial DMSA Is Negative for Scar

Two studies report risk <5 %, and one study, 11 %, for renal scarring with recurrent UTI when an earlier DMSA was negative for scar after UTI.

A study identified 429 children ages 3 and 4 years at time of prior assessment for UTI who had a normal renal US and a negative DMSA scan. These children were contacted 2–11 years later (at ages 6–15 years) for another follow-up DMSA, and participating parents were asked the number of UTIs that occurred after the initial scan. Over 80 % of patients participated. One or more recurrent UTIs were reported by 103 patients, with new DMSA scars found in four (4 %), all with three or more additional infections. One other patient who did not report recurrent UTI had a scar (Vernon et al. 1997).

A retrospective analysis of 138 children with VUR included acute DMSA with subsequent DMSA 4–6 months later for abnormal findings, and another late DMSA 4–6 months after recurrent UTI. Recurrences were found in 118, but only 16 had more than one recurrence and only 26 were described as fUTI. Of these, 2/71 (3 %) without scar during first evaluation later had scar formation, versus 13/67 (19 %) with new/progressive scarring after an earlier study with scarring (Soylu et al. 2008).

The Swedish reflux trial included 203 patients with mean age 1.8 years (1–2) with grades 3–4 VUR. Number of fUTI prior to entry was not stated, but baseline DMSA was positive in 124 (61 %). New defects in those with negative DMSA occurred in 9/79 (11 %). Timing of DMSA and number of recurrent UTIs were not stated (Brandstrom et al. 2010).

References

AAP (American Academy of Pediatrics). Committee on Quality Improvement. Subcommittee on Urinary Tract Infection. Practice parameter: the diagnosis, treatment, and evaluation of the initial urinary tract infection in febrile infants and young children. Pediatrics. 1999;103(4 Pt 1):843–52.

Afshar K, Stothers L, Scott H, Macneily AE. Cranberry juice for the prevention of pediatric urinary tract infection: a randomized controlled trial. J Urol. 2012;188 (4 Suppl):1584–7.

Agras K, Ortapamuk H, Naldoken S, Tuncel A, Atan A. Resolution of cortical lesions on serial renal scans in children with acute pyelonephritis. Pediatric Radiol. 2007;37(2):153–8.

Barroso Jr U, Barroso VA, de Bessa J, Jr CAA, Zerati FM. Predictive factors for contralateral reflux in patients with conservatively treated unilateral vesicoureteral reflux. J Urol. 2008;180(1):297–9.

Bouissou F, Munzer C, Decramer S, Roussel B, Novo R, Morin D, et al. Prospective, randomized trial comparing short and long intravenous antibiotic treatment of acute pyelonephritis in children: dimercaptosuccinic acid scintigraphic evaluation at 9 months. Pediatrics. 2008;121(3):e553–60.

Brandstrom P, Esbjorner E, Herthelius M, Swerkersson S, Jodal U, Hansson S. The Swedish reflux trial in children: III. Urinary tract infection pattern. J Urol. 2010;184(1):286–91.

Chen JJ, Mao W, Homayoon K, Steinhardt GF. A multivariate analysis of dysfunctional elimination syndrome, and its relationships with gender, urinary tract

infection and vesicoureteral reflux in children. J Urol. 2004;171(5):1907–10.
Cheng YW, Wong SN. Diagnosing symptomatic urinary tract infections in infants by catheter urine culture. J Paediatr Child Health. 2005;41(8):437–40.
Conway PH, Cnaan A, Zaoutis T, Henry BV, Grundmeier RW, Keren R. Recurrent urinary tract infections in children: risk factors and association with prophylactic antimicrobials. JAMA. 2007;298(2):179–86.
Craig JC, Irwig LM, Knight JF, Sureshkumar P, Roy LP. Symptomatic urinary tract infection in preschool Australian children. J Paediatr Child Health. 1998; 34(2):154–9.
Craig JC, Simpson JM, Williams GJ, Lowe A, Reynolds GJ, McTaggart SJ, et al. Antibiotic prophylaxis and recurrent urinary tract infection in children. N Engl J Med. 2009;361(18):1748–59.
Dias CS, Silva JM, Diniz JS, Lima EM, Marciano RC, Lana LG, et al. Risk factors for recurrent urinary tract infections in a cohort of patients with primary vesicoureteral reflux. Pediatr Infect Dis J. 2010;29(2): 139–44.
Doganis D, Siafas K, Mavrikou M, Issaris G, Martirosova A, Perperidis G, et al. Does early treatment of urinary tract infection prevent renal damage? Pediatrics. 2007;120(4):e922–8.
Ferrara P, Romaniello L, Vitelli O, Gatto A, Serva M, Cataldi L. Cranberry juice for the prevention of recurrent urinary tract infections: a randomized controlled trial in children. Scand J Urol Nephrol. 2009;43(5): 369–72.
Garin EH, Olavarria F, Garcia Nieto V, Valenciano B, Campos A, Young L. Clinical significance of primary vesicoureteral reflux and urinary antibiotic prophylaxis after acute pyelonephritis: a multicenter, randomized, controlled study. Pediatrics. 2006;117(3):626–32.
Gelfand MJ, Koch BL, Elgazzar AH, Gylys-Morin VM, Gartside PS, Torgerson CL. Cyclic cystography: diagnostic yield in selected pediatric populations. Radiology. 1999;213(1):118–20.
Giorgi Jr LJ, Bratslavsky G, Kogan BA. Febrile urinary tract infections in infants: renal ultrasound remains necessary. J Urol. 2005;173(2):568–70.
Gorelick MH, Shaw KN. Screening tests for urinary tract infection in children: A meta-analysis. Pediatrics. 1999;104(5):e54.
Herz D, Merguerian P, McQuiston L, Danielson C, Gheen M, Brenfleck L. 5-year prospective results of dimercapto-succinic acid imaging in children with febrile urinary tract infection: proof that the top-down approach works. J Urol. 2010;184(4 Suppl):1703–9.
Hewitt IK, Zucchetta P, Rigon L, Maschio F, Molinari PP, Tomasi L, et al. Early treatment of acute pyelonephritis in children fails to reduce renal scarring: data from the Italian Renal Infection Study Trials. Pediatrics. 2008;122(3):486–90.
Hoberman A, Wald ER, Hickey RW, Baskin M, Charron M, Majd M, et al. Oral versus initial intravenous therapy for urinary tract infections in young febrile children. Pediatrics. 1999;104(1 Pt 1):79–86.
Hoberman A, Charron M, Hickey RW, Baskin M, Kearney DH, Wald ER. Imaging studies after a first febrile urinary tract infection in young children. N Engl J Med. 2003;348(3):195–202.
Hodson EM, Willis NS, Craig JC. Interventions for idiopathic steroid-resistant nephrotic syndrome in children. Cochrane Database Syst Rev (Online). 2010(11): CD003594.
Hoebeke P, Van Laecke E, Van Camp C, Raes A, Van De Walle J. One thousand video-urodynamic studies in children with non-neurogenic bladder sphincter dysfunction. BJU Int. 2001;87(6):575–80.
Ismaili K, Wissing KM, Lolin K, Le PQ, Christophe C, Lepage P, et al. Characteristics of first urinary tract infection with fever in children: a prospective clinical and imaging study. Pediatr Infect Dis J. 2011; 30(5):371–4.
Jodal U. The natural history of bacteriuria in childhood. Infect Dis Clin North Am. 1987;1(4):713–29.
Lau AY, Wong SN, Yip KT, Fong KW, Li SP, Que TL. A comparative study on bacterial cultures of urine samples obtained by clean-void technique versus urethral catheterization. Acta Paediatr. 2007;96(3): 432–6.
Loening-Baucke V. Urinary incontinence and urinary tract infection and their resolution with treatment of chronic constipation of childhood. Pediatrics. 1997;100 (2 Pt 1):228–32.
Montini G, Zucchetta P, Tomasi L, Talenti E, Rigamonti W, Picco G, et al. Value of imaging studies after a first febrile urinary tract infection in young children: data from Italian renal infection study 1. Pediatrics. 2009; 123(2):e239–46.
Mori R, Yonemoto N, Fitzgerald A, Tullus K, Verrier-Jones K, Lakhanpaul M. Diagnostic performance of urine dipstick testing in children with suspected UTI: a systematic review of relationship with age and comparison with microscopy. Acta Paediatr. 2009;99(4): 581–4.
Neumann PZ, DeDomenico IJ, Nogrady MB. Constipation and urinary tract infection. Pediatrics. 1973;52(2): 241–5.
Nuutinen M, Uhari M. Recurrence and follow-up after urinary tract infection under the age of 1 year. Pediatr Nephrol (Berlin, Germany). 2001;16(1):69–72.
Panaretto K, Craig J, Knight J, Howman-Giles R, Sureshkumar P, Roy L. Risk factors for recurrent urinary tract infection in preschool children. J Paediatr Child Health. 1999;35(5):454–9.
Papadopoulou F, Efremidis SC, Oiconomou A, Badouraki M, Panteleli M, Papachristou F, et al. Cyclic voiding cystourethrography: is vesicoureteral reflux missed with standard voiding cystourethrography? Eur Radiol. 2002;12(3):666–70.
Parvex P, Willi JP, Kossovsky MP, Girardin E. Longitudinal analyses of renal lesions due to acute pyelonephritis in children and their impact on renal growth. J Urol. 2008;180(6):2602–6. discussion 6.
Pecile P, Miorin E, Romanello C, Vidal E, Contardo M, Valent F, et al. Age-related renal parenchymal lesions

in children with first febrile urinary tract infections. Pediatrics. 2009;124(1):23–9.

Pennesi M, Travan L, Peratoner L, Bordugo A, Cattaneo A, Ronfani L, et al. Is antibiotic prophylaxis in children with vesicoureteral reflux effective in preventing pyelonephritis and renal scars? A randomized, controlled trial. Pediatrics. 2009;121(6):e1489–94.

Polito C, Rambaldi PF, La Manna A, Mansi L, Di Toro R. Enhanced detection of vesicoureteric reflux with isotopic cystography. Pediatr Nephrol (Berlin, Germany). 2000;14(8–9):827–30.

Preda I, Jodal U, Sixt R, Stokland E, Hansson S. Normal dimercaptosuccinic acid scintigraphy makes voiding cystourethrography unnecessary after urinary tract infection. J Pediatr. 2007;151(6):581–4. 4 e1.

Roussey-Kesler G, Gadjos V, Idres N, Horen B, Ichay L, Leclair MD, et al. Antibiotic prophylaxis for the prevention of recurrent urinary tract infection in children with low grade vesicoureteral reflux: results from a prospective randomized study. J Urol. 2008;179(2): 674–9. discussion 9.

Salo J, Uhari M, Helminen M, Korppi M, Nieminen T, Pokka T, et al. Cranberry juice for the prevention of recurrences of urinary tract infections in children: a randomized placebo-controlled trial. Clin Infect Dis. 2011;54(3):340–6.

Schoen EJ, Colby CJ, Ray GT. Newborn circumcision decreases incidence and costs of urinary tract infections during the first year of life. Pediatrics. 2000;105(4 Pt 1):789–93.

Shaikh N, Morone NE, Bost JE, Farrell MH. Prevalence of urinary tract infection in childhood: a meta-analysis. Pediatr Infect Dis J. 2008;27(4):302–8.

Shaikh N, Ewing AL, Bhatnagar S, Hoberman A. Risk of renal scarring in children with a first urinary tract infection: a systematic review. Pediatrics. 2010;126(6): 1084–91.

Singh-Grewal D, Macdessi J, Craig J. Circumcision for the prevention of urinary tract infection in boys: a systematic review of randomised trials and observational studies. Arch Dis Child. 2005;90(8):853–8.

Siomou E, Giapros V, Fotopoulos A, Aasioti M, Papadopoulou F, Serbis A, et al. Implications of 99mTc-DMSA scintigraphy performed during urinary tract infection in neonates. Pediatrics. 2009;124(3):881–7.

Snodgrass W. Relationship of voiding dysfunction to urinary tract infection and vesicoureteral reflux in children. Urology. 1991;38(4):341–4.

Snodgrass W, Shah A, Yang M, Kwon J, Villanueva C, Traylor J, et al. Prevalence and risk factors for renal scars in children with febrile UTI and/or VUR: a cross-sectional observational study of 565 consecutive patients. J Pediatr Urol. (2013), http://dx.doi.org/10.1016/j.jpurol.2012.11.019.

Soylu A, Demir BK, Turkmen M, Bekem O, Saygi M, Cakmakci H, et al. Predictors of renal scar in children with urinary infection and vesicoureteral reflux. Pediatr Nephrol (Berlin, Germany). 2008;23(12): 2227–32.

Tabbers MM, Boluyt N, Berger MY, Benninga MA. Clinical practice: diagnosis and treatment of functional constipation. Eur J Pediatr. 2011;170(8): 955–63.

To T, Agha M, Dick PT, Feldman W. Cohort study on circumcision of newborn boys and subsequent risk of urinary-tract infection. Lancet. 1998;352(9143):1813–6.

Vernon SJ, Coulthard MG, Lambert HJ, Keir MJ, Matthews JN. New renal scarring in children who at age 3 and 4 years had had normal scans with dimercaptosuccinic acid: follow up study. BMJ (Clinical Research Ed). 1997;315(7113):905–8.

Whiting P, Westwood M, Watt I, Cooper J, Kleijnen J. Rapid tests and urine sampling techniques for the diagnosis of urinary tract infection (UTI) in children under five years: a systematic review. BMC Pediatr. 2005;5(1):4.

2 Vesicoureteral Reflux

Warren T. Snodgrass and Nicol C. Bush

Primary aims in the diagnosis and management of vesicoureteral reflux (VUR):

1. **Reduce recurrent febrile urinary tract infection (fUTI).**
2. **Prevent acquired renal damage.**

Summary of evidence for these aims:

Children with VUR have been assumed to have high risk for renal scarring and recurrent fUTI, justifying therapy in most patients. However:

- **RCTs indicate only approximately one-third of patients with VUR will have recurrent UTI within 2 years of diagnosis**
- **Acquired renal scarring occurs in approximately 15 % of children with VUR after fUTI.**
- **If DMSA scan for renal scar is negative, risk subsequent fUTI will cause renal damage is ≤10 %.**
- **No randomized controlled trial (RCT) has been done to determine if VUR therapy (medical or surgical) decreases additional acquired renal damage in children with renal scar at presentation.**
- **Antibiotic prophylaxis is no more effective than placebo to prevent recurrent UTI in children 1–24 months of age with grades 1–4 VUR.**
- **There are no data regarding benefit of antibiotic prophylaxis in children >2 years of age with VUR, with VUR and no history of UTI, with grade 5 VUR, or with recurrent UTI.**
- **Surgical correction of VUR (reimplantation or endoscopic injection) reduces recurrent fUTI.**
- **Identification and treatment of voiding dysfunction in children with VUR has not been clearly demonstrated to improve resolution or reduce fUTI.**

The two indications to diagnose and treat VUR are to decrease likelihood for recurrent fUTI and renal scarring. The association of VUR to fUTI and renal scarring has prompted investigations not only to diagnose VUR after UTI, but also in siblings or offspring of patients with VUR, and in newborns with prenatal hydronephrosis. However, recent prospective trials and observational studies indicate most children with VUR will not have frequently recurrent infections after their initial one, and most will not develop renal scarring. Furthermore, these studies also challenge the foundation of VUR management, questioning efficacy of continuous antibiotic prophylaxis to prevent recurrent UTI in children with VUR.

W.T. Snodgrass, M.D. (✉) • N.C. Bush, M.D., M.S.C.S.
Department of Pediatric Urology,
University of Texas Southwestern Medical Center
and Children's Medical Center Dallas,
1935 Medical District Drive, MS F4.04,
Dallas, TX 75235, USA
e-mail: warren.snodgrass@childrens.com

W.T. Snodgrass (ed.), *Pediatric Urology: Evidence for Optimal Patient Management*,
DOI 10.1007/978-1-4614-6910-0_2, © Springer Science+Business Media New York 2013

VUR Prevalence

After Febrile UTI

VUR is diagnosed in one-third or fewer of patients less than approximately 2 years of age following fUTI. Grades 1–3 account for over 75 % of cases, and are equally distributed between genders, while grades 4 and 5 are more common in males.

Several prospective studies have reported VUR incidence after first known symptomatic UTI:

- 302 children (33 boys) ages 1–24 months underwent VCUG after first fUTI. VUR occurred in 117 (39 %), grade 1 in 25, grade 2 in 42, grade 3 in 45, grade 4 in 5, and grade 5 in 0 children. Therefore, 96 % of VUR cases were grades 1–3. Note the small percentage of males in the study, who are more likely than females to have the higher VUR grades (Hoberman et al. 2003).
- 297 consecutive children (169 boys) under age 5 years with first symptomatic UTI (fUTI in 242) reported reflux in 28 %, but did not state the grades (Craig et al. 1998).
- 209 children with first symptomatic UTI at median age 10 months (0.2–204) had 53 (25 %) cases of VUR. Of these, 45 (85 %) were grades 1–3, while 8 (15 %) were grades 4 and 5 (gender not stated) (Ismaili et al. 2011).
- 72 term neonates 0–28 days of age with symptomatic UTI (fever, vomiting, poor feeding, failure to thrive) underwent VCUG, with VUR reported by renal units occurring in 22 % found equally in males and females. Of 144 renal units, there were grades 1 and 2 in 13 (9 %), grade 3 in 10 (7 %), and grades 4 and 5 in 8 (5.5 %). Grades 4 and 5, which accounted for 25 % of detected VUR, were found only in boys (Siomou et al. 2009).

Sibling and Offspring Screening

Siblings and offspring of affected patients have similar prevalence of VUR, approximately one-third of those screened.

Most detected VUR is low grade, with approximately 10 children per 100 screened having grades 3–5.

Prevalence of VUR decreases with age.

Meta-analysis of 22 published articles by the AUA Reflux Guidelines panel found data regarding VUR in siblings ($n=2{,}957$) and offspring ($n=244$), reporting the following:

- 100 % concordance in identical twins.
- 35–50 % prevalence in fraternal twins.
- Overall incidence was 27.4 (95 % CI 2.9–51.9)/100 screened siblings.
- Detected VUR grade was reported as "low grade" 1 and 2 vs. "high grade" 3–5. Most was low grade, with a mean prevalence of grades 3–5 in 9.8 (95 % CI 5.3–17.4)/100 siblings screened.
- Males and females were equally affected.
- Incidence in offspring was 35.7 (95 % CI 16.4–61)/100 screened.

Likelihood for VUR in screened persons decreased with age at a rate of 4 % per year (Skoog et al. 2010).

Prenatal Hydronephrosis

VUR is found in 16 % of infants diagnosed with prenatal hydronephrosis.

Prevalence is not influenced by extent of prenatal dilation, and it remains unchanged even if postnatal ultrasound (US) is normal.

Two-thirds of detected VUR are grades 1–3.

There are no data to determine if antibiotic prophylaxis to prevent first UTI in neonates with VUR is more effective than no treatment.

Meta-analysis by the AUA Reflux Guidelines panel to determine prevalence of VUR in newborns with prenatal HN included 34 studies in which the mean percentage of screened patients was 78 % (11–100 %), reporting the following:

- VUR occurred in an average of 16 % (7–35 %) with cystography.
- Grade distribution was approximately one-third each for grades 1–2, 3, and 4–5.
- VUR occurred in the non-dilated kidney in 25 % of cases.
- Prevalence was 18 % even if postnatal US was negative for HN.

- Extent of prenatal dilation did not predict likelihood for postnatal VUR.

Relative risk for UTI posed by this VUR could not be assessed from literature review, nor could possible impact, if any, of antibiotic prophylaxis (Skoog et al. 2010).

Likelihood for Recurrent fUTI

Less than one-third of children diagnosed with VUR after first fUTI receiving no therapy will have a second fUTI in the following 2 years.

Of those with recurrent infection, most will have a single recurrence, with less than 10 % of patients having three or more recurrences within 1–2 years.

The following is a summary of recurrent fUTI rates in patients with VUR from prospective studies:

- 225 children (69 boys, "most" not circumcised) ages 1 month to 3 years with first fUTI found to have grades 1–3 VUR were followed for 18 months. Recurrent fUTI developed in 32 (14 %) (Roussey-Kesler et al. 2008).
- 100 children (48 boys) <30 months of age with first fUTI and found to have VUR grades 2–4 were followed for 2 years. Recurrent fUTI occurred in 33 %, one episode in 11, two episodes in 3, and three or more episodes in 2 (Pennesi et al. 2008).
- 87 children (22 boys) 3 months to 12 years of age with grades 1–3 VUR were enrolled after fUTI (number of UTIs prior to enrollment was not stated). Recurrent fUTI occurred in 8 (9 %) during 1-year follow-up (Garin et al. 2006).
- 68 children (26 boys) ages 1–2 years with grades 3 and 4 VUR were observed without treatment for 2 years. Number of fUTIs before enrollment was not stated. Recurrent fUTI developed in 25(37 %) (Brandstrom et al. 2010).

Renal Scarring

VUR increases likelihood of renal scar by approximately 2.5 times, with increasing risk associated with increasing reflux grade, especially grades 4 and 5.

Presumed congenital reflux nephropathy was found in 4 % and focal scars in 19 % of referred patients with VUR in one study.

Meta-analysis to determine risk for renal scarring in children with UTI included 33 studies and reported scar by follow-up DMSA scan in 15 % (95 % CI 11–18). VUR had significantly increased relative risk for scar (RR 2.6 [95 % CI 1.7–3.9]), based on four studies (Shaikh et al. 2010).

A prospective study of 565 consecutive children referred for urologic assessment after fUTI and/or VUR diagnosis included DMSA scintigraphy ≥3 months after infection (mean 7.4 months; median 4 months), if present. Presumed congenital reflux nephropathy (≤44 % ipsilateral function and no cortical defects) was found in 24 (4 %), while focal cortical defects likely representing scars were found in 84/541 (15.5 %) remaining study patients. Of 340 patients with VUR, excluding those with congenital nephropathy, 65 (19 %) had focal scar. This comprised 12 % of patients with grades 1–2, 15 % with grade 3, and 50 % for grades 4–5. The OR for focal DMSA abnormalities by VUR grade were grade 1, 3.94 (95 % CI 1.05–14.85); grade 2, 3.12 (95 % CI 1.35–7.21); grade 3, 3.93 (95 % CI 1.68–9.22); grade 4, 28.91 (95 % CI 10.73–77.86); and grade 5, 77.37 (95 % CI 16.62–360.20) (see Table 1.2) (Snodgrass et al. 2012).

New Renal Scars After Prior Negative DMSA

Our review found one RCT and one retrospective review that reported 11 and 3 % of patients with VUR and a prior negative DMSA scan developed renal scar with recurrent UTI.

The IRS reported 15 % of patients and 4 % of kidneys with normal DMSA at entry developed focal defects and/or renal function decrease, but related events (fUTI, obstruction after reimplantation) were not specifically described for these children versus those with abnormal DMSA at entry.

The European branch of the IRS obtained DMSA at entry and again during follow-up at a duration of 5 years (timing of second scan not clearly stated). There were 306 children, median age 3.5 years, with DMSA studies completed and/or of sufficient quality for review in 287. All had UTI before entry, and initial DMSA was done afterwards at <2 months in 6 %, between 2 and 6 months in 40 %, and at >6 months in 54 %. During follow-up, 95 % of DMSA were obtained >6 months after last UTI. Entry DMSA was normal in 52 patients, and during follow-up 8 (15 %) showed deterioration; of 246 normal kidneys at entry, 11 (4 %) showed deterioration. There was no difference in changes based on randomization to medical versus surgical therapy. Details regarding these patients with initially normal scans who developed cortical defects or renal function loss were not specifically described. Overall DMSA changes occurred in 48 children, including 9 who developed obstruction after reimplantation and 32 stated to not have UTI during management (Piepsz et al. 1998).

The Swedish reflux trial included 203 patients with mean age 1.8 years (1–2) with grades 3 and 4 VUR. Number of fUTI prior to entry was not stated, but baseline DMSA was positive in 124 (61 %). New defects in those with negative DMSA occurred in 9/79 (11 %). Timing of DMSA and number of recurrent UTIs were not stated (Brandstrom et al. 2010).

A retrospective analysis of 138 children (53 boys) with VUR grades 1–5 included acute DMSA with subsequent DMSA 4–6 months later for abnormal findings, and another late DMSA 4–6 months after recurrent UTI. Recurrences developed in 118, but only 26 were described as fUTI and only 16 involved more than one recurrent episode. Of these, 2/71 (3 %) without scar during first evaluation were found to have new scar formation (Soylu et al. 2008).

Natural History

VUR may spontaneously resolve, with likelihood influenced by grade, laterality (unilateral versus bilateral), and patient age at diagnosis.

Initially diagnosed unilateral VUR is found in up to 20 % of cases to have contralateral VUR on subsequent cystography.

Spontaneous Resolution

Graphs summarizing VUR resolution during medical therapy were published by the first AUA Reflux Guidelines panel. These 10 resolution curves for grades 1–4 were constructed using data from three articles that comprised a total of 587 patients, of which 250 (43 %) had grade 2 (Elder et al. 1997). Subgroups with included patient numbers and percent chance for resolution in 1–5 years are found in Table 2.1.

Nomograms for VUR resolution were also constructed from a longitudinal database maintained from 1998 and analyzed in 2006 containing 2,462 children. Annual cystography was done following diagnosis, with resolution defined as one negative study. Spontaneous resolution occurred in 51 % during mean follow-up 1.95 ± 1.37 years: 72 %, grade 1; 61 %, grade 2; 49 %, grade 3; and 32 %, grades 4–5. Another 23 % had ongoing VUR at mean follow-up 2.6 ± 1.6 years, and the remaining 26 % underwent surgery at 2.3 ± 1.6 years. Multivariable analysis showed increased spontaneous resolution for the following:

- Age <1 year (HR 1.31 [95 % CI 1.16–1.48])
- Prenatal HN of sibling VUR (HR 1.24 [95 % CI 1.08–1.42])
- Single ureter (vs. duplication) (HR 1.55 [95 % CI 1.24–1.9])
- Male gender/unilateral female (HR 1.42 [95 % CI 1.26–1.59])

As a group, males and those females with unilateral VUR resolved faster than females with bilateral VUR (Estrada et al. 2009)

Internet-based calculators have been developed to predict spontaneous resolution in individual patients based on a variety of clinical data points. Each was created using different methods based upon retrospective data, including a logistic regression model, a neural network, and literature meta-analysis. A study inputting identical theoretic patient characteristics into each reported statistically significantly different predictions for spontaneous resolution (Routh et al. 2010).

New Contralateral VUR

A retrospective review was done in 167 children (33 boys) diagnosed at mean age 55 months (2–169) with unilateral VUR from 1986 to 2004. Two-cycle VCUGs were performed. All patients

Table 2.1 Percent chance of VUR resolution[a]

Risk category (age in months)(number of patients on which estimates are based)	Percent chance (95 % confidence interval)				
	1 year	2 years	3 years	4 years	5 years
Grade I[b] ($n=15$)	39.3 (24.6–51.1)	63.1 (43.2–76.1)	77.6 (57.2–88.3)	86.4 (67.7–94.3)	91.8 (75.7–97.2)
Grade II[b] ($n=250$)	28 (24.1–31.7)	48.1 (42.3–53.4)	62.7 (56.2–68.1)	73.1 (66.8–78.2)	80.6 (74.8–85.1)
Grade III, unilateral, age 0–24 ($n=27$)	21.4 (10.8–30.8)	38.2 (20.4–52.1)	51.5 (29–66.8)	61.9 (36.6–77.1)	70 (43.5–84.1)
Grade III, unilateral, age 25–60 ($n=27$)	13.4 (4.6–21.4)	25 (8.9–38.3)	35.1 (13.1–51.5)	43.8 (17.1–61.9)	51.3 (20.9–70.1)
Grade III, unilateral, age 61–120 ($n=15$)	10.8 (3.5–17.5)	20.5 (6.9–32)	29.1 (10.2–43.9)	36.7 (13.4–53.8)	43.6 (16.5–61.9)
Grade III, bilateral, age 0–24 ($n=62$)	12.7 (7–18.1)	23.8 (13.5–32.9)	33.5 (19.5–45)	41.9 (25.1–55)	49.3 (30.3–63.1)
Grade III, bilateral, age 25–60 ($n=53$)	7 (3.1–10.8)	13.5 (6.1–20.4)	19.6 (9–28.9)	25.2 (11.8–36.6)	30.5 (14.6–43.4)
Grade III, bilateral, age 61–120 ($n=14$)	2.6 (0.7–4.5)	5.2 (1.4–8.8)	7.7 (2.1–13)	10.1 (2.8–16.9)	12.5 (3.5–20.7)
Grade IV, unilateral[c] ($n=28$)	16.1 (8.5–23.1)	29.7 (16.4–40.8)	41 (23.5–54.5)	50.5 (30–65)	58.5 (36–73.1)
Grade IV, bilateral[c] ($n=96$)	4.5 (1–7.9)	6.4 (2–15.1)	7.8 (3–21.8)	8.9 (4–28)	9.9 (4.9–33.7)

[a]Reproduced with permission from Jack S. Elder, MD; Craig Andrew Peters, MD; Billy S. Arant, Jr., MD; David H. Ewalt, MD; Charles E. Hawtrey, MD; Richard S. Hurwitz, MD; Thomas S. Parrott, MD; Howard M. Snyder, III, MD; Robert A. Weiss, MD. AUA Pediatric Vesicoureteral Reflux Clinical Guidelines Panel: The Management of Primary Vesicoureteral Reflux in Children. American Urological Association Education and Research, Inc., © 1997. http://www.auanet.org/content/guidelines-and-quality-care/clinical-guidelines/archived-guidelines/vesi_reflux07.pdf. The yearly rate of reflux resolution remains constant for each group
[b]No difference shown by age or laterality (unilateral/bilateral); therefore, these categories were combined
[c]Estimates only apply to the time of diagnosis and are not age-specific

had at least two cystograms, with 84 having three to seven studies. Contralateral VUR not seen on the initial VCUG occurred in 33 (21 %) in patients with a mean 3.5 ± 1.4 cystograms. This VUR was grade 1 in 4, 2 in 18, 3 in 9, and 4 in 1 patient. Variables analyzed included gender, side, age, VUR grade, and voiding dysfunction. Of these, only higher VUR grade was predictive, with contralateral VUR found in 12/91 (13 %) of grades 1–2 vs. 21/62 (34 %) with grades 3–5, $p = 0.006$ (Barroso et al. 2008).

Voiding Dysfunction

Few studies report impact of treatment for voiding dysfunction on VUR outcomes.

Our review found only one retrospective analysis stating breakthrough UTI was significantly more likely, despite AC in females with VUR and urge syndrome versus those without voiding dysfunction.

One report found no difference in VUR resolution at 3 years in patients with versus without detrusor instability.

Two others reported spontaneous resolution in approximately 60 % of ureters with mostly grades 1 and 2 VUR in 6–12 months with biofeedback, but had no control groups.

The 2010 AUA Reflux Guidelines reported the following observations about VUR and bladder/bowel dysfunction (BBD):

- BBD increases risk for fUTI in children with VUR on antibiotic prophylaxis (44 % with BBD vs. 13 % without)
- Spontaneous VUR resolution is less at 24 months in children with BBD (31 % with vs. 61 % without)
- The rate of postoperative UTI after VUR surgery is greater with BBD (22 % vs. 5 %)

Despite these observations, the panel stated there are few data regarding the impact of treatment for BBD on VUR outcomes (Peters et al. 2010).

A retrospective study of females ages 3–10 years old with VUR systematically obtained history for voiding dysfunction, found in 36/94 (40 %) presenting after UTI (characterized as 1–2 or ≥3 in the preceding 12 months; febrile vs. nonfebrile not stated). Those with symptoms of frequency, urgency, holding maneuvers, and/or diurnal incontinence for at least 6 months were treated with timed voiding and oxybutynin 2.5–5.0 mg/dose 3 times daily at 6-month intervals until symptoms did not recur off medication. All patients also received antibiotic prophylaxis. All were considered to have a satisfactory response to AC (not defined). Breakthrough UTI occurred in a total of 23/86 (27 %) with follow-up of 1 year, 18 (78 %) with urge syndrome. Breakthrough UTI was significantly more likely in females with treated urge syndrome versus those without symptoms, 18/42 (43 %) vs. 5/44 (11 %), $p = 0.001$, despite similar age and VUR grades (Snodgrass 1998).

One-hundred one children, 67 % females, mean age 5 years (6 week to 15 year) with recurrent UTI (febrile vs. nonfebrile; number of infections not stated) underwent UD with fluoroscopy that identified VUR. Grades were 1 ($n = 1$), 2 ($n = 14$), 3 ($n = 13$), 4 ($n = 10$), and 5 ($n = 1$). Of these patients, detrusor instability was diagnosed in 41 (41 %). Treatment comprised AC, and all children had antibiotic prophylaxis. Reimplantation was done as initial therapy in some patients and within 1 year in others (in ≤4 patients for recurrent UTI), leaving 30 patients (39 ureters) with detrusor instability with medical management and follow-up a mean of 3 years. Resolution occurred in 15/39 (38 %), vs. 27/57 (47 %) ureters in 42 patients with a stable bladder, $p = 0.4$. UTI following treatment was not clearly described (Scholtmeijer and Nijman 1994).

Twenty-five females, mean age 9 years (6–10), with VUR and dysfunctional voiding underwent a mean of seven biofeedback sessions (2–20) weekly–biweekly with repeat VCUG 1 year later. VUR grade was 1 ($n = 10$), 2 ($n = 15$), 3 ($n = 5$), and 4 ($n = 1$). Resolution occurred in 17/31(55 %) ureters. Correlation to dysfunctional voiding was not described, except to state that all children with resolved VUR had resolved or improved symptoms and decreased PVR from a mean 40–10 % voided volume (Palmer et al. 2002).

Seventy-eight children, 90 % females, mean age 9 years (5–14), were diagnosed with dysfunctional voiding (uroflow with pelvic floor EMG) and VUR, which was grade 1 ($n = 26$), 2 ($n = 32$), 3 ($n = 28$), and 4 ($n = 12$). All received urotherapy ("proper toilet posture," hydration, timed voiding) and biofeedback for a median 6 (2–14) sessions. At 6 months follow-up, subjective reduction in symptoms of ≥90 % was reported for diurnal incontinence in 70 % and frequency in 76 %, and normalization of uroflow patterns occurred in 80 %. VUR resolved in 63 % of affected renal units (96 and 81 % of grades 1 and 2, 36 % of grade 3, and 8 % of grade 4). UTI was not discussed (Kibar et al. 2007).

Impact of VUR on Pregnancy

There are limited data regarding pregnancy risks from uncorrected VUR.

One literature review reported the primary risk factor for pregnancy complications, including UTI, gestational hypertension, preeclampsia, or fetal morbidity, was renal scarring.

The first AUA Reflux Guidelines panel reviewed published literature on this subject and concluded available data were insufficient to determine actual risk of uncorrected VUR during pregnancy. They reviewed five studies that demonstrated renal insufficiency increased toxemia, preterm labor, fetal growth retardation, and fetal demise (Elder et al. 1997).

Literature review regarding impact of VUR on pregnancy identified 15 articles for inclusion, reporting the following:

- fUTI in pregnancy (four studies) ranged from 3 to 37 %; fUTI in patients with childhood ureteral reimplantation (two studies) occurred in 25/141 (18 %) and 5/77 (7 %).
- Hypertension in pregnancy (three studies) was not increased by history of VUR with no renal scarring; hypertension occurred in 31 and 42 % with renal scarring (extent of renal damage not described).
- Preeclampsia (five studies) was increased by renal scarring; two studies reported no increased preeclampsia without renal scarring in a total of 23 women.
- No study reported history of VUR impacted fetal outcomes; one reported 8/39 pregnancies with renal scarring had low birth weight (Hollowell 2008).

Management

VUR management aims to reduce recurrent fUTI and renal scarring.

Historically, risk for fUTI and renal scar have been assumed present in all children with VUR, with management based on the general assumption that reflux should resolve or be surgically corrected, especially in girls.

Few studies specifically address impact of treatment on recurrent UTI and/or renal scarring.

Continuous Antibiotic Prophylaxis

Continuous antibiotic prophylaxis (CAP) has been routinely recommended in children with VUR while awaiting spontaneous reflux resolution.

Meta-analysis of six RCTs by the 2011 AAP UTI Guidelines panel concluded antibiotic prophylaxis is no more effective than no therapy to prevent recurrent fUTI in children 1–24 months of age with grades 1–4 VUR.

Overall fUTI recurrence was 19 % in 1–2 years, with increasing percentage recurrence with increasing VUR grade.

There are no data regarding efficacy of CAP to reduce recurrent fUTI in patients with grade 5 VUR.

There are no data to determine if antibiotic prophylaxis is effective to prevent initial fUTI in children with VUR detected by sibling or prenatal hydronephrosis screening.

There are no data to determine efficacy of antibiotic prophylaxis in patients presenting with recurrent UTI.

Meta-analysis was done on data provided by six RCTs to determine efficacy of CAP to prevent recurrent fUTI versus no treatment in infants 2–24 months of age with VUR. Findings are shown in Table 2.2. There was no benefit of CAP versus no treatment for any grade of VUR, based on a sample

Table 2.2 Recurrence of febrile UTI/pyelonephritis in infants 2–24 months of age with and without antimicrobial prophylaxis, according to grade of VUR[a]

	Prophylaxis		No prophylaxis		
Reflux grade	No. of recurrences	Total *n*	No. of recurrences	Total *n*	*p*
None	7	210	11	163	0.15
I	2	37	2	35	1.00
II	11	133	10	124	0.95
III	31	140	40	145	0.29
IV	16	55	21	49	0.14

[a]Reproduced with permission from Pediatrics, Vol.128, Page 604, Copyright 2011 by the AAP

size of 718 patients: 72, grade 1; 257, grade 2; 285, grade 3; and 104, grade 4. Recurrent fUTI occurred in 133 (19 %); percentage fUTI recurrences by grade were 6 %, grade 1; 8 %. grade 2; 25 %, grade 3; and 36 %, grade 4 (AAP 2011).

Compliance with drug therapy has been raised as a potential confounder in these data, specifically that patients assigned to antibiotic might not have taken the medication, which likely would be representative of clinical practice. Of these six RCTs:

- Craig et al. assessed adherence by counting pills and direct questioning during visits. Sixteen percent of study patients discontinued therapy by 3 months, and 31 % at 12 months, with no difference in placebo versus drug treatment groups.
- Montini et al. tested antibiotic activity in routine urine cultures, with 71 % positive in the drug treatment group.
- Penesi et al. reported 6/50 (12 %) did not take prophylaxis.
- Brandstrom et al. stated 2/67 (3 %) admitted to noncompliance.
- Garin et al. excluded patients who self-admitted to noncompliance.
- Roussley-Kessler et al. did not assess compliance.

The AAP review limited analysis of antibiotic prophylaxis to children <2 years of age with grades 0–4 VUR after one febrile UTI. Our review found no reports concerning antibiotic prophylaxis in other scenarios:

- Grade 5 VUR
- Children with VUR and no history of UTI
- Children with recurrent UTI at diagnosis

Surgical Correction of VUR: Primary Outcomes

The two desired outcomes from surgical VUR correction are reduction in fUTI and renal scarring.

One RCT demonstrated ureteral reimplantation in children with VUR grades 3 and 4 significantly decreased recurrent fUTI over antibiotic prophylaxis (8 % surgical vs. 22 % medical therapy).

Three studies reported that recurrent fUTI after endoscopic injection occurs in ≤ approximately 10 % of patients. Odds for recurrence were 8.5 times greater in patients having more than three versus one febrile infection within 1 year before injection.

Recurrent febrile UTI after initially successful Dx/HA injection is associated with recurrent VUR in approximately 50 % of cases. Cystography for febrile UTI after reimplantation has not been reported.

There are no RCTs demonstrating VUR correction reduces renal scarring.

Ureteral Reimplantation

The International Reflux Study randomized children less than 11 years of age with grades 3 and 4 VUR to either antibiotic prophylaxis or ureteral reimplantation (Politano-Leadbetter, Lich-Grigoir, Cohen, based on surgeon preference). The US arm comprised 62 patients, 24 with unilateral and 38 with bilateral VUR, while the

European arm had 151 patients, 33 with unilateral and 118 with bilateral reflux. While overall UTI rates were similar between medical and surgical patients, fUTI occurred significantly less often after reimplantation (22 % medical vs. 8–10 % surgical, RR 0.43[95 % CI 0.27–0.70]) (Wheeler et al. 2003).

The European arm of the IRS obtained DMSA at entry and during 5-year follow-up in 287 children median age 3.5 years with grades 3 or 4 VUR. Of these, 52 (18 %) were initially normal. Follow-up DMSA was considered to show deterioration (new or larger cortical defect and/or renal function decrease >3 %) in 48 (17 %) children, including 8 (15 %) initially normal. There was no difference in these changes between those treated medically or surgically (Piepsz et al. 1998).

One study reported preoperative and postoperative DMSA scan in 143 children (45 boys) with VUR undergoing ureteral reimplantation at median age 2 years (2.5 month to 14 years). Maximum grade was 2–5 in 18, 59, 27, and 4 %. Preoperative scintigraphy was obtained less than 3 months after last UTI in 31 % of cases and not documented in 12 %, while 10 % had no history of UTI. Interval from DMSA scan to surgery was a mean 1.4 months (1 day to 1.5 years). Preoperative DMSA findings included congenital reflux nephropathy in 12 (8 %) and at least one kidney had abnormal findings in 94 (72 %) of the remainder. Postoperative DMSA was obtained at median 3 years (1–9). Postoperative UTI was known to have occurred in 12 %. One male developed a cortical defect, but he had UTI after his preoperative DMSA and before reimplantation, and another postoperatively 3 weeks before the last DMSA, so designation as scar and timing of injury was uncertain. Two other patients had new scars: one male with no preoperative UTI but "a scarred kidney" had one UTI postoperatively, while one female with preoperative scarring had recurrent postoperative UTI and a new scar. Timing of last DMSA in relation to last UTI was not stated. Overall mean change in ipsilateral renal function was 2.5 %, with nine kidneys in nine children having a 13–48 % decrease. There was no mention of postoperative UTI occurrence in these patients. UTIs were not characterized as febrile or not (Webster et al. 2000).

Another retrospective study found that preoperative and postoperative DMSA scans had been obtained in 74 children (45 boys) out of 223 undergoing reimplantation from 1985 to 1997. These scans had been done a median 2 months (10 day to 58 months) before and a median 19 months (5–44) after surgery. fUTI occurred in only two patients after operation. No new scars were diagnosed (Choi et al. 1999).

Endoscopic Injection

Meta-analysis of reported outcomes in 12 studies after endoscopic injection stated recurrent fUTI occurred in 0.75 % (95 % CI 0.18–3.09) of patients. Incidence and frequency of pre-injection fUTI were not described, nor was duration of post-injection follow-up (Elder et al. 2006).

One study comprising 167 children with initially successful Dx/HA injection involved chart review and phone calls to both parents and PCP to determine incidence of recurrent infection. At median follow-up of 32 months (7–53), 12 % had recurrent fUTI, of which half had recurrent VUR on subsequent cystography. Multivariable analysis showed the number of preoperative fUTIs within 1 year of injection predicted UTI recurrence:

- Two to three preoperative infections, OR 3 (95 % CI 1.1–8.2) for postoperative fUTI
- Three preoperative infections, OR 8.5 (95 % CI 3.3–22) for postoperative fUTI (Chi et al. 2008)

Another retrospective study included 100 patients mean age 3.8 ± 0.3 years (24 % boys) after successful Dx/HA injection followed a mean of 15 months. A fivefold reduction in UTIs/year (febrile vs. nonfebrile not stated) was noted, from a mean 0.68 ± 0.09 pre-injection to 0.12 ± 0.04 post-injection. Recurrent infection occurred in 13 %, of which half had recurrent VUR (Wadie et al. 2007).

A third retrospective analysis reported Dx/HA injection in 311 children (41 boys) at mean age 5.7 years, of which 253 had negative cycled

VCUG post-injection. During mean follow-up of 2.6 years, 7 (3 %) developed fUTI. VCUG was repeated in five, and each demonstrated recurrent VUR (Traxel et al. 2009).

Correction of VUR: Secondary Outcomes

Reimplantation: Reflux Resolution

Published literature reviews indicate initial success for ureteral reimplantation to correct VUR in ≥95 % of ureters on cystography performed ≤6 months postoperatively.

The International Reflux Study reported VUR resolution 6 months after surgery in 94 and 89 % of US and European arms, respectively.

The European arm reported recurrent VUR in 3 % of patients at 5-year cystography.

There are few other data regarding recurrent VUR after reimplantation in either symptomatic or asymptomatic children to verify common opinion that surgical success is durable in the long term.

The first AUA Reflux Guidelines panel reviewed 86 articles providing reimplantation outcomes (published between 1965 and 1994) in 6,472 patients and 8,563 ureters. It reported overall success was 95 % of patients, and >98 % of ureters for VUR grades 1–4 and 81 % for grade 5. Techniques reviewed and date of last cystography after surgery were not stated (Elder et al. 1997).

A review of published outcomes for case series involving at least 100 reimplanted ureters analyzed 19 articles and the authors' own data comprising 3,346 patients and 5,008 ureters. Techniques used included Cohen, Politano-Leadbetter, Glenn-Anderson, and Lich-Gregoir. Overall VUR resolution occurred in 99 % of ureters. Five series reported failed reimplantation in a total of 40/1,116 (4 %) ureters on initial postoperative cystography, with spontaneous resolution in 1–5 years in 34 (85 %) (Bisignani and Decter 1997).

The US arm of the International Reflux Study included surgery in 87 patients and 157 ureters with grade 3–4 VUR done using the Cohen technique in 52 %, Politano-Leadbetter in 28 %, Glenn-Anderson in 10 % and "other modifications" in 9 % (of patients). VUR persisted in five (6 %) patients, ultimately resolving spontaneously in all but one case at a mean of 20 months after surgery. There were no obstructions from surgery (Duckett et al. 1992).

The European arm operated on 150 patients (36 boys) and 237 ureters, using Politano-Leadbetter in 55 %, Lich-Grigoir in 26 %, and Cohen in 18 % (of patients). Persistent VUR was found at 6 months cystography in 15 % of bilateral and 6 % of unilateral reimplanted children, that resolved by 5-year cystography in 13/17 (76 %). Of 134 patients with negative 6-month postoperative cystograms, recurrent VUR was found during repeat cystography at 5 years in 4 (3 %). Obstruction developed in 10 (7 %) children, including 3 undergoing Politano-Leadbetter who had the ureter passed through the intestinal wall (Hjalmas et al. 1992).

Reimplantation: Intravesical Versus Extravesical

Extravesical reimplantation creates less gross hematuria and subjective bladder spasm than intravesical repairs.

Bilateral extravesical reimplantation can result in temporary postoperative urinary retention in ≤10 % of patients; this is not seen with intravesical techniques.

One RCT randomized 44 children with unilateral VUR grades 2–4 to either extravesical Lich-Gregoir or intravesical Politano-Leadbetter reimplantation (method used to randomize was not stated). Mean age of patients in the two groups was similar (69.7 months [18–110] vs. 62.1 months [8–110]). Extravesical operations were done through an ipsilateral inguinal incision, whereas intravesical procedures used a Pfannenstiel incision. All patients had postoperative catheter drainage for 48 h, urethral for extravesical reimplants, and suprapubic for intravesical repairs. Postoperative pain was assessed using an objective scale, and episodes of bladder spasm quantified. The authors did not state who performed these evaluations, and there is no mention of blinding. They found that extravesical reimplantation had significantly less bladder spasm and no gross hematuria. Objective pain scale scores were significantly less after extravesical surgery (potentially related in part to the smaller incision), but opioid use was not different. There was no difference in mean postoperative post-void residual urine volumes (time of assessment not stated) (Schwentner et al. 2006).

A prospective study involved 237 patients undergoing extravesical reimplantation, of which 144 were bilateral. Mean age for the entire series was 5.5 years (2 months to 15 years), and all operations were done with a Pfannenstiel incision with postoperative urethral catheter drainage for 12–36 h (reason for varying intervals not stated). Short-term urinary retention developed in 8 % after bilateral reimplantation that did not occur in unilateral cases. This retention resolved within 1 week in all affected patients (Lapointe et al. 1998).

A retrospective review evaluated 220 patients, mean age approximately 5.5 years, who underwent bilateral extravesical reimplantation with postoperative urethral catheterization for 24–48 h from 1991 to 1997. Complete inability to void after catheter removal occurred in 23 (10 %), treated with catheter replacement for another 7–10 days. Retention resolved in 22 during catheterization, while one had clean intermittent catheterization (CIC) for 4 months. Univariate analysis reported grades 4–5 VUR, age ≤3 years and male gender, but not treated preoperative voiding dysfunction (not defined) correlated with urinary retention (Barrieras et al. 1999).

Overnight Foley drainage was used in a retrospective series of 50 consecutive toilet-trained children (13 boys), mean age 5 years (2–13 years), undergoing bilateral extravesical reimplantation for VUR grades 1–5. There was no case of postoperative urinary retention (McAchran and Palmer 2005).

Another retrospective study included 41 children with mean age 38 months (16–81) who had bilateral robotic extravesical reimplantation for VUR grades 3–5. All had overnight catheterization followed by post-void bladder scan that found a mean residual of 13 mL. None developed urinary retention (Casale et al. 2008).

Contralateral VUR After Unilateral Reimplantation

Meta-analysis reported approximately 10 % of patients undergoing unilateral reimplantation will have contralateral VUR on postoperative cystography.

One review stated new contralateral VUR ranged from grades 1–5.

Potential risk factors, including one versus more than one and cycled versus non-cycled preoperative cystography, grade of ipsilateral VUR, and history of resolved contralateral VUR, have not been analyzed.

Most this reflux resolves within 1 year of diagnosis.

The first AUA Reflux Guidelines panel reported its review of literature from 1965 to 1994 and indicated that an average of 9 % of unilateral reimplantations demonstrated contralateral VUR postoperatively. Repeat surgery was not recommended for at least 1 year, because most reported new contralateral VUR resolved during that time. Risk factors for contralateral VUR were not reported (Elder et al. 1997).

A retrospective review after either unilateral Cohen or Glenn-Anderson reimplantation found 20 (19 %) of 120 patients had new contralateral VUR. Seventy percent of patients had more than one preoperative VCUG. The authors implied all subjects had only unilateral VUR diagnosed preoperatively. New contralateral VUR was grade 1 in nine, grade 2 in nine, grades 3 and 4 in two each, and grade 5 in one patient. This reflux resolved in 12 (67 %) of 18 with grades 1–2, in 1 with grade 3, and persisted in all with grades 4–5 by 3 years follow-up. Reoperation to reimplant the contralateral ureter was done in 3 (15 %) (Hoenig et al. 1996).

Another retrospective study of 43 unilateral Lich-Gregoir reimplants found new contralateral VUR in 5 (12 %) patients. Of these, four had known prior bilateral VUR with unilateral resolution. The number of preoperative cystograms for the entire group was not stated; nor was the grade of new contralateral reflux. Spontaneous resolution occurred in four of five cases within 1 year (Burno et al. 1998).

Endoscopic Injection: Reflux Resolution

Endoscopic injection is less effective than reimplantation for VUR correction.

Results are best predicted by VUR grade, success diminishing with increasing grade.

Creation of an elevated, coapted mound correlates with VUR resolution, regardless of injection technique (STING vs. intraorifice vs. HIT) or injected volume.

Failures usually are found to have mound loss or shift from under the orifice.

Failure rates of 13–26 % have been reported at repeat cystographymore than 12 months after initially successful injection. One report found likelihood for recurrence increased according to initial VUR grade.

Meta-analysis of published results from 63 articles including 5,527 patients and 8,101 ureters reported probability for resolving VUR (defined as negative cystography ≥1 month post-injection) with one or more injections using primarily polytetrafluoroethylene, collagen, or Dx/HA was 87 % of patients and 85 % of ureters, with significantly less success in duplicated versus single systems (50 % vs. 73 %).

One injection success probability was as follows:

- 67 % of patients (95 % CI 53.61–78.33)
- 76 % of ureters (95 % CI 70.62–80.10)
- Success by grade: 79 % for grades 1 and 2, 72 % grade 3, 63 % grade 4, 51 % grade 5.

Second injection success probability was as follows:

- 54 % of patients (95 % CI 39.97–68.10)
- 68 % of ureters (95 % CI 61.04–74.29)

Third injection success probability was as follows:

- 34 % of ureters (95 % CI 20.24–50.89) (Elder et al. 2006).

A systematic review of 47 articles and 7,303 ureters regarding Dx/HA injection found similar outcomes, resolution in 77 % of ureters (95 % CI: 76–78 %). The most predictive factor for outcome was VUR grade, with success in 81 % of grade 1 vs. 62 % of grade 5, $p<0.001$ (Routh et al. 2010).

A prospective study reported a single Dx/HA injection resolved reflux on a 3-month post-injection cystogram in 70 % of 168 patients and 78 % of 259 ureters having grades 1–5 VUR. Patients failing the initial injection were offered a second, with 61 % of those performed successful, achieving overall reflux resolution in the series in 82 %. The initial 80 children had STING injection technique, whereas the remainder had intraorifice injection—in all cases with the intention to elevate and coapt the orifice. Mean injected volume was 0.54 cc (SD 0.27). Multivariable analysis of factors potentially impacting outcomes (gender, unilateral vs. bilateral VUR, duplicated vs. single system refluxing ureters, VUR grade, injection technique, volume injected, satisfactory versus unsatisfactory post-injection mound morphology) found results independently predicted by the following:

- VUR grade (OR 0.46 [95 % CI .29–72])
- Injected volume <0.5 cc vs. >0.5 cc (OR 0.3 [95 % CI 0.09–0.98])
- Desired mound morphology (OR 11.5 [95 % CI 5.3–25])

Increasing VUR grade predicted less success, with a single injection resolving reflux in 100 % grade 1, 83 % grade 2, 73 % grade 3, 53 % grade 4, and 29 % grade 5 ureters. "Satisfactory" mound created in 196 of 243 ureters correlated with 89 % success, while an unsatisfactory mound in 47 ureters resolved reflux in only 36 % (Yucel et al. 2007).

A prospective study compared outcomes in ureters after intraorifice or HIT in consecutive patients treated by a single surgeon. The first 96 ureters had intraorifice injection, while the last 52 had HIT, with single-injection VUR resolution in 86.5 % vs. 79 %, $p=0.23$. HIT resulted in significantly increased injection volumes versus intraorifice injection (0.68 cc vs. 0.51 cc, $p=0.002$) (Gupta and Snodgrass 2008).

A retrospective review compared STING to HIT in 301 children and 453 ureters performed by five surgeons. Multivariable analysis found only the surgeon and increasing VUR grade, but not injection technique or volume < or >1 cc, predicted results (Routh et al. 2007).

A multicenter retrospective analysis reported 87 % of 97 ureters failing Dx/HA injection with a mean 0.86 cc (0.3–2) were found to have mound volume loss and/or shifting of the implant from under the orifice (Higham-Kessler et al. 2007).

There are limited data regarding recurrent VUR after initial resolution by bulking agents, but available reports indicate success diminishes with time:

- In a report of Dx/HA injection of 334 ureters, 94 % with grades 3–4 VUR, 45 with VUR resolution had subsequent cystography 2–5 years later. Recurrent VUR was noted in six (13 %), four with grade 2 and one each with grades 3 and 4 (Lackgren et al. 2001).
- Another retrospective review of 337 injected ureters reported initial success in 246 (73 %) at 3-month cystography. Of these, 150 (61 %) underwent repeat cystography at 12 months and 39 (26 %) had recurrent VUR, found in 0 % of those originally with grade 1, 19 % of grade 2, 37 % of grade 3, 33 % of grade 4, and 60 % of grade 5 (Lee et al. 2009).

Contralateral VUR After Unilateral Injection

Two studies reported approximately 10 % of children will have new contralateral VUR after unilateral endoscopic injection.

Grade of new VUR ranged from 1 to 4.

Pre-injection VUR grade did not correlate with likelihood for new contralateral VUR.

One study reported a similar average of approximately two pre-injection cystograms in those with and without new VUR.

A retrospective review included 662 children (203 boys) with endoscopic treatment for unilateral VUR using polytetrafluoroethylene or Dx/HA at mean age of 3 years. VUR resolution occurred in all, 83 % with one, 14 % with two, and 3 % with three injections. New contralateral VUR occurred after resolution in 67 (10 %), grade 1 in 16, grade 2 in 17, grade 3 in 27, and grade 4 in 7. There was no correlation between initial VUR grade and likelihood for contralateral VUR. The number of cystograms performed pre- and post-injection in those with versus without new VUR was not stated (Menezes et al. 2007).

Another retrospective report included 126 children (30 boys) with unilateral Dx/HA injection, after excluding those with a history of resolved contralateral VUR. New contralateral VUR was found in 17 patients (13 %) during VCUG 12 weeks post-injection, grade 1 in 9, grade 2 in 6, and grade 3 in 2. There was no difference in mean patient age, mean number of pre-injection VCUGs (1.9 vs. 1.8) or mean VUR grade (2.5 vs. 2.7) in those with and without new contralateral VUR (Elmore et al. 2006).

A third retrospective report analyzed cystoscopic assessment of the contralateral orifice to guide decision-making in unilateral VUR, performing bilateral injection when it had a stadium or worse configuration and/or ≥ grade 2 hydrodistention. There were 146 patients with median of 3 (1–6) pre-injection cystograms. Of these, 101 (69 %) were judged to have an abnormal orifice and received bilateral injection versus 45 who were not injected. New contralateral reflux occurred in 8 and 13 %, which was not significantly different (Routh et al. 2008).

References

AAP 2011. Roberts KB, Subcommittee on Urinary Tract Infection, Steering Committee on Quality Improvement and Management. Urinary tract infection: clinical practice guideline for the diagnosis and management of the initial UTI in febrile infants and children 2 to 24 months. Pediatrics. 2011;128(3):595–610.

Barrieras D, Lapointe S, Reddy PP, Williot P, McLorie GA, Bagli D, et al. Urinary retention after bilateral extravesical ureteral reimplantation: does dissection distal to the ureteral orifice have a role? J Urol. 1999;162(3 Pt 2):1197–200.

Barroso Jr U, Barroso VA, de Bessa J, Jr CAA, Zerati FM. Predictive factors for contralateral reflux in patients with conservatively treated unilateral vesicoureteral reflux. J Urol. 2008;180(1):297–9. discussion 9.

Bisignani G, Decter RM. Voiding cystourethrography after uncomplicated ureteral reimplantation in children: is it necessary? J Urol. 1997;158(3 Pt 2): 1229–31.

Brandstrom P, Esbjorner E, Herthelius M, Swerkersson S, Jodal U, Hansson S. The Swedish reflux trial in children: III. Urinary tract infection pattern. J Urol. 2010;184(1):286–91.

Burno DK, Glazier DB, Zaontz MR. Lessons learned about contralateral reflux after unilateral extravesical

ureteral advancement in children. J Urol. 1998;160(3 Pt 2):995–7. discussion 1038.
Casale P, Patel RP, Kolon TF. Nerve sparing robotic extravesical ureteral reimplantation. J Urol. 2008;179(5): 1987–9. discussion 90.
Chi A, Gupta A, Snodgrass W. Urinary tract infection following successful dextranomer/hyaluronic acid injection for vesicoureteral reflux. J Urol. 2008;179(5): 1966–9.
Choi H, Oh SJ, So Y, Lee DS, Lee A, Kim KM. No further development of renal scarring after antireflux surgery in children with primary vesicoureteral reflux: review of the results of 99mtechnetium dimercapto-succinic acid renal scan. J Urol. 1999;162(3 Pt 2):1189–92.
Craig JC, Irwig LM, Knight JF, Sureshkumar P, Roy LP. Symptomatic urinary tract infection in preschool Australian children. J Paediatr Child Health. 1998; 34(2):154–9.
Duckett JW, Walker RD, Weiss R. Surgical results: International Reflux Study in Children–United States branch. J Urol. 1992;148(5 Pt 2):1674–5.
Elder JS, Peters CA, Arant Jr BS, Ewalt DH, Hawtrey CE, Hurwitz RS, et al. Pediatric Vesicoureteral Reflux Guidelines Panel summary report on the management of primary vesicoureteral reflux in children. J Urol. 1997;157(5):1846–51.
Elder JS, Diaz M, Caldamone AA, Cendron M, Greenfield S, Hurwitz R, et al. Endoscopic therapy for vesicoureteral reflux: a meta-analysis. I Reflux resolution and urinary tract infection J Urol. 2006;175(2): 716–22.
Elmore JM, Kirsch AJ, Lyles RH, Perez-Brayfield MR, Scherz HC. New contralateral vesicoureteral reflux following dextranomer/hyaluronic Acid implantation: incidence and identification of a high risk group. J Urol. 2006;175(3 Pt 1):1097–100. discussion 100–1.
Estrada Jr CR, Passerotti CC, Graham DA, Peters CA, Bauer SB, Diamond DA, et al. Nomograms for predicting annual resolution rate of primary vesicoureteral reflux: results from 2,462 children. J Urol. 2009;182(4): 1535–41.
Garin EH, Olavarria F, Garcia Nieto V, Valenciano B, Campos A, Young L. Clinical significance of primary vesicoureteral reflux and urinary antibiotic prophylaxis after acute pyelonephritis: a multicenter, randomized, controlled study. Pediatrics. 2006;117(3): 626–32.
Gupta A, Snodgrass W. Intra-orifice versus hydrodistention implantation technique in dextranomer/hyaluronic acid injection for vesicoureteral reflux. J Urol. 2008;180(4 Suppl):1589–92. discussion 92–3.
Higham-Kessler J, Reinert SE, Snodgrass WT, Hensle TW, Koyle MA, Hurwitz RS, et al. A review of failures of endoscopic treatment of vesicoureteral reflux with dextranomer microspheres. J Urol. 2007;177(2): 710–4. discussion 4–5.
Hjalmas K, Lohr G, Tamminen-Mobius T, Seppanen J, Olbing H, Wikstrom S. Surgical results in the International Reflux Study in Children (Europe). J Urol. 1992;148(5 Pt 2):1657–61.
Hoberman A, Charron M, Hickey RW, Baskin M, Kearney DH, Wald ER. Imaging studies after a first febrile urinary tract infection in young children. N Engl J Med. 2003;348(3):195–202.
Hoenig DM, Diamond DA, Rabinowitz R, Caldamone AA. Contralateral reflux after unilateral ureteral reimplantation. J Urol. 1996;156(1):196–7.
Hollowell JG. Outcome of pregnancy in women with a history of vesico-ureteric reflux. BJU Int. 2008;102(7):780–4.
Ismaili K, Lolin K, Damry N, Alexander M, Lepage P, Hall M. Febrile urinary tract infections in 0- to 3-month-old infants: a prospective follow-up study. J Pediatr. 2011;158(1):91–4.
Kibar Y, Ors O, Demir E, Kalman S, Sakallioglu O, Dayanc M. Results of biofeedback treatment on reflux resolution rates in children with dysfunctional voiding and vesicoureteral reflux. Urology. 2007;70(3):563–6. discussion 6–7.
Lackgren G, Wahlin N, Skoldenberg E, Stenberg A. Long-term followup of children treated with dextranomer/hyaluronic acid copolymer for vesicoureteral reflux. J Urol. 2001;166(5):1887–92.
Lapointe SP, Barrieras D, Leblanc B, Williot P. Modified Lich-Gregoir ureteral reimplantation: experience of a Canadian center. J Urol. 1998;159(5):1662–4.
Lee EK, Gatti JM, Demarco RT, Murphy JP. Long-term followup of dextranomer/hyaluronic acid injection for vesicoureteral reflux: late failure warrants continued followup. J Urol. 2009;181(4):1869–74. discussion 74–5.
McAchran SE, Palmer JS. Bilateral extravesical ureteral reimplantation in toilet trained children: Is 1-day hospitalization without urinary retention possible? J Urol. 2005;174(5):1991–3. discussion 3.
Menezes M, Mohanan N, Haroun J, Colhoun E, Puri P. New contralateral vesicoureteral reflux after endoscopic correction of unilateral reflux–is routine contralateral injection indicated at initial treatment? J Urol. 2007;178(4 Pt 2):1711–3.
Palmer LS, Franco I, Rotario P, Reda EF, Friedman SC, Kolligian ME, et al. Biofeedback therapy expedites the resolution of reflux in older children. J Urol. 2002;168(4 Pt 2):1699–702. discussion 702–3.
Pennesi M, Travan L, Peratoner L, Bordugo A, Cattaneo A, Ronfani L, et al. Is antibiotic prophylaxis in children with vesicoureteral reflux effective in preventing pyelonephritis and renal scars? A randomized, controlled trial. Pediatrics. 2008;121(6):e1489–94.
Peters CA, Skoog SJ, Arant Jr BS, Copp HL, Elder JS, Hudson RG, et al. Summary of the AUA Guideline on Management of Primary Vesicoureteral Reflux in Children. J Urol. 2010;184(3):1134–44.
Piepsz A, Tamminen-Mobius T, Reiners C, Heikkila J, Kivisaari A, Nilsson NJ, et al. Five-year study of medical or surgical treatment in children with severe vesico-ureteral reflux dimercaptosuccinic acid findings. International Reflux Study Group in Europe Eur J Pediatr. 1998;157(9):753–8.
Roussey-Kesler G, Gadjos V, Idres N, Horen B, Ichay L, Leclair MD, et al. Antibiotic prophylaxis for the

prevention of recurrent urinary tract infection in children with low grade vesicoureteral reflux: results from a prospective randomized study. J Urol. 2008; 179(2):674–9. discussion 9.

Routh JC, Inman BA, Ashley RA, Vandersteen DR, Reinberg Y, Wolpert JJ, et al. Unilateral vesicoureteral reflux: does endoscopic injection based on the cystoscopic appearance of the ureteral orifice decrease the incidence of de-novo contralateral reflux? J Pediatr Urol. 2008;4(4):260–4.

Routh JC, Reinberg Y, Ashley RA, Inman BA, Wolpert JJ, Vandersteen DR, et al. Multivariate comparison of the efficacy of intraureteral versus subtrigonal techniques of dextranomer/hyaluronic acid injection. J Urol. 2007;178(4 Pt 2):1702–5. discussion 5–6.

Routh JC, Inman BA, Reinberg Y. Dextranomer/hyaluronic acid for pediatric vesicoureteral reflux: systematic review. Pediatrics. 2010;125(5):1010–9.

Scholtmeijer RJ, Nijman RJ. Vesicoureteric reflux and videourodynamic studies: results of a prospective study after three years of follow-up. Urology. 1994; 43(5):714–8.

Schwentner C, Gozzi C, Lunacek A, Rehder P, Bartsch G, Oswald J, et al. Interim outcome of the single stage dorsal inlay skin graft for complex hypospadias reoperations. J Urol. 2006;175(5):1872–6. discussion 6–7.

Shaikh N, Ewing AL, Bhatnagar S, Hoberman A. Risk of renal scarring in children with a first urinary tract infection: a systematic review. Pediatrics. 2010; 126(6):1084–91.

Siomou E, Giapros V, Fotopoulos A, Aasioti M, Papadopoulou F, Serbis A, et al. Implications of 99mTc-DMSA scintigraphy performed during urinary tract infection in neonates. Pediatrics. 2009;124(3):881–7.

Skoog SJ, Peters CA, Arant Jr BS, Copp HL, Elder JS, Hudson RG, et al. Pediatric Vesicoureteral Reflux Guidelines Panel Summary Report: Clinical Practice Guidelines for Screening Siblings of Children With Vesicoureteral Reflux and Neonates/Infants with Prenatal Hydronephrosis. J Urol. 2010;184(3):1145–51.

Snodgrass W. The impact of treated dysfunctional voiding on the nonsurgical management of vesicoureteral reflux. J Urol. 1998;160(5):1823–5.

Snodgrass W, Shah A, Yang M, Kwon J, Villanueva C, Traylor J, et al. Prevalence and risk factors for renal scars in children with febrile UTI and/or VUR: a cross-sectional observational study of 565 consecutive patients. J Pediatr Urol. (2012), http://dx.doi.org/10.1016/j.jpurol.2012.11.019.

Soylu A, Demir BK, Turkmen M, Bekem O, Saygi M, Cakmakci H, et al. Predictors of renal scar in children with urinary infection and vesicoureteral reflux. Pediatr Nephrol (Berlin, Germany). 2008;23(12): 2227–32.

Traxel E, DeFoor W, Reddy P, Sheldon C, Minevich E. Risk factors for urinary tract infection after dextranomer/hyaluronic acid endoscopic injection. J Urol. 2009;182(4 Suppl):1708–12.

Wadie GM, Tirabassi MV, Courtney RA, Moriarty KP. The deflux procedure reduces the incidence of urinary tract infections in patients with vesicoureteral reflux. J Laparoendosc Adv Surg Tech A. 2007;17(3): 353–9.

Webster RI, Smith G, Farnsworth RH, Rossleigh MA, Rosenberg AR, Kainer G. Low incidence of new renal scars after ureteral reimplantation for vesicoureteral reflux in children: a prospective study. J Urol. 2000; 163(6):1915–8.

Wheeler D, Vimalachandra D, Hodson EM, Roy LP, Smith G, Craig JC. Antibiotics and surgery for vesicoureteric reflux: a meta-analysis of randomised controlled trials. Arch Dis Child. 2003;88(8):688–94.

Yucel S, Gupta A, Snodgrass W. Multivariate analysis of factors predicting success with dextranomer/hyaluronic acid injection for vesicoureteral reflux. J Urol. 2007;177(4):1505–9.

3 Bladder and Bowel Dysfunction

Nicol C. Bush

Primary goals in diagnosis and treatment of functional bladder disorders:

1. **Stop urinary incontinence.**
2. **Reduce associated UTI.**

A secondary aim is to reduce behavior dysfunction associated with incontinence.

Summary of evidence for these goals:

- **Several studies indicate placebo results in cure or improvement of symptoms in approximately 40 % of children with voiding dysfunction.**
- **There is little evidence that biofeedback, AC, or alpha-blockers are more effective than urotherapy or placebo to reduce diurnal incontinence. One trial demonstrated an alarm watch is better than timed voiding.**
- **Several small series indicate botulinum A injection in patients with refractory overactive bladder (OAB) stops incontinence in approximately 50 %, with an average response duration of 6 months.**
- **Two small series report transcutaneous electrical nerve stimulation (TENS) or Interstim devices improve symptoms in children refractory to other treatments.**
- **While urinary symptoms improve during treatment for constipation, one RCT found no added benefit to polyethylene glycol versus placebo, and another study reported improvement in diurnal incontinence in patients both with and without improved stooling.**
- **Our review found no evidence that the voiding dysfunction treatment reduces UTI. Two studies reported recurrent UTI within 1 year in approximately 40 % of females despite various treatments (urotherapy, biofeedback, AC).**
- **While children with voiding dysfunction also have increased behavioral problems, our review found only one study that reports impact of therapy, finding decreased problems in those with dysfunctional voiding but not urge syndrome. One case–control study found improved self-esteem in patients after incontinence therapy.**

ICCS Definitions

Subgroups listed below apply to children who have attained bladder control or are ≥5 years of age. The general phrase for voiding symptoms in children is now similar to that in adults, "lower urinary tract symptoms" (LUTS), which replaces the phrase "dysfunctional voiding." The ICCS defines urinary frequency as ≥8 voids/day and decreased frequency as ≤3 voids/day (Neveus et al. 2006).

Overactive bladder (OAB). urinary urgency, defined as a sudden and unexpected need to void. Concomitant urinary frequency and/or

N.C. Bush, M.D., M.S.C.S. (✉)
Department of Pediatric Urology,
University of Texas Southwestern Medical Center
and Children's Medical Center Dallas,
1935 Medical District Drive, MS F4.04,
Dallas, TX 75235, USA
e-mail: nicol.bush@childrens.com

W.T. Snodgrass (ed.), *Pediatric Urology: Evidence for Optimal Patient Management*,
DOI 10.1007/978-1-4614-6910-0_3,

Table 3.1 Criteria for Diagnosis Commonly Referenced

	Rome II (Rasquin-Weber et al. 1999)	Rome III (Rasquin et al. 2006)	PACCT (Benninga et al. 2005)
Age	Infant–16 years	Developmental age ≥4 years	Not specified
Duration of symptoms	Not specified	≥2 months	≥8 weeks
No. of symptom/exam findings to meet criteria	At least 2	At least 2	At least 2
Diagnostic criteria	Majority of stools scybalous, pebble-like, hard	≤2 defecations per week	<3 defecations per week
	Firm stools ≤2×/week	≥1 episode of fecal incontinence/week	>1 episode of fecal incontinence/week
	No metabolic, endocrine, structural disease	Stool-retentive posturing	Large fecal mass in rectum or palpable in abdomen
		Hard or painful bowel movements	Large-diameter stools that could obstruct the toilet
		Large-diameter stools that could obstruct the toilet	Stool-retentive posturing
		Large fecal mass in rectum	Hard or painful bowel movements

incontinence may be present but are not prerequisites. Children with OAB should not be diagnosed with detrusor overactivity without cystometric confirmation (Neveus et al. 2006).

Urge syndrome. frequent attacks of urinary urgency with squatting or other holding maneuvers, voiding frequency >7×/day, and urge incontinence (Bael et al. 2008a). While the ICCS has adopted adult terminology in using "OAB" to describe children with urgency, others continue to use "urge syndrome" to define children with a characteristic pattern of urinary frequency and urgency ± incontinence.

Extraordinary daytime urinary frequency. daytime voiding ≥1×/h with small volumes ≤50 % estimated capacity for age, usually without incontinence and with normal nocturnal bladder behavior.

Underactive bladder. low voiding frequency and straining to initiate, maintain, or complete voiding.

Voiding postponement. daytime incontinence associated with low micturition frequency and holding maneuvers.

Giggle incontinence. complete voiding occurring during or immediately after laughing in a child with normal bladder function when not laughing.

Dysfunctional voiding. habitual contraction of the urethral sphincter during voiding verified with repeated uroflows demonstrating a staccato pattern on UD.

Hinman's syndrome. constellation of findings including diurnal urinary ± fecal incontinence, bladder trabeculation in the absence of outlet obstruction or neurologic disease, and upper tract changes including VUR and/or hydronephrosis. The term was used by the editors of the Journal of Urology to replace "nonneurogenic neurogenic bladder" and was not included in 2006 ICCS terminology (Hinman 1986).

Constipation. the ICCS notes "there are no good definitions of constipation." Table 3.1 lists criteria for diagnoses commonly referenced (Rome II, Rome III and PACCT). The Bristol Stool Form Scale has not been validated for the diagnosis of constipation in children. It was originally developed as a measure of gastrointestinal transit time in adults with various bowel pathologies.

Retrospective chart review of 336 children mean age 6±3.5 years referred for defecation disorder compared Rome II and Rome III criteria; 34 % versus 87 % ($p<0.001$) met criteria for functional constipation using these diagnostic recommendations, respectively (Burgers et al. 2012).

A prospective longitudinal study of 128 consecutive children mean age 67±46 months referred to a tertiary constipation clinic compared Rome II to PACCT criteria. Functional defecation disorders (functional constipation, fecal retention, or fecal soiling without retention) were diagnosed in 48 % versus 89 %, $p=0.001$. There was poor agreement (Kappa=0.173), implying these two sets of criteria identify different patient groups. Among those diagnosed with constipation, 80 % had straining and pebble-like stools, 66 % had painful defecation, and 63 % had large-diameter stools (Boccia et al. 2007).

Our review found no report concerning prevalence of the various categories of voiding dysfunction or constipation in unselected children referred for urologic evaluation.

Prevalence

Population-based surveys found that reported LUTS and, specifically, OAB, decreases with age, with <20 % of children 7 years old having daytime incontinence, which occurred daily in <1 %.

Prevalence of the various clinical conditions that together comprise functional bladder disorders has not been reported in consecutive (unselected) patients.

Constipation was reported in ≤20 % of children with LUTS.

The Avon Longitudinal Study of Parents and Children, a prospective population-based study with 14,000 children followed since birth, queried parents about daytime urinary incontinence (DUI) in children at ages 4.5, 5.5, 6.5, 7.5, and 9.5 years. Data were available for 10,819 children (Swithinbank et al. 2010):

- DUI was present in 15.5 % at 4.5 years and decreased to 4.5 % at 9.5 years, with girls exhibiting slightly higher rates at all time points; daytime wetting >2×/week was present in 1.9, 1.5, 1.0, 1.0, and 0.5 % at the above-listed ages.
- At age 7.5 years, DUI frequency was <1 episode per week in 9 %, 2–5 episodes per week in 0.5 %, and nearly daily in 0.3 %.
- Voiding frequency was significantly less in those without DUI, <5×/daily in 43 % and 5–9×/daily in 56 % versus 36 % and 61.5 % in incontinent children. Boys and those with DUI>5 episodes/week had higher voiding frequency.
- Both constipation and soiling were significantly more likely in those with DUI versus no incontinence (13 and 29 % vs. 10 and 5 %).

A validated questionnaire about bowel and bladder habits was completed by the parents of 2,856 children (mean 7±1 year) in a cross-sectional, population-based study. Daytime incontinence (>1×/prior 6 months) was reported in 17 % of children, constipation (Rome II criteria) in 6 %, and encopresis in 10 % (Sureshkumar et al. 2009).

A survey was done in 1,982 among 3,627 children entering school at age 7 years, with school nurses asking about voiding dysfunctions. Positive answers prompted an additional phone call to parents from the study team. Incontinence was defined as one or more episodes of wetting in 3 months. Daytime incontinence was reported by 5 %, which was less than 1×/week in 2 %, and 3–7×/week in 0.7 % (Hellstrom et al. 1990).

OAB (urgency±urge incontinence during the past 3 months) was present in 2,740 (17 %) Korean children in a population-based, cross-sectional parental survey of 16,516 children. Of children with urgency, 739/2,740 (27 %) had urge incontinence. Prevalence of urgency decreased with age (23 % at age 5 decreasing to 12 % at age 13, $p=0.0001$), and was evenly split between boys and girls (1,435 [52 %] boys and 1,305 [48 %] girls) (Chung et al. 2010).

Similar OAB prevalence of 18 % was reported in Japan despite older mean age of 9±2 years. Among 5,282 children in this cross-sectional, population-based survey, 19 % boys and 17 % girls experienced OAB, defined as increased daytime frequency (>1 SD beyond the average number voids/day for age)±urge in the past month (i.e., urge was not a prerequisite). Daytime frequency decreased with increasing age. Constipation (<3x/week) was present in 971 (18.5 %) children, of which symptoms of OAB were equally present in those with and without constipation (20 % vs. 17.5 %, $p>0.05$) (Kajiwara et al. 2006).

Diagnostic Instruments

History

The ICCS recommends that a detailed history be taken from the child when possible, but stated "literature on this topic is sparse" (Hoebeke et al. 2010).

Questionnaires

Four validated questionnaires have been developed—two answered by children, one by their parents, one by either, depending on patient age—that distinguish children with voiding dysfunctions from normal children.

A scoring system was validated comparing parent responses in 86 children (1.5:1 females to males, mean age 8 years, range 4–10) with "various wetting and daytime voiding problems" to 265 controls of similar age without urinary symptoms. The questionnaire had 13 questions with potential scores ranging from 0 to 35. Median scores in patients versus controls were 18.6 versus 2.9. Receiver operating characteristic plotting showed the optimal cutoff score of 8.5 distinguished children with "voiding abnormalities" from normal children with 90 % sensitivity and specificity (Akbal et al. 2005).

The dysfunctional voiding symptom score was adapted from the International Prostate Symptom Score to include ten questions (potential scores 0–30) relevant to children and designed to be answered by children. Validation compared 104 consecutive patients (4:1 female to male) between ages 3 and 10 years with a history of diurnal incontinence, "abnormal voiding habits," or UTI to 54 age-matched children (1.3:1 female to male) without urologic complaints. Using receiver operating characteristics, the optimal cutoff score for "dysfunctional voiding" was 6 in females (93 % sensitivity, 87 % specificity) and 9 in males (81 % sensitivity, 91 % specificity) (Farhat et al. 2000). Among a subset of 48 patients who underwent a bladder behavioral modification program for "dysfunctional voiding," follow-up DVSS scores improved from 14.5 to >6.0 among the 28 patients whose parents indicated they were compliant with the program versus no significant change (14.5 to >11.0) among the 20 patients who were reportedly not compliant (Farhat et al. 2001).

The Incontinence Symptom Index-Pediatric is a validated 11-item instrument with subdomains for stress incontinence, urge incontinence, insensate incontinence, enuresis, and pad use designed for children 11–17 years of age to answer independently. Scores were significantly different in 19 patients (with incontinence) versus controls (well-child exams) for the full instrument and subdomains (Nelson et al. 2007).

Evaluation of these three instruments was done, with 37 children 4–10 years of age using the DVSS (answered by patients) and Akbar questionnaire (scored by parents), and 35 children 11–17 years old answering the Nelson survey. These scores were compared to blinded physician rating using a scoring sheet. Physician rating correlated with all three instruments, but was best with patient reporting using either the DVSS or Nelson surveys (Schneider et al. 2011).

A fourth instrument uses 14 questions to be answered by children ≥9 years old, or by parents of younger patients, concerning bowel and bladder dysfunctions. A Likert scale scores each from 0 to 4, for a maximum score of 56. It was validated in 62 patients median age 8 years (4–16) and 50 healthy controls, with a median 14 in patients and 6 in controls, $p=0.001$. ROC curve indicated that a score of 11 was the optimum threshold with AUC 0.9 (95 % CI 0.8–0.9) (Afshar et al. 2009).

Voiding Diary/Pad Tests

One study reported parent responses to the questionnaire underestimated incontinence and overestimated frequency when compared to a 72-h voiding diary.

Two studies report pad tests did not record wetting in approximately one-third of subjects reporting incontinence.

Two hundred two children ages 6–12 enrolled in the EBDS had pretreatment questionnaires regarding voiding frequency, volume, and diurnal incontinence completed by their parents. A 72-h voiding diary was then obtained, and a 12-h pad test was used to measure urinary loss at home. Parents were found to underestimate incontinence and to overestimate frequency when answering the questionnaire. The 12-h pad test provided quantitative data but had poor sensitivity (64 %) in those with incontinence, because it missed wetting in 36 % of children. Specificity for those without incontinence was 91 % (Bael et al. 2007).

Fifty children (39 females, mean age 9 years, range 6–14) with urinary incontinence had pad testing done in a 2-h clinic setting and at home. For clinic testing, an oral fluid load 13 mL/kg was given over 15 min and then various exercises were done. The 12-h pad testing was used for home, changing pads every hour, with or without a similar fluid provocation. An increase in pad weight of 0.5 g was considered "significant urine leak." Results were as folows: 35/50 (70 %) had a positive clinic test, 34 (68 %) a positive home test, and 16/20 (80 %) a positive provocative fluid intake home test, with eight positive only in the clinic and eight positive only at home. The authors concluded clinic testing was not needed (Hellstrom et al. 1986).

Uroflowometry

One prospective trial reported uroflow patterns did not correlate with clinical diagnosis of either urge syndrome or dysfunctional voiding.

Several studies report uroflow parameter (Q_{max}, curve shape) improved with treatment, but did not consistently correlate with clinical outcomes.

One study found uroflow pattern (bell-shaped vs. other) did not predict past history or future development of UTI.

The EBDS included 97 children with clinically diagnosed urge syndrome and 105 with clinically diagnosed dysfunctional voiding. Uroflowometry was described by patterns as "normal bell-shaped," "steep tower-shaped," or "staccato or fractionated." Voided volumes were not reported, nor was the minimum volume for an acceptable test. Among 66 patients with urge syndrome, 29 % had bell, 20 % had tower, and 51 % had staccato or fractionated patterns. Patterns for 78 patients with dysfunctional voiding were 18 % bell, 6 % tower, and 76 % staccato or fractionated. Patterns for neither condition predicted clinical results of therapy (Bael et al. 2008b).

A prospective trial included 86 children referred for dysfunctional voiding after failure of timed voiding and constipation management for 3 months. Inclusion criteria were symptoms (incontinence, straining, intermittent and/or weak stream) and three consecutive staccato and/or interrupted uroflows with positive EMG activity during voiding. Following therapy, urinary incontinence stopped in 22 and persisted in 20 who had post-treatment uroflowometry; 18/22 (82 %) cured had a bell-shaped curve versus 5/20 (25 %) not cured, $p<0.001$. Staccato/interrupted curve persisted in 3/22 (14 %) cured versus 7/20 (35 %) still incontinent, $p=0.15$ (Vesna et al. 2010).

A retrospective review was done in 81 consecutive patients, 80 % female, mean age 8 years (4–17) treated with biofeedback for voiding dysfunction with incontinence and/or recurrent UTI. Baseline uroflows were obtained, but timing for uroflow during or after treatment was not stated. There was significant improvement in Q_{max}, decrease in PVR, and normalization of uroflow curves, but no significant differences when patients were stratified as cured or unchanged (Nelson et al. 2004).

A retrospective review of 23 children with dysfunctional voiding treated with tamsulosin obtained baseline uroflowometry with two-thirds bladder capacity and repeated the study at 1 month on therapy. Mean Q_{max}, mean voided volume, and mean PVR all showed significant improvement, while the proportion with a non-bell-shaped curve decreased from 100 to 50 %. Results were only presented as means for the study group, without dividing them according to responders versus nonresponders (Vanderbrink et al. 2009).

A review of 148 consecutive toilet-trained patients, 69 % female, mean age 9 years (4–18) with voiding dysfunction analyzed uroflow patterns (bell-shaped vs. other) and recurrent UTI. Of 78 baseline studies, 61 (78 %) were abnormal. No correlation was seen in abnormal pattern and the number of prior or subsequent UTIs (Shaikh et al. 2005).

Bladder Wall Thickness/Post-void Residual

There is no consensus regarding the ultrasound (US) method to measure bladder wall thickness, for example, with the bladder nearly empty versus filled. Clinical usefulness was limited in one study by overlap in normal and abnormal patients.

One study found that post-void residual (PVR) >10 % bladder capacity for age (1998 ICCS definition of abnormal) increased risk for recurrent UTI, but was not strongly predictive, as 50 % of patients with residuals did not have infection.

Nomograms were developed from observations in 3,376 consecutive children undergoing US for non-urologic indications, from which bladder volume wall thickness index values were calculated. Bladder wall thickness was measured in the transverse plane with the bladder nearly empty (after voiding), averaging anteriorlateral, posteriorlateral, and lateral measurements. A trend of increasing thickness for increasing age was noted (Leung et al. 2007).

A retrospective study evaluated 139 children (69 % girls, 7 months to 16 years) who underwent UD for various indications and compared US measurements of bladder wall thickness at maximum UD-determined capacity. Bladder wall thickness (mm) varied according to diagnostic category defined by 1998 ICCS criteria: normal UD 1.3 ± 0.5 in 46 children; urge syndrome 2.0 ± 0.7 in 52 children; dysfunctional voiding 2.6 ± 0.5 in 33 children; and lazy bladder (bladder underactivity) 0.9 ± 0.1 in 4 children, $p < 0.05$ for all mean comparisons except normal versus underactive bladder. However, there was wide overlap in the bladder wall thickness between groups such that a cutoff value was not possible (Cvitkovic-Kuzmic et al. 2002).

The retrospective review by Shaikh et al. (2005) mentioned above analyzed elevated PVR (>10 % bladder capacity for age) with number of UTIs. Fifteen percent had elevated PVR, with 9/18 having subsequent UTI during follow-up at a mean of 19 months (7–30). There was a positive correlation between PVR and the number of subsequent UTIs ($r = 0.3$, $p < 0.002$), even when controlling for female gender, VUR, and UTIs prior to study. However, the risk for children to develop UTI could not be predicted by elevated PVR, as 50 % of those with PVR did not have recurrent infection.

Urodynamics

Cochrane review found no trial comparing clinical versus UD-based diagnosis or treatment in children with incontinence.

The EBDS reported 28 % of children with clinical urge syndrome had either no or "slight" detrusor overactivity by UD, and 7 % of children with a clinical diagnosis of dysfunctional voiding had normal UD patch EMG activity during voiding.

One study reported poor agreement between blinded versus unblinded UD interpretation for detrusor overactivity.

Two studies performing UD in selected referred patients with voiding dysfunctions both reported detrusor overactivity in over 50 % of cases, followed by dysfunctional voiding in ≥25 %, "lazy bladder" in 4 %, and normal in 6–17 %. Neither correlated UD findings to clinical diagnoses.

Cochrane Review was done to determine if treatment for incontinence according to UD-based diagnosis versus clinical diagnosis is more effective. Seven trials were included, with the following findings:

- No trial included children.
- There was no evidence that UD improved treatment of adult females; the proportion with persistent incontinence after 1 year, 70 %, was with versus 62 % without UD, RR 1.23 (95 % CI 0.6–2.6).
- There was discordance regarding usefulness of UD in clinical management. Two studies reported that a patient with UD was more likely to receive drugs, but in three studies they were not more likely to have surgery (Glazener and Lapitan 2012).

The EBDS described above also performed UD in patients clinically diagnosed with urge syndrome and dysfunctional voiding. Detrusor overactivity expected in children with urge syndrome was absent or "slight" in 25/88 (28 %), only occurred "before voiding" in 35 (40 %), and occurred throughout filling in 28 (32 %). Pelvic floor relaxation determined by patch electrodes was considered normal in 6/91 (7 %) children with a clinical diagnosis of voiding dysfunction and reported as incompletely relaxed in another 22 (24 %). The remainder had increased pelvic floor activity during voiding. Inclusion in the trial was based on clinical history rather than UD results (Bael et al. 2008b).

The EBDS also reported agreement in UD interpretation between the unblinded reviewer who performed the study versus a blinded committee of three other reviewers. All UD were performed in the same manner following a consensus 3-day workshop before the study began, and a standardized scoring sheet was used for interpretations. Among 247 UD tracings, concordance for detrusor overactivity during filling was 37 %. Concordance for pelvic floor relaxation was greater at 81 %. The authors concluded investigator bias in UD interpretation could only be overcome with blinded reviews (Bael et al. 2009).

UD was done in 366 of more than 500 referred patients with dysfunctional voiding symptoms, excluding those "too young, those who refused, and those with infrequent voiding responding to behavioral modification." Patients had diurnal incontinence ± enuresis and/or recurrent UTI. UD diagnoses were detrusor overactivity in 52 %, voiding dysfunction (bladder/sphincter dysfunction) in 25 %, normal in 17 %, and lazy bladder in 4 % (despite exclusion of these). The authors did not correlate UD findings to clinical symptoms (Schulman et al. 1999).

A subsequent study performed UD in 1,000 children, 48 % female, with "history of UTI, small bladder capacity despite urotherapy, repeated dysfunctional uroflow, US abnormalities, or resistance to therapy," from a population of 3,500 patients seen for incontinence. UD diagnosis was urge syndrome (detrusor overactivity) in 58 %, dysfunctional voiding in 32 %, lazy bladder (voiding postponement) in 4 %, and normal in 6 %, which also were not correlated to clinical symptoms (Hoebeke et al. 2000).

KUB

Systematic review did not support use of KUB to assist in the diagnosis of constipation.

One study reported poor interrater reliability using three fecal loading scoring systems (Barr, Blethyn, Leech).

Another trial found Blethyn and Leech scores did not correlate to clinical symptoms before or after polyethylene glycol treatment.

Systematic review was done to determine the association between KUB and signs and symptoms of constipation, limited to controlled observational studies in children 1–18 years old. Six articles were included, of which only one was designed to determine whether clinical variables identified patients with radiologically diagnosed constipation. Findings included the following:

- One study found a clinical diagnosis existed 1.2× more often than the radiologic diagnosis, LR 1.2 (95 % CI 1.0–1.4).
- Four studies examined whether KUB could discriminate children with versus without clinical symptoms of constipation, with only one reporting significant discriminative value, LR 3.0 (95 % CI 1.6–4.3).
- All but one study reported moderate to excellent interobserver reliability (K 0.63–0.95); intraobserver reliability reported by three studies was moderate to excellent (K 0.52–0.85).

- There was conflicting evidence for the correlation of radiologic versus clinical diagnosis of constipation, meaning there was no evidence supporting use of KUB in the case of doubt for constipation in a child (Reuchlin-Vroklage et al. 2005).

Another study had two pediatric urologists, a pediatric radiologist, and three pediatric nurse practitioners score KUBs from children 4–12 years of age who had "lower urinary tract dysfunction symptoms" and age-matched controls with radiographs after foreign-body ingestion, using three methods: Barr, Blethyn, and Leech. Interrater reliability was poor to marginally good using all three rating systems (kappa range Barr, 0.049–0.481; Blethyn, 0.045–0.451; Leech, 0.119–0.273; with kappa values of >0.75 indicating excellent, 0.4–0.75 good, and <0.4 poor reliability). Similarly, intraclass correlations (which describe the reproducibility of measurements made by different observers rating the same image) were poor for all three rating systems (Barr, 0.026; Blethyn, 0.201; and Leech, 0.331). None of the scoring systems provided reliable results between observers in grading constipation (Moylan et al. 2010).

One RCT used KUB scored using Leech and Blethyn systems in 138 children mean age 7 years, 62 % female, with OAB. Baseline urinary and bowel symptom questionnaires were used, with minimal bowel symptoms reported, yet 61(47 %) had KUB-defined constipation using either scale. There was no correlation of urinary urge and bowel symptoms. Patients were then randomized to placebo versus polyethylene glycol for 1 month. Complete response to urge symptoms occurred in 11/71(15 %) completers, and overall 45 % had improvement (>20 % decrease in urge symptoms) in both cohorts, but KUB scores did not change (Bush et al. 2012).

Ultrasound-Determined Rectal Diameter

Three studies reported constipated children have a larger transverse rectal ampulla diameter on pelvic US than normal controls.

Two suggesting a 3 cm diameter as the threshold for constipation stated that 25–44 % of constipated and 4–25 % of normal children would be misdiagnosed by this criteria.

One study compared rectal diameter behind the bladder in 82 normal children (no history of constipation), median age 5.5 years, and 95 patients, median age 6.5 years, with chronic constipation for at least 6 months. Median rectal diameter in controls was 2.4 cm (1.3–4.2) versus 3.4 cm (2.1–7) in patients, $p<0.001$. Age was a significant confounder; the older the child, the larger the rectal diameter, but no adjustment values were described. The authors recommended 3 cm as the threshold to diagnose rectal distention, although use of that cutoff would result in mis-classification of 25 % of both controls and patients (Singh et al. 2005).

A second study compared 120 children, mean age 6 years (1.5–18) with constipation by Rome II criteria to 105 controls, mean age 8 years, with "a normal defecation pattern." Results were reported as the ratio between the diameter of the rectal ampulla and pelvic width (distance between the anterior superior iliac spines). There were significantly greater ratios in patients than controls when analyzed by age groups <3, 3–6, 6–12, and >12 years. To compare to other publications, the authors added that patients have a mean 4.3 cm (3–8.2 cm) rectal diameter (Bijos et al. 2007).

Another study included 51 children ages 4–12 years, 27 having constipation according to Rome III criteria and the other 24 considered normal. US was done using a 7.5-MHz probe to measure the rectal diameter. Constipated children had a larger diameter than controls, 4 ± 1 cm versus 2 ± 0.6 cm, $p<0.001$. When normal was considered the mean +2 SD of controls, a cutoff value for constipation was 3 cm, the authors noting that this would misdiagnose 12/27 (44 %) patients and 1/24 (4 %) controls. Disimpaction and 4 weeks of polyethylene glycol significantly reduced rectal diameter in patients to mean 3 ± 0.5 cm, $p<0.001$ (Joensson et al. 2008).

Spinal Cord MRI

Less than 10 % of imaged patients with normal neurologic examinations, no sacral skin lesions, and persistent incontinence have

abnormal MRI findings (tethered cord, thick filum, syrinx, lipoma).

A prospective trial that enrolled 176 children with functional urinary and bowel problems (enuresis, diurnal incontinence, urinary frequency, UTI, VUR, chronic constipation, encopresis) referred to a center after unsuccessful management—88 with spina bifida occulta on KUB and the other 88 age- and gender-matched controls. None had known neurologic conditions. MRI was abnormal in 12 (7 %) with tethered cord ($n=5$), syrinx ($n=4$), club-shaped conus ($n=2$), and thick filum ($n=1$); there was no difference in abnormal findings in those with versus those without spina bifida occulta (Nejat et al. 2008).

Another prospective study included 114 children, median age 9 years (5–14), with UTI and/or voiding dysfunction symptoms. All had 6 months of therapy, mostly AC, with resolution of voiding symptoms in 46 %, none of which had abnormal sacral skin lesions. The other 61 who did not respond had MRI, and included 19 (31 %) with sacral skin lesions, including "macula, lipoma, dimple, or hyertrichosis"; 7/19 (36 %) with skin lesions and 2/42 (5 %) without skin lesions had abnormal MRI with tethered cord ($n=8$), lipoma ($n=2$), and diastematomyelia ($n=1$) (Tarcan et al. 2012).

A retrospective study included 23 children, 3–17 years of age, with persistent incontinence despite treatment a mean of 29 months with timed voiding, anticholinergics, and constipation management. Six also had intermittent back or leg pain, but all had normal neurologic examinations. MRI was normal in 21 (91 %), showed a thoracic spine syrinx in one, and spinal cord tethering in one (Ritchey et al. 1994).

A retrospective study of 456 patients with day and night incontinence revealed spina bifida occulta in 48 children among the subset of 127 (28 %) who underwent X-rays of the spine. The outcomes of those with known spina bifida occulta were compared to the 79 children with normal spine X-rays during mean follow-up of 3 years in both groups. Most patients resolved the incontinence with timed voiding ± AC, with similar results between groups. Of the 48 with spina bifida occulta, MRI or US of the spine was performed in ten, and lipoma with tethered cord was found in one (Ritchey et al. 1994).

Associated Conditions

One study reported that a history of fUTI at age <2 years did not increase likelihood for dysfunctional elimination after toilet training, which occurred in 22 %. There was no difference in prevalence of dysfunctional elimination in those with versus those without VUR.

One study using UD-based categorization of voiding dysfunction reported 34 % of all patients had a history of UTI and 14 % had VUR.

UTI/VUR (See Also Chap. 2)

Dysfunctional elimination, variously defined, was reported in from 14 to 51 % of children with VUR and 34–43 % with UTI.

One study found no difference in prevalence of dysfunctional voiding in patients with versus those without a prior history of UTI before age 2.

Children enrolled in the European branch of the International Reflux Study in Children underwent a questionnaire of voiding symptoms. Among these 310 children, all of whom had grade III or IV VUR, 255 (82 %) were considered to have normal bladder/sphincter function, with 26 (8 %) exhibiting symptoms of OAB, 4 (1 %) staccato voiding, 14 (5 %) incomplete voiding, 3 (1 %) voiding postponement, and 8 (3 %) "unclassifiable" voiding dysfunction by blinded review of the questionnaires by two experienced pediatric nephrologists. However, exclusion criteria for the study included "overt dysfunctional voiding" (van Gool et al. 1992).

One study collected prospective data for 2,759 consecutive children who underwent VCUG. "Dysfunctional elimination syndrome" (DES) was defined as daytime wetting beyond 3.5 years for girls/4.0 years for boys, or three of six criteria: thick-walled bladder on US, trabeculated bladder on VCUG, >30 % bladder capacity for age on VCUG, spinning top deformity on VCUG, Vincent's curtsy, and/or voiding <3x/day. They reported the following:

- DES among 32 % of children with VUR, indicating most VUR patients did not have DES.

- DES occurred in 43 % of children with UTI (not further defined), also indicating most UTI patients did not have DES (Chen et al., 2004).

The study of 1,000 UD by Hoebeke et al. (2000) described the above reported history of UTI (not defined) in 34 %, and VUR in 14 %. Among subgroups defined by ICCS criteria, VUR was identified in 88/582 (15 %) patients with OAB, 46/316 (15 %) with dysfunctional voiding, and 4/40 (10 %) with underactive bladder.

A prospective study evaluated 143 children, 73 % female, age not stated, who had VUR for "dysfunctional elimination syndrome" (DES): bladder instability (urge ± incontinence), infrequent voiding (<4×/day), and/or constipation (≤3×/week, encopresis, or stool on X-ray). Sixty-six (46 %) had DES, including OAB in 18, infrequent voiding in 15, and constipation in 33 (Koff et al. 1998).

A retrospective study evaluated 128 children, 84 % female, 3–10 years old, with VUR in whom history for voiding dysfunction was systematically obtained. Symptoms of frequency, urgency, holding maneuvers, and/or diurnal incontinence for at least 6 months were diagnosed with voiding dysfunction. Of females with a history of UTI (characterized as 1–2 or ≥3 in the preceding 12 months; febrile vs. non-febrile not stated), 38/94 (40 %) had voiding dysfunction. Of 128 children with VUR, 66 (51 %) had voiding dysfunction (Snodgrass 1998).

The dysfunctional voiding symptom score questionnaire (described above) was administered to 123 children with a history of fUTI before age 2 years and 125 controls without UTI, with no difference in the two cohorts based on gender, age (mean 7 years), or ethnicity. Dysfunctional elimination was diagnosed by a score >6 in females and >9 in males. Symptoms of dysfunctional voiding did not differ between the two groups; they were present in 22 % with and 21 % without UTI. Among patients with UTI history, there was no difference in dysfunctional elimination in those with versus those without VUR (18 % with vs. 25 %, $p=0.52$) (Shaikh et al. 2003).

Therapy

Placebo/Timed Voiding/Urotherapy

One study reported that 45 % of children with OAB given placebo had significant symptom reduction. Cochrane meta-analysis found approximately 40 % symptom improvement among adults with OAB taking placebo.

One RCT found children using a daytime alarm watch to have significantly greater resolution of diurnal incontinence than those with timed voiding.

Another trial reported no benefit (to reduce recurrent UTI or incontinence) in urotherapy plus uroflowmetry to produce bell-shaped voiding patterns over urotherapy alone.

Cochrane meta-analysis of adults assigned to placebo versus anticholinergics for symptoms of OAB found that 41 % of patients assigned placebo reported cure or improvement in symptoms (Nabi et al. 2006).

One double-blinded RCT randomized children with OAB to 1 month of placebo versus polyethylene glycol with no discussion of voiding modification. Urinary symptom questionnaires modified from DVSS for OAB were administered at baseline and repeated at 1 month, with improvement defined as ≥20 % decrease in score. Symptom improvement occurred in 17/38 (45 %) given placebo, including complete symptom resolution in five (Bush et al. 2012).

Our review found no RCT comparing no treatment to timed voiding.

A RCT enrolled 60 children at mean age 7 years with diurnal urge incontinence and OAB without constipation (Rome III criteria) to first undergo "standard urotherapy" for 1 month (>1,200 mL fluid equally distributed through the day, timed voiding every 2 h). Forty-eight hour voiding diaries confirmed frequency and incontinence. Ninety-five percent of patients had previously failed urotherapy (not described). Two had a complete response (no diurnal incontinence); the remainder were randomized to continue standard urotherapy versus standard urotherapy using an alarm watch for timed voiding for 12 additional weeks. Using the alarm watch, 9/30 (30 %) had a complete response versus 0/28 using standard time voiding, $p = 0.002$ (Hagstroem et al. 2010).

Another trial included 143 children at mean age 8 years with dysfunctional voiding who had "clear peaks and declines" in two uroflows with ≥100 cm^3, PVR ≥10 %, and recurrent UTI (not defined). These were allocated to three treatment groups for 2 months: "standard treatment" (education, "proper voiding pattern," "good toilet positioning") standard treatment with video instructions (reemphasizing voiding pattern and toilet positioning, watched daily), and standard treatment with uroflowometry (and instructions to produce a bell-shaped curve 4× daily). All received antibiotic prophylaxis for 24 weeks. The endpoint was no infections and no incontinence at 52 weeks. There was no difference in results between the groups; there were no further UTIs in 71/130 (55 %) and no incontinence in 66/95 (69 %) (Klijn et al. 2006).

Biofeedback

One RCT reported no benefit to biofeedback using pelvic floor EMG during voiding versus pelvic floor contraction/relaxation exercises alone.

Another found no benefit to urotherapy plus biofeedback over urotherapy plus placebo.

A RCT recruited patients from a dysfunctional voiding clinic with incontinence who failed prior treatment in their clinic with timed voiding, "hydration, proper hygiene and constipation management," and, in some cases, AC. Fifty-six children, 66 % female, ages 6–15 years (mean 10), were allocated to pelvic floor contraction/relaxation exercises versus biofeedback plus pelvic floor exercises (generating an EMG tracing). Patients were evaluated at 1, 6, and 12 months for reduction in incontinent episodes, cure being defined as no incontinence over 4 weeks. There was no difference in outcomes between the two groups, with cures noted at 1 and 12 months in 43 % and 71 % with exercises alone versus 30 % and 75 % with additional biofeedback (Vasconcelos et al. 2006).

The EBDS described above identified 97 children with clinically diagnosed urge syndrome and incontinence who all then received urotherapy (education, adequate fluid intake, voiding diaries, proper voiding posture, and personal hygiene). In addition, patients were randomized to biofeedback (12 sessions of uroflow/EMG) versus double blinded pharmacotherapy using placebo or oxybutynin (0.3 mg/kg/day). There were outcomes data at 6 months for 64 patients, reported before medication cohorts were unblinded. Cure was defined as no incontinence, and did not significantly vary by therapy. Nine of 23 (39 %) with biofeedback, and 14/20 (70 %) and 9/21 (43 %) with either placebo or oxybutynin were cured, indicating a placebo effect (or spontaneous resolution) of at least 43 % and no additional benefit to biofeedback (Misselwitz et al. 1999).

Anticholinergics

One placebo-controlled trial in children with urge syndrome reported cure in 43 % only receiving urotherapy.

Cochrane review of OAB in adults also reported a 42 % placebo response for cure or improvement.

One trial comparing urotherapy, placebo, and tolterodine found significant decrease in DVSS scores with both tolterodine and placebo.

The study by Misselwitz et al. (1999) described above had not unblinded placebo versus AC treatment groups at time of reporting (both receiving urotherapy). Fourteen of 20 (70 %) and 9/21 (43 %) with either placebo or oxybutynin were cured at 6-month follow-up.

Another trial included 71 children (49 % females), ages 4–12 years (mean 8), with voiding dysfunction defined as "incontinence, frequency, urgency or obstructive symptoms ± non-febrile UTI, with PVR < 20 mL" who scored >6 (females) or >9 (males) on the DVSS (described above). All were trained in timed voiding, double voiding, and pelvic floor relaxation during voiding. Patients were then randomized to no additional treatment, placebo, or tolterodine 1 mg 2× daily with repeated DVSS scoring at 1 and 3 months. Outcomes were determined using only 4 of the 10 DVSS questions that the authors considered relevant to OAB, and reported the decrease in mean scores was significantly greater with tolterodine (9 vs. 3.5, $p<0.001$) than placebo (9 vs. 5, $p<0.05$) or behavioral modification (8 vs. 7). There was no change from baseline in those with urotherapy, but a significant reduction also occurred with placebo (Ayan et al. 2005).

Cochrane review of AC for OAB treatment in adults analyzed 13 studies and 1,770 patients typically treated for 3–12 weeks. Symptomatic improvement during treatment was greater with AC versus bladder training (gradual increase in intervals between voiding, voiding diaries), RR 0.73 (95 % CI 0.59–0.90), and with AC + bladder training versus bladder training alone, RR 0.55 (95 % CI 0.32–0.93) (Alhasso et al. 2006).

Another Cochrane review considered AC versus placebo for OAB in adults, analyzing 61 trials and 11,956 patients. Cure or improvement, difference in 24-h incontinent episodes and number of voids in 24 h all favored AC. However, placebo response was 42 % (cure or improvement), with AC giving an additional 15 % response with number needed to treat of seven (Nabi et al. 2006).

Alpha-Adrenergic Blockers

One retrospective study reported decreased frequency and incontinence with tamsulosin, while one RCT reported a nonsignificant reduction in incontinence versus placebo.

A RCT evaluated doxazosin versus placebo for 1 month as primary therapy for voiding dysfunction (diurnal incontinence with frequency and urgency) in 28 children 5–16 years old. There was a nonsignificant decrease in median incontinent episodes/week with doxazosin (18–4 vs. 14 in placebo, $p=0.13$) (Kramer et al. 2005).

A retrospective study reviewed 23 children mean age 9 years (5–16), 52 % females, with dysfunctional voiding (not defined) refractory to 3-h timed voiding and "bowel hygiene" who received tamsulosin (0.2–0.4 mg nightly). All had a non-bell-shaped uroflow pattern and pelvic floor EMG without "excessive" activity during voiding. Three-day voiding diaries were completed before therapy and at ≤4 weeks follow-up while on medication. Mean number of voids and incontinent episodes decreased from baseline 11.5 ± 7.6 and 5.6 ± 1.9 to 7 ± 1 and 0.8 ± 1, $p<0.05$ (Vanderbrink et al. 2009).

Nerve Stimulation

One RCT using TENS reported no cure and partial response in 60 % of children with refractory urge incontinence.

One trial using Interstim reported complete resolution of diurnal incontinence in 75 %, but complete relief of all symptoms without medication in 25 %.

A RCT enrolled 25 children, 60 % females, 5–14 years old (mean 9), with diurnal urge incontinence at least 2×/week refractory to urotherapy (hydration and timed voiding), alarm timed voiding, and AC, and randomized them to sacral TENS versus sham for 4 weeks. All had pretreatment UD demonstrating detrusor overactivity. No child had complete cure of incontinence. Partial response occurred in 61 % of TENS versus 17 % of sham TENS patients, $p<0.05$ (Hagstroem et al. 2009).

A cohort of 20 patients, 75 % female, mean age 11 years (8–17) had sacral nerve stimulation (Interstim) after failure of prior medical therapies. Of these, 16 had diurnal incontinence and at follow-up at a median of 27 months, 12 (75 %) reported complete resolution. Urgency in 13 children completely resolved in 9 (69 %). However, complete resolution of all symptoms (day and night incontinence, urgency, frequency, constipation) only occurred in five patients (25 %), and only six were able to stop all other medications. Two patients had deactivation without recurrent symptoms, while three others had prompt recurrent symptoms and 18 continued with the device (Roth et al. 2008).

Botulinum A Toxin Injection

Complete resolution of OAB in three trials using botulinum A injections occurred in approximately 40–60 %, durable to at least 6 months.

A prospective study identified 21 children, 52 % females, mean age 11 years (8–14), with OAB and UD-demonstrated detrusor overactivity refractory to AC and urotherapy. These were injected with 100 μ Botox (Allergan, Irvine, CA, USA) at 15 sites sparing the trigone. There was follow-up in 15 at 6 months, with 9 (60 %) having a complete response (no incontinence or urgency). Eight had continued complete response at 12 months. Side effects included urinary retention for 10 days in one, flank pain with voiding for 2 weeks in one, and UTI in two (Hoebeke et al. 2006).

Another prospective trial included 13 children (8 females) at median age 11 years (7–19) with urge incontinence refractory to timed voiding and AC. Twelve had detrusor overactivity on UD pretreatment. Primary injections used 50–100 IU botulinum A at 20–30 sites, sparing the trigone. Complete response was no incontinence reported at follow-up at a mean of 1.5 months later (0.3–2.8), which occurred in five (38 %) and persisted at 6 months in 30 % and 12 months in 33 % (Lahdes-Vasama et al. 2011).

A retrospective review included 57 children, 39 % female, with OAB who failed AC or had side effects precluding further treatment. Injection was done using 12 IU/kg Dysport (Ipsen, Paris, France) to maximum of 480 IU. Complete response (no voiding symptoms and no incontinence) was achieved in 38 (67 %) with mean duration of 6 months (2–18). No side effects were reported (McDowell et al. 2012).

Constipation Management

One RCT reported 45 % of patients had improvement in urge syndrome symptoms with placebo, and no added benefit to polyethylene glycol.

One study of patients referred to an encopresis clinic, mostly males, reported a significant decrease in diurnal incontinence with successful stool management (≥3 stools/week without soiling), but a significant reduction in urinary symptoms also occurred in those with persistent constipation.

Prospective assessment was done for voiding symptoms in 234 consecutive children, mean age 9 years (5–18), 25 % female, with constipation and encopresis referred to a university encopresis clinic. Day incontinence was diagnosed if occurring ≥1 episode/week, and was found in 46 %. Treatment included education, disimpaction, high-fiber diet, timed toilet sitting, daily laxatives (mostly milk of magnesia), and stooling diaries continued for "several months" and then decreased to maintain daily stooling without soiling. Follow-up evaluation was at ≥12 months (mean 15), mostly by a questionnaire mailed to families that included questions regarding urinary incontinence. Constipation was rated successfully treated if a patient had ≥3 stools weekly without soiling. Daytime incontinence significantly decreased in those with successful constipation treatment from 28/121 (23 %) to 3/121 (2 %) and in those without successful bowel management from 36/113 (32 %) to 14/113 (12 %) (Loening-Baucke 1997).

A RCT assumed constipation diagnosis might be inaccurate in children presenting with urge syndrome, and so randomized all patients to initial therapy by polyethylene glycol versus placebo for 1 month. The endpoint was ≥20 % reduction in symptom score using a modified DVSS (for urge syndrome). Among 71 completers, improvement occurred in 45 % assigned to placebo and 48.5 % receiving medication, demonstrating no added benefit to polyethylene glycol in either intention to treat ($p = 0.77$) or per-protocol ($p = 0.84$) analysis (Bush et al. 2012).

Impact of Voiding Dysfunction on Behavior

Children with urge syndrome, dysfunctional voiding, and voiding postponement have been found to have increased behavioral problems.

Two studies found that severity of bladder or bowel dysfunction did not correlate with quality of life in one study.

One quality-of-life assessment reported children do not report less self-esteem or quality of life versus controls, but their parents score them lower.

One study reported that treatment for dysfunctional voiding, but not urge syndrome, resulted in improved behavior. Presence of behavior problems did not reduce treatment efficacy.

Another study found improved self-esteem in children following treatment for day and/or night urinary incontinence.

A 2011 ICCS consensus statement recommends screening all incontinent children for psychological symptoms with validated questionnaires such as the Child Behavior Checklist or the Short Screening Instrument for Psychological Problems in Enuresis (von Gontard et al. 2011). No data are available whether such widespread screening would improve either psychological or urological outcomes.

Prospective evaluation was done in 94 incontinent children clinically diagnosed with urge syndrome ($n=42$) and with voiding postponement (<5 voids/day, incontinence while watching television or playing) ($n=52$) recruited at presentation from pediatric and psychiatric clinics in Germany. Parents answered the Achenback Child Behavioral Checklist and a structured interview was done with the child regarding body image and interpretation of wetting. There were significantly more females with urge syndrome (62 %) and more boys with voiding postponement (65 %), with mean age in both 7 years. Parents scored significantly more behavioral problems in those with voiding postponement (37 vs. 14 %). There were no differences in child responses based on clinical diagnosis, with only 11 % responding they had an illness, although 70 % knew the reason for their evaluation. Thirty percent did not know the origin of urine (von Gontard et al. 1998).

In a subsequent study, consecutive children, 5–13 years old, with urge syndrome ($n=22$) or voiding postponement ($n=27$) and 32 age-matched controls had health-related quality-of-life and self-esteem assessments using standardized and validated instruments. Thirty percent of children with both conditions also had encopresis, versus none in controls. Patients had significantly more behavioral problems, but there was no difference in quality of life or self-esteem versus controls. However, parents rated quality of life lower in patients than controls, especially those with voiding postponement (Natale et al. 2009).

A study of 138 children with incontinence of various etiologies who were referred to a tertiary clinic completed the PINQ (quality of life) and the Akbal (urinary symptom) questionnaire. Children with non-white race, older age, and female gender had lower quality of life scores on the PINQ; severity of urinary symptoms based on the Akbal score ($r=0.15$, $p=0.09$) did not correlate with worse quality of life (Deshpande et al. 2011).

Another study in 103 children referred for incontinence using a validated health-related quality-of-life questionnaire showed type and severity of urinary or fecal incontinence was not correlated with total scores, and that overall quality of life among children referred for incontinence were similar to reference samples of children with other chronic conditions such as asthma, cystic fibrosis, and epilepsy (Bachmann et al. 2009).

The EBDS included the Achenbach's Child Behavioral Checklist (a validated checklist documenting social competence and problem behavior) at enrollment and 12 months after treatment, answered by parents. Of 202 patients, 188 completed forms at entry and 111 at 1 year. Overall, 19 % had abnormal behavioral scores, which after treatment decreased to 11 %, the authors commenting that this approximates prevalence in a normal population. However, this improvement occurred in patients with dysfunctional voiding, whereas those with urge syndrome did not change. Similarly, externalizing problems found in 12 % of children decreased significantly after treatment, but only in those with dysfunctional voiding. Internalizing problems occurred in 16 % overall, with no significant change in either subgroup with therapy. The presence of behavioral problems at entry did not influence treatment success for either urge syndrome or dysfunctional voiding (Bael et al. 2008a).

Sixty-six children identified through school-based questionnaire to have day and/or night wetting scored lower than age-matched controls on a Swedish validated self-esteem scale (12.5 vs. 19.4, $p<0.001$). Treatment of the incontinence increased self-esteem levels to that of controls at 6 months (19.5), with scores higher in those who achieved dryness versus those still wetting (23.1 vs. 17.3, $p<0.001$) (Hagglof et al. 1998).

References

Afshar K, Mirbagheri A, Scott H, MacNeily AE. Development of a symptom score for dysfunctional elimination syndrome. J Urol. 2009;182(4 Suppl): 1939–43.

Akbal C, Genc Y, Burgu B, Ozden E, Tekgul S. Dysfunctional voiding and incontinence scoring system: quantitative evaluation of incontinence symptoms in pediatric population. J Urol. 2005;173(3):969–73.

Alhasso AA, McKinlay J, Patrick K, Stewart L. Anticholinergic drugs versus non-drug active therapies for overactive bladder syndrome in adults. Cochrane Database Syst Rev. 2006;18(4): CD003193.

Ayan S, Kaya K, Topsakal K, Kilicarslan H, Gokce G, Gultekin Y. Efficacy of tolterodine as a first-line treatment for non-neurogenic voiding dysfunction in children. BJU Int. 2005;96(3):411–4.

Bachmann C, Lehr D, Janhsen E, Sambach H, Muehlan H, von Gontard A, et al. Health related quality of life of a tertiary referral center population with urinary incontinence using the DCGM-10 questionnaire. J Urol. 2009;182(4 Suppl):2000–6.

Bael AM, Lax H, Hirche H, Gabel E, Winkler P, Hellstrom AL, et al. Self-reported urinary incontinence, voiding frequency, voided volume and pad-test results: variables in a prospective study in children. BJU Int. 2007;100(3):651–6.

Bael A, Winkler P, Lax H, Hirche H, Gabel E, Vijverberg M, et al. Behavior profiles in children with functional urinary incontinence before and after incontinence treatment. Pediatrics. 2008a;121(5):e1196–200.

Bael A, Lax H, de Jong TP, Hoebeke P, Nijman RJ, Sixt R, et al. The relevance of urodynamic studies for Urge syndrome and dysfunctional voiding: a multicenter controlled trial in children. J Urol. 2008b;180(4): 1486–93.

Bael A, Verhulst J, Lax H, Hirche H, van Gool JD. Investigator bias in urodynamic studies for functional urinary incontinence. J Urol. 2009;182(4 Suppl): 1949–52.

Benninga M, Candy DC, Catto-Smith AG, Clayden G, Loening-Baucke V, Di Lorenzo C, et al. The Paris consensus on childhood constipation terminology (PACCT) group. J Pediatr Gastroenterol Nutr. 2005; 40(3):273–5.

Bijos A, Czerwionka-Szaflarska M, Mazur A, Romanczuk W. The usefulness of ultrasound examination of the bowel as a method of assessment of functional chronic constipation in children. Pediatr Radiol. 2007;37(12): 1247–52.

Boccia G, Manguso F, Coccorullo P, Masi P, Pensabene L, Staiano A. Functional defecation disorders in children: PACCT criteria versus Rome II criteria. J Pediatr. 2007;151(4):394–8. 8 e1.

Burgers R, Levin AD, Di Lorenzo C, Dijkgraaf MG, Benninga MA. Functional defecation disorders in children: comparing the Rome II with the Rome III criteria. J Pediatr. 2012;161(4):615–20.e1.

Bush NC, Shah A, Barber T, Yang M, Bernstein I, Snodgrass W. Randomized, double-blind, placebo-controlled trial of polyethylene glycol (MiraLAX((R))) for urinary urge symptoms. J Pediatr Urol. 2012, http://dx.doi.org/10.1016/j.jpurol.2012.10.011.

Chen JJ, Mao W, Homayoon K, Steinhardt GF. A multivariate analysis of dysfunctional elimination syndrome, and its relationships with gender, urinary tract infection and vesicoureteral reflux in children. J Urol. 2004;171(5):1907–10.

Chung JM, Lee SD, Kang DI, Kwon DD, Kim KS, Kim SY, et al. An epidemiologic study of voiding and bowel habits in Korean children: a nationwide multicenter study. Urology. 2010;76(1):215–9.

Cvitkovic-Kuzmic A, Brkljacic B, Ivankovic D, Grga A. Ultrasound assessment of detrusor muscle thickness in children with non-neuropathic bladder/sphincter dysfunction. Eur Urol. 2002;41(2):214–8.

Deshpande AV, Craig JC, Smith GH, Caldwell PH. Factors influencing quality of life in children with urinary incontinence. J Urol. 2011;186(3):1048–52.

Farhat W, Bagli DJ, Capolicchio G, O'Reilly S, Merguerian PA, Khoury A, et al. The dysfunctional voiding scoring system: quantitative standardization of dysfunctional voiding symptoms in children. J Urol. 2000; 164(3 Pt 2):1011–5.

Farhat W, McLorie GA, O'Reilly S, Khoury A, Bagli DJ. Reliability of the pediatric dysfunctional voiding symptom score in monitoring response to behavioral modification. Can J Urol. 2001;8(6):1401–5.

Glazener CM, Lapitan MC. Urodynamic studies for management of urinary incontinence in children and adults. Cochrane Database Syst Rev. 2012;1:CD003195.

Hagglof B, Andren O, Bergstrom E, Marklund L, Wendelius M. Self-esteem in children with nocturnal enuresis and urinary incontinence: improvement of self-esteem after treatment. Eur Urol. 1998;33 Suppl 3Suppl 3:16–9.

Hagstroem S, Mahler B, Madsen B, Djurhuus JC, Rittig S. Transcutaneous electrical nerve stimulation for refractory daytime urinary urge incontinence. J Urol. 2009;182(4 Suppl):2072–8.

Hagstroem S, Rittig S, Kamperis K, Djurhuus JC. Timer watch assisted urotherapy in children: a randomized controlled trial. J Urol. 2010;184(4):1482–8.

Hellstrom AL, Andersson K, Hjalmas K, Jodal U. Pad tests in children with incontinence. Scand J Urol Nephrol. 1986;20(1):47–50.

Hellstrom AL, Hanson E, Hansson S, Hjalmas K, Jodal U. Micturition habits and incontinence in 7-year-old Swedish school entrants. Eur J Pediatr. 1990;149(6): 434–7.

Hinman Jr F. Nonneurogenic neurogenic bladder (the Hinman syndrome)–15 years later. J Urol. 1986; 136(4):769–77.

Hoebeke P, De Kuyper P, Goeminne H, Van Laecke E, Everaert K. Bladder neck closure for treating pediatric incontinence. Eur Urol. 2000;38(4):453–6.

Hoebeke P, De Caestecker K, Vande Walle J, Dehoorne J, Raes A, Verleyen P, et al. The effect of botulinum-A toxin in incontinent children with therapy resistant overactive detrusor. J Urol. 2006;176(1):328–30.

Hoebeke P, Bower W, Combs A, De Jong T, Yang S. Diagnostic evaluation of children with daytime incontinence. J Urol. 2010;183(2):699–703.

Joensson IM, Siggaard C, Rittig S, Hagstroem S, Djurhuus JC. Transabdominal ultrasound of rectum as a diagnostic tool in childhood constipation. J Urol. 2008; 179(5):1997–2002.

Kajiwara M, Inoue K, Kato M, Usui A, Kurihara M, Usui T. Nocturnal enuresis and overactive bladder in children: an epidemiological study. Int J Urol. 2006; 13(1):36–41.

Klijn AJ, Uiterwaal CS, Vijverberg MA, Winkler PL, Dik P, de Jong TP. Home uroflowmetry biofeedback in behavioral training for dysfunctional voiding in school-age children: a randomized controlled study. J Urol. 2006;175(6):2263–8.

Koff SA, Wagner TT, Jayanthi VR. The relationship among dysfunctional elimination syndromes, primary vesicoureteral reflux and urinary tract infections in children. J Urol. 1998;160(3 Pt 2):1019–22.

Kramer SA, Rathbun SR, Elkins D, Karnes RJ, Husmann DA. Double-blind placebo controlled study of alpha-adrenergic receptor antagonists (doxazosin) for treatment of voiding dysfunction in the pediatric population. J Urol. 2005;173(6):2121–4.

Lahdes-Vasama TT, Anttila A, Wahl E, Taskinen S. Urodynamic assessment of children treated with botulinum toxin A injections for urge incontinence: a pilot study. Scand J Urol Nephrol. 2011;45(6):397–400.

Leung VY, Chu WC, Yeung CK, Sreedhar B, Liu JX, Wong EM, et al. Nomograms of total renal volume, urinary bladder volume and bladder wall thickness index in 3,376 children with a normal urinary tract. Pediatr Radiol. 2007;37(2):181–8.

Loening-Baucke V. Urinary incontinence and urinary tract infection and their resolution with treatment of chronic constipation of childhood. Pediatrics. 1997;100 (2 Pt 1):228–32.

McDowell DT, Noone D, Tareen F, Waldron M, Quinn F. Urinary incontinence in children: botulinum toxin is a safe and effective treatment option. Pediatr Surg Int. 2012;28(3):315–20.

Misselwitz J, Ulrike J, Tamminen-Mobius T, Lax-Gross H, Hirche H, Van Gool J, et al., editors. Oxybutynine-HCI versus placebo in children with urodynamically proven urge syndrome—a placebo-controlled study. Denver, CO: International Continence Society; 1999.

Moylan S, Armstrong J, Diaz-Saldano D, Saker M, Yerkes EB, Lindgren BW. Are abdominal x-rays a reliable way to assess for constipation? J Urol. 2010;184 (4 Suppl):1692–8.

Nabi G, Cody JD, Ellis G, Herbison P, Hay-Smith J. Anticholinergic drugs versus placebo for overactive bladder syndrome in adults. Cochrane Database Syst Rev. 2006;18(4):CD003781.

Natale N, Kuhn S, Siemer S, Stockle M, von Gontard A. Quality of life and self-esteem for children with urinary urge incontinence and voiding postponement. J Urol. 2009;182(2):692–8.

Nejat F, Radmanesh F, Ansari S, Tajik P, Kajbafzadeh A, El KM. Spina bifida occulta: is it a predictor of underlying spinal cord abnormality in patients with lower urinary tract dysfunction? J Neurosurg Pediatr. 2008;1(2):114–7.

Nelson JD, Cooper CS, Boyt MA, Hawtrey CE, Austin JC. Improved uroflow parameters and post-void residual following biofeedback therapy in pediatric patients with dysfunctional voiding does not correspond to outcome. J Urol. 2004;172(4 Pt 2):1653–6.

Nelson CP, Park JM, Bloom DA, Wan J, Dunn RL, Wei JT. Incontinence Symptom Index-Pediatric: development and initial validation of a urinary incontinence instrument for the older pediatric population. J Urol. 2007;178(4 Pt 2):1763–7.

Neveus T, von Gontard A, Hoebeke P, Hjalmas K, Bauer S, Bower W, et al. The standardization of terminology of lower urinary tract function in children and adolescents: report from the Standardisation Committee of the International Children's Continence Society. J Urol. 2006;176(1):314–24.

Rasquin A, Di Lorenzo C, Forbes D, Guiraldes E, Hyams JS, Staiano A, et al. Childhood functional gastrointestinal disorders: child/adolescent. Gastroenterology. 2006;130(5):1527–37.

Rasquin-Weber A, Hyman PE, Cucchiara S, Fleisher DR, Hyams JS, Milla PJ, et al. Childhood functional gastrointestinal disorders. Gut. 1999;45 Suppl 2Suppl 2:II60–8.

Reuchlin-Vroklage LM, Bierma-Zeinstra S, Benninga MA, Berger MY. Diagnostic value of abdominal radiography in constipated children: a systematic review. Arch Pediatr Adolesc Med. 2005;159(7):671–8.

Ritchey ML, Sinha A, DiPietro MA, Huang C, Flood H, Bloom DA. Significance of spina bifida occulta in children with diurnal enuresis. J Urol. 1994;152(2 Pt 2):815–8.

Roth TJ, Vandersteen DR, Hollatz P, Inman BA, Reinberg YE. Sacral neuromodulation for the dysfunctional elimination syndrome: a single center experience with 20 children. J Urol. 2008;180(1):306–11.

Schneider D, Yamamoto A, Barone JG. Evaluation of consistency between physician clinical impression and 3 validated survey instruments for measuring lower urinary tract symptoms in children. J Urol. 2011;186(1):261–5.

Schulman SL, Quinn CK, Plachter N, Kodman-Jones C. Comprehensive management of dysfunctional voiding. Pediatrics. 1999;103(3):E31.

Shaikh N, Hoberman A, Wise B, Kurs-Lasky M, Kearney D, Naylor S, et al. Dysfunctional elimination syndrome: is it related to urinary tract infection or vesicoureteral reflux diagnosed early in life? Pediatrics. 2003;112(5):1134–7.

Shaikh N, Abedin S, Docimo SG. Can ultrasonography or uroflowmetry predict which children with voiding dysfunction will have recurrent urinary tract infections? J Urol. 2005;174(4 Pt 2):1620–2.

Singh SJ, Gibbons NJ, Vincent MV, Sithole J, Nwokoma NJ, Alagarswami KV. Use of pelvic ultrasound in the diagnosis of megarectum in children with constipation. J Pediatr Surg. 2005;40(12):1941–4.

Snodgrass W. The impact of treated dysfunctional voiding on the nonsurgical management of vesicoureteral reflux. J Urol. 1998;160(5):1823–5.

Sureshkumar P, Jones M, Cumming R, Craig J. A population based study of 2,856 school-age children with urinary incontinence. J Urol. 2009;181(2):808–15.

Swithinbank LV, Heron J, von Gontard A, Abrams P. The natural history of daytime urinary incontinence in children: a large British cohort. Acta Paediatr. 2010;99(7):1031–6.

Tarcan T, Tinay I, Temiz Y, Alpay H, Ozek M, Simsek F. The value of sacral skin lesions in predicting occult spinal dysraphism in children with voiding dysfunction and normal neurological examination. J Pediatr Urol. 2012;8(1):55–8.

van Gool JD, Hjalmas K, Tamminen-Mobius T, Olbing H. Historical clues to the complex of dysfunctional voiding, urinary tract infection and vesicoureteral reflux. The International Reflux Study in Children. J Urol. 1992;148(5 Pt 2):1699–702.

Vanderbrink BA, Gitlin J, Toro S, Palmer LS. Effect of tamsulosin on systemic blood pressure and nonneurogenic dysfunctional voiding in children. J Urol. 2009;181(2):817–22.

Vasconcelos M, Lima E, Caiafa L, Noronha A, Cangussu R, Gomes S, et al. Voiding dysfunction in children. Pelvic-floor exercises or biofeedback therapy: a randomized study. Pediatr Nephrol. 2006;21(12):1858–64.

Vesna Z, Milica L, Marina V, Andjelka S, Lidija D. Correlation between uroflowmetry parameters and treatment outcome in children with dysfunctional voiding. J Pediatr Urol. 2010;6(4):396–402.

von Gontard A, Lettgen B, Olbing H, Heiken-Lowenau C, Gaebel E, Schmitz I. Behavioural problems in children with urge incontinence and voiding postponement: a comparison of a paediatric and child psychiatric sample. Br J Urol. 1998;81 Suppl 3Suppl 3:100–6.

von Gontard A, Baeyens D, Van Hoecke E, Warzak WJ, Bachmann C. Psychological and psychiatric issues in urinary and fecal incontinence. J Urol. 2011;185(4):1432–6.

Nocturnal Enuresis

4

Nicol C. Bush

The primary reason to diagnose and treat nocturnal enuresis is to achieve dryness. A secondary aim is to improve body image and/or low self-esteem associated with nocturnal enuresis.

Primary outcome measures for therapy of nocturnal enuresis have been defined as follows:

- **Short-term success: dryness for 14 consecutive nights**
- **Long-term success: dryness for 6 consecutive months**
- **Adverse treatment events**

Secondary outcome measures include psychological and quality-of-life assessments.

Summary of evidence for these goals:

- **Alarms achieve dryness for 14 consecutive nights during use in 50–75 % of enuretic children. Half of these maintain dryness when therapy stops.**
- **Desmopressin achieves dryness for 14 consecutive nights in approximately 20 % of treated children. Nearly all resume wetting when therapy stops.**
- **Desmopressin plus tolterodine was more effective than desmopressin plus placebo in one trial enrolling children with mono-symptomatic enuresis who failed desmopressin alone.**
- **Imipramine achieves dryness for 14 consecutive nights in 20–33 % of treated children. Approximately two-thirds relapse when treatment stops after 3 months.**
- **There are few data regarding efficacy of long-term medication use.**
- **Our review found no reports regarding 6-month dryness in treated patients.**
- **Children with enuresis have greater behavioral problems than non-bedwetters. However, successful treatment of enuresis is reported to not impact behavior significantly.**
- **One study reported improved self-concept with treatment.**

N.C. Bush, M.D., M.S.C.S. (✉)
Department of Pediatric Urology, University of Texas Southwestern Medical Center and Children's Medical Center Dallas, 1935 Medical District Drive, MS F4.04, Dallas, TX 75235, USA
e-mail: nicol.bush@childrens.com

Definitions

Infrequent bedwetting: <2 nights per week.

Enuresis: involuntary voiding during sleep ≥2 nights per week for at least three consecutive months and/or causing significant distress/impairment in a child >5 years old without CNS defects (DSM-IV).

Mono-symptomatic nocturnal enuresis: wetting only when asleep.

Non-mono-symptomatic (or poly-symptomatic) nocturnal enuresis: nighttime incontinence associated with daytime symptoms such as incontinence, urgency, and/or frequency.

Secondary enuresis: previously dry for more than six consecutive months.

W.T. Snodgrass (ed.), *Pediatric Urology: Evidence for Optimal Patient Management*,
DOI 10.1007/978-1-4614-6910-0_4,

Prevalence

Infrequent Bedwetting

Bedwetting <2 nights/week occurs in ≤20 % of 5-year-olds and diminishes to 2 % by 19 years of age.

Infrequent bedwetting is more common in boys than girls.

The Avon Longitudinal Study of Parents and Children (ALSPAC) is an ongoing, prospective, population-based cohort study in the UK that includes 13,973 children born in 1992–1993 and followed at regular intervals. Questionnaires that included questions about enuresis were administered at regular intervals between 54 and 115 months of age. Infrequent bedwetting was present in 22 % at 4.5 years; 16 % at 5.4 years; 13 % at 7.5 years, and 8 % at 9.5 years. Boys had a greater prevalence of infrequent bedwetting than girls at all ages up to 115 months (roughly two times), with identical rates of decline for both males and females. At age 7.5 years, 15 % of boys versus 8 % of girls had infrequent bedwetting, which declined to 10 % of boys at age 9.5 years versus 5 % of girls (Butler and Heron 2008).

In an epidemiologic cross-sectional survey of 16,512 children aged 5–19 years in Hong Kong, bedwetting more than once every 3 months was present in 16 % at 5 years, 10 % at 7 years, and 2 % at 19 years, with boys more likely to have bedwetting than girls at all ages (Yeung et al. 2006).

Mono-symptomatic Nocturnal Enuresis

Enuresis occurs in approximately 8 % of children age 5 years, decreasing to 1–3 % by age 10 years.

Boys have ≥2 times greater risk for enuresis at all ages than girls.

A higher proportion of older children have bedwetting ≥3 nights/week.

Prevalence estimates from 13,973 children in the UK prospective cohort study (ALSPAC) demonstrated enuresis in 8 % of children at 4.5 years, 3 % at 7.5 years, and 1.5 % at 9.5 years. Boys were more likely to have enuresis at all ages than girls (4 vs. 2 % at age 7.5 years) (Butler and Heron 2008).

In the cross-sectional survey of 16,512 children aged 5–19 years in Hong Kong mentioned above, enuresis ≥3 nights/week occurred in 7 % at age 5 years, 3 % at age 7.5 years, and 2 % at age 9.5 years. More frequent bedwetting (≥3 nights/week) occurred in a higher proportion of patients as age increased, such that 82 % of patients with bedwetting aged >10 years had ≥3 wet nights/week versus 42 % of patients aged 5–10 years ($p<0.0001$); 14.3 % of children aged 5 years had enuresis 7 nights/week compared to 48.3 % of 19-year-olds ($p<0.0001$) (Yeung et al. 2006). While bedwetting (infrequent plus frequent) was more common in boys than girls at all ages, data were not gender-stratified for those meeting DSM-IV criteria for enuresis.

Data from 1,136 US children aged 8–11 years in a cross-sectional, nationally representative sample of children participating in the National Health and Nutrition Examination Survey (NHANES) demonstrated enuresis in 8 % of children at 8 years, decreasing to 3 % at 11 years. Enuresis was more prevalent in boys than girls (6 vs. 2.5 %), with a 2.7-fold risk of enuresis among 8- to 11-year-old boys (OR2.69 [95 % CI 1.37–5.2]) (Shreeram et al. 2009).

Poly-symptomatic Enuresis

Prospective epidemiologic studies report daytime symptoms occurred in approximately 20–40 % of children with enuresis.

Of consecutive children referred to an enuresis clinic, daytime symptoms occurred in over 80 %.

The ALSPAC prospective cohort study of 13,973 children mentioned above described 1,260 (15.5 %) children with bedwetting (infrequent plus frequent), comprising mono-symptomatic enuresis in 12 %, and day and nighttime wetting in 3 %. Only 0.2 % experienced frequent (>2×/week) wetting episodes both during the day and night. Of children with nighttime wetting, 29 % had daytime urge symptoms, with increased likelihood with increasing frequency of enuresis (Butler et al. 2005).

In the cross-sectional epidemiological study reported by Yeung et al. (2006) above, daytime incontinence was present in 106 (21 %) of the 512 patients with bedwetting (>1x/3 months), including 38 (14 %) of 279 children aged 5–10 years and 68 (29 %) of 233 adolescents >10 years (Yeung et al. 2006).

Another cross-sectional study of 5,282 Japanese school children mean age 9 years (7–12) found bedwetting (>1x/month) in 6 %. Daytime symptoms, including frequency >8x/day and/or urge incontinence >1x/month, occurred in 41 % of these. The prevalence of poly-symptomatic enuresis was 3 % at age 7 years, and decreased to 0.8 % at age 12 years (Kajiwara et al. 2006).

An Australian cross-sectional study involved a random sample of 2,856 children from elementary schools with a mean age of 7.3 years (SD 1.3), reporting enuresis in 6 %. Daytime incontinence occurred in 17 %, associated with mild, moderate, and severe enuresis (1–6x/month; >7x/month but < nightly; 7x/week) in univariate analysis and multivariate logistic regression (adjusted OR [95 % CI]: 3.0 [2.1–4.2], 2.6 [1.3–5.2], and 4.8 [2.9–7.9]), respectively (Sureshkumar et al. 2009).

Among 170 patients with nocturnal enuresis (quantity not specified) enrolled into a prospective study of consecutive children aged ≥3.5 years presenting to a referral clinic for enuresis, 83 % experienced "urinary urgency" (not defined). Daytime wetting was present in 84 %, urinary frequency (>8x/day) in 39 %, and squatting maneuvers in 35 % of girls (Robson et al. 2005).

Secondary Enuresis

Approximately one-third of enuretics have onset after a dry period, comprising secondary enuresis.

One study found no difference in daytime symptoms in secondary versus primary enuretics.

Two studies reported life stressors such as divorce, birth of siblings, and school problems associated with secondary versus primary enuresis.

The prospective case–control study of 170 referred patients to an enuresis clinic mentioned above (Robson et al. 2005) reported primary enuresis in 123 (72 %) and secondary enuresis in 47 (28 %). Of the studied characteristics (demographic information, urologic history, uroflowmetry, and post-void residual), the only difference in those with secondary enuresis was the increased presence of constipation (diagnosed with palpable stool on abdominal exam and/or abdominal radiograph), in 75 % with primary versus 56 % with secondary enuresis (OR 2.17 [95 % CI 1.07–4.41]). Daytime symptoms, including incontinence, which was reported by 85 %, had similar frequency in both groups.

A prospective birth cohort study of 1,265 New Zealand children determined that the rate of nocturnal enuresis in 8-year-olds was 7 %, which the authors estimated represented secondary enuresis in one-third to one-half. Children exposed in any given year from ages 2–8 years to multiple life stressors, defined as change of parents or residence and/or other events from a 20-item Social Readjustment Rating Scale, were more likely to develop secondary enuresis (OR 2.56 [95 % CI 1.18–5.50]). This likelihood for secondary enuresis also related to age at which nighttime dryness was first achieved, with children not dry until age 5 years more susceptible than those dry at age ≤3 years (OR 3.39 [95 % CI 1.76–6.56]) (Fergusson et al. 1990).

A prospective study of 110 consecutive children with primary (82, 75 %) versus secondary (28, 25 %) enuresis that performed semi-structured child interviews and parental questionnaires found a higher rate of behavioral disorders (primarily internalizing) and/or life stressors (divorce, birth of sibling, school problems) in those with secondary enuresis (von Gontard et al. 1996).

Family History

One study of consecutive patients referred to a specialty enuresis clinic reported a positive family history in first- or second-degree relatives in 62 %.

A prospective cohort study found approximately 20 % of children with enuresis had a

parent with a history of bedwetting beyond age 5 years, equally affecting mothers and fathers.

Cross-sectional epidemiologic studies found increased likelihood for a child having enuresis if either mother or father reported bedwetting.

One study found sibling enuresis an independent risk factor compared to parental history.

Two twin studies report concordance in identical twins more than fraternal twins, suggesting a strong genetic component.

A prospective study evaluated family history among 167 consecutive children aged 5–10 years attending an outpatient enuresis clinic, of whom 110 had mono-symptomatic enuresis. A positive family history (parent, sibling, aunt, uncle, cousin) was reported by 67 (62 %), including 21 % of mothers, 23 % of fathers, and 17.5 % siblings (von Gontard et al. 1996).

A cross-sectional study of 3,206 Finnish 7-year-olds, of whom 8 % experienced bedwetting, found a positive family history in 37 %, with the risk of enuresis in a child 7.1 times greater (95 % CI 5.1–9.8) when the father had bedwetting beyond 4 years of age, and 5.2 times greater (95 % CI 3.9–7.0) when the mother did (Jarvelin et al. 1988).

Enuresis occurred in 159 (10 %) of 1,694 Turkish school children mean age 9 years (7–11 years) responding to a school-based cross-sectional survey. Univariate analysis found higher rates of parents and siblings with a history of treatment for enuresis among children with enuresis compared to those without enuresis (parental history: 68.5 vs. 4.6 %, $p<0.001$; sibling history: 34.6 vs. 2.3 %, $p<0.001$). Multiple logistic regression demonstrated that parental and sibling history of enuresis were both independent risk factors for enuresis (parent: OR 12.17, 95 % CI 4.05–36.61; sibling: OR 3.79, 95 % CI 1.23–11.68) (Inan et al. 2007).

In the ALSPAC prospective birth cohort study of 13,973 UK children mentioned above, detailed family history was obtained during the pregnancy of the enrolled child. Parents were asked if they experienced nighttime incontinence beyond the age of 5 years; a positive history was reported by 9 % of both mothers and fathers. Parent/child pairs were constructed based on frequency of bedwetting, and odds ratios were calculated to determine risk of enuresis. Rates of enuresis (>2 nights/week) at age 7.5 years were 3.63 and 1.85 times higher among children with a family history of maternal or paternal bedwetting, respectively (von Gontard et al. 2011a).

A prospective study in New Zealand followed children from birth to age 8 years, and obtained information regarding family history of enuresis from mothers of the children at the 5-year visit, recorded as number of first-degree relatives with nocturnal enuresis. The mean age of attaining bladder control ("regularly remained dry throughout the night") in children with zero, one, and two first-degree relatives with nocturnal enuresis were 3.7, 4.4, and 5.2 years, respectively ($p<0.0001$). On multivariate analysis, the number of first-degree relatives was the strongest predictor of age to attain bladder control, which on average occurred 1.5 years later when two first-degree relatives had nocturnal enuresis compared to those without a family history (Fergusson et al. 1986).

Among 338 pairs of twins prospectively enrolled in a study to evaluate "various behavior disorders," including bedwetting, thumb-sucking, and nail-biting, 146/676 (22 %) had enuresis, defined as wetting repeatedly >4 years of age. A positive history for a parent having had bedwetting was obtained in 85 %, equally involving mothers and fathers (Bakwin 1971).

Enuresis in the above-mentioned study reported that of the twins with enuresis, 68 % were monozygmatic versus 36 % dizygomatic, further supporting a strong genetic component (Bakwin 1971).

Similarly, a nationwide Finnish Twin Cohort of over 11,000 patients demonstrated a higher concordance rate of nocturnal enuresis in childhood among identical versus fraternal twins (43 vs. 19 %) (Hublin et al. 1998).

Associated Disorders

Constipation

Three prospective studies reported that encopresis, but not constipation, was a risk factor for nocturnal enuresis.

Two stated that fecal incontinence was associated with enuresis; it was found in 11 % of enuretics in one study.

The Australian cross-sectional study of 2,856 children described above categorized "severe" (nightly the past 1 month), "moderate" (≥7 episodes in past month), and "mild" (1–6 episodes the past month) enuresis. Constipation as defined by ROME-II criteria was not associated with mild, moderate, or severe enuresis (OR 0.7 [95 % CI 0.4–1.2], 1.5 [95 % CI 0.7–3.6], and 0.7 [95 % CI 0.3–1.9], respectively). However, encopresis was more likely with severe enuresis in multivariate logistic regression adjusting for age (OR 2.7 [95 % CI 1.6–4.4]), and marginally associated with mild and moderate enuresis (OR 1.6 [95 % CI 1.0–2.4] and 2.1 [95 % CI 1.1–4.3], respectively) (Sureshkumar et al. 2009).

The survey of Turkish school children reporting enuresis in 10 % mentioned above defined constipation as ≥2 of the following: bowel movement <3×/week, fecal incontinence >1×/week, palpable stools, stopping up toilet, withholding maneuvers, and/or pain with defecation. Univariable analysis reported both fecal incontinence and constipation more likely in enuretic versus non-enuretic children, but multivariate analysis demonstrated that only fecal incontinence, which occurred in 11 % with bedwetting, was an independent risk factor for enuresis (OR 6.13 [95 % CI 1.46–43.83]) (Inan et al. 2007).

The cross-sectional study of 5,282 Japanese school children reported above defined constipation as <3 bowel movements/week. There was no difference in rates of mono-symptomatic enuresis (6 %) in children with and without constipation, while poly-symptomatic urinary incontinence was more likely with constipation (3 % with vs. 2 % without, $p<0.05$) (Kajiwara et al. 2006).

A retrospective review of 30 consecutive patients mean age 9 years (5–15) with a "chief complaint of nocturnal enuresis" found 10 % reported constipation (bowel movement < every other day). Using a novel measurement of the ratio of the widest point of rectal diameter to pelvic outlet diameter on abdominal radiograph, all children had "fecal rectal distention" Therapy with polyethylene glycol for ≥2 weeks cured the enuresis in 25 (83 %) (Hodges and Anthony 2012). The number of wet nights/week before bowel therapy was not stated, and it was unclear if these patients had daytime incontinence. The indications for radiography and the number of other patients with enuresis not undergoing x-rays also were not stated.

Sleep-Disordered Breathing

A systematic review reported that approximately 33 % of children with sleep-disordered breathing (snoring, obstructive sleep apnea) also had enuresis.

Several population-based surveys report enuresis in 7–22 % of children who report sleep-disordered breathing, which is significantly greater than in children without snoring or sleep apnea (2–16 %).

Systematic review found tonsillectomy and adenoidectomy (T&A) reduced enuresis during median follow-up of 6 months.

A systematic review of 12 articles published from 1998 to 2010 included 3,550 children with sleep-disordered breathing, of which 1,113 (33 %) also had enuresis (not separated into primary versus secondary). Patient age ranged from 2 to 19 years. The authors commented that their finding that 33 % of patients age 6 years with sleep-disordered breathing also had enuresis suggests a relationship, given the usual prevalence of <15 % enuresis reported for this age. Seven articles with 1,360 patients (enuresis in 426, 31 %) had data regarding enuresis after T&A, finding that postoperative prevalence with median follow-up of 6 months was reduced to 16 % ($p=0.002$) (Jeyakumar et al. 2012).

Among 17,646 children aged 5–7 years in Kentucky completing a questionnaire about sleep habits, enuresis (defined as >2×/month) was present in 531/1976 (27 %) with habitual snoring (>3 nights/week and medium to loud on a loudness scale) versus 1,821/15,670 (12 %) without snoring ($p<0.00001$, OR 2.79 [95 % CI 2.50–3.13]). A random sample of 378 children at risk for sleep apnea based on these questionnaires underwent overnight polysomnography.

Of these, enuresis ≥3×/week was present in 33/149 (22 %) with obstructive sleep apnea and 36/229 (16 %) with habitual snoring but not obstructive sleep apnea. Severity of sleep disturbance did not correlate with severity of enuresis (Capdevila et al. 2008).

Two additional population-based cross-sectional studies also found increased rates of enuresis among children with snoring. Of 2,746 5–13-year-old children in Istanbul, children with occasional and habitual snoring had higher rates of nocturnal enuresis (quantity not specified) versus non-snorers (10 and 15 % vs. 7.5 %, $p=0.005$, OR 2.2 [95 % CI 1.2–3.5]) (Ersu et al. 2004).

Among 1,821 children aged 5–14 years in Greece, children with habitual snoring (>3 nights/week) were more likely to have primary nocturnal enuresis (>1×/week) versus non-snorers (7.4 vs. 2 %, OR=4.00 [95 % CI 1.93–8.32]) (Alexopoulos et al. 2006).

A case–control study compared 149 children in a sleep-disorders clinic to 139 controls from general pediatric practice, and found that children with obstructive sleep apnea had higher odds of having mono-symptomatic enuresis (quantity not specified) (OR=5.29 [95 % CI 2.25–12.45]) (Barone et al. 2009).

Another case–control study included 270 children referred to a sleep center for enuresis and 274 gender- and age-matched healthy children without enuresis as controls. Significant differences in sleep patterns occurred in enuretic versus healthy controls, as measured by the validated sleep disturbance scale for children (Carotenuto et al. 2011).

Attention Deficit/Hyperactivity Disorder

One literature survey reported a co-occurrence rate of attention deficit/hyperactivity disorder (ADHD)/behavioral problems and enuresis of 16–32 %.

One population-based US study found ADHD increased in children with enuresis (12 %), while a similar study of German children reported enuresis was not related to ADHD.

A literature survey concerned the co-occurrence of ADHD and enuresis in "recent studies" characterized as epidemiological ($n=6$) versus clinical ($n=12$), reporting ADHD/behavioral problems occurred in approximately 16–29 % of enuretics. Four other studies reported that enuresis occurred in 21–32 % of children with ADHD (Baeyens et al. 2005).

A population-based, nationally representative cross-sectional cohort of 1,136 US children found enuresis (defined by DSM-IV criteria and present within the past 12 months before the survey) in 4 % children aged 8–11 years. Using a validated structured diagnostic interview that elicits DSM-IV criteria for both enuresis and ADHD, nearly 10 % of children met DSM-IV criteria for ADHD. Enuretic children were more likely than non-enuretics to have ADHD: 12.5 vs. 4 % without, $p=0.001$. There was a 2.9-fold risk for ADHD among children with enuresis, OR 2.88 (95 % CI 1.26–6.57) (Shreeram et al. 2009).

The ALSPAC prospective birth cohort mentioned above demonstrated higher rates of parent-reported psychological problems, including attention problems, in children with any bedwetting and combined day and night wetting versus in those without wetting at age 7.5 years, bedwetting OR 1.58 (95 % CI 1.32–1.90), and combined wetting OR 2.23 (95 % CI 1.64–3.05) (Joinson et al. 2007).

Another cross-sectional study that controlled for developmental delay among a cohort of 1,379 children undergoing a mandatory school entry medical examination in Germany demonstrated that nocturnal enuresis alone was not a significant risk factor for symptoms of ADHD, whereas daytime incontinence with or without nocturnal enuresis strongly increased the odds of ADHD symptoms, OR 4.6 (95 % CI 1.6–13.0) (von Gontard et al. 2011b).

A cross-sectional study of 344 children enrolled in a genetic study of ADHD demonstrated a 17 % prevalence of enuresis (not quantified), which localized to the inattentive ADHD phenotype, but genome-wide analysis of 51 of these children did not identify an association with chromosomal regions previously linked to enuresis (Elia et al. 2009).

Psychologic Impact of Enuresis

One study reported children age 9 years considered bedwetting a social problem that ranked fourth of 21 difficult life events.

As noted earlier, behavioral problems are increased in children with both primary and secondary enuresis.

As part of the ALSPAC population-based study concerning health and development of children, questionnaires were sent to 10,985 children age 9 years, with 8,209 returns (75 % response) equally distributed between genders. They were asked to rate perceived difficulty of life events from a list of 21 items, as "not at all," "a little difficult," "quite difficult," and "really difficult." The top four most difficult events were "don't have friends," "being teased," "left out of things," and "wet the bed." Those rated less severe included "often ill," "move to a new school," "always in trouble," and "don't like how they look." Enuretic children (≥2 nights per week) comprised 1 % of respondents, and reported bedwetting a more difficult event than non-wetters. Nevertheless, 36 % of children dry at night rated bedwetting a "really difficult" problem. The fact that children rated bedwetting a more difficult problem than physical illness was interpreted by the authors to indicate that they perceive this a social, rather than medical, issue (Butler and Heron 2007).

Another ALSPAC questionnaire study concerned parental attitudes regarding combined bedwetting and daytime incontinence in children approximately 7.5 years old. Parents reported more psychological problems in children with combined wetting than those with only bedwetting or no wetting, as already mentioned in the section above (Joinson et al. 2007).

One-hundred ten consecutive children presenting to an enuresis clinic were diagnosed as having primary ($n=82$) or secondary bedwetting. Evaluation included a "full child psychiatric and psychological assessment," and parent questionnaires for life events they considered to have caused enuresis. Patients with secondary enuresis had significantly higher rates of behavioral disorders and psychological risk factors (such as divorce, sibling birth, entering kindergarten) (von Gontard et al. 1996).

Natural History

Spontaneous Resolution

Our review found no longitudinal study assessing spontaneous resolution rates of enuresis in a population of untreated children.

Short-term dryness (within 2–22 weeks) in nine RCTs was achieved in only 4 % of untreated controls.

No longitudinal study reports spontaneous resolution of bedwetting in untreated children.

The 15 % annual spontaneous resolution rate commonly quoted was derived from patients failing at least two drug treatments and behavioral modifications.

A questionnaire-based study of 1,129 (of 1,483) patients evaluated in an enuresis clinic in Belfast between 1952 and 1959 reported approximately 15 % "spontaneous" resolution per year in patients aged 5–19 years, with 33 (3 %) having continued enuresis after age 20 years (Forsythe and Redmond 1974). This study is frequently referenced in review articles of enuresis for the often-quoted 15 % rate of "spontaneous resolution" in children not treated with a bedwetting alarm. However, all these patients failed therapy with ≥2 drugs and many also failed various behavioral modifications, and so are not representative of untreated children. Furthermore, the numbers of patients evaluated at different ages to calculate annual resolution rates was not stated, and length of time of follow-up was not taken into account. Duration of time without wetting considered "cure" was not stated.

A Cochrane systematic review found no treatment or placebo arms of RCTs demonstrate <10 % of patients achieve 14 consecutive nights of dryness during the study periods (ranging from 2 to 22 weeks), and only 1–2 % remain dry. This pooled analysis of nine trials reporting data for bedwetting alarm versus no treatment reported failure (<14 consecutive dry nights) in 250 of 260 (96 %) controls (Glazener et al. 2009a).

Our review did not find any long-term longitudinal cohort studies of enuretic patients reporting spontaneous resolution without medical, behavioral, and/or alarm therapy. Enuresis rates at various ages in population-based, cross-sectional studies such as those described provide prevalence rates at various ages, but it is unknown or not specified how many of these children received therapy to alleviate enuresis at any given point in time, and so these studies cannot be used to estimate true spontaneous resolution.

Evaluation

No laboratory, radiologic, or urodynamic testing is needed after history and physical examination in children with mono-symptomatic enuresis.

The following is a summary of current guidelines for evaluation of enuresis.

NICE guidelines (2010), derived from "best available evidence" by a team selected by the National Clinical Guidelines Centre, recommend the following:

- Urinalysis when there is a suspicion of diabetes or UTI, secondary enuresis, and/or daytime symptoms
- Voiding and fluid-intake diaries
- No radiographic studies

European Association of Urology guidelines, derived primarily from expert consensus, recommend the following:

- Diagnosis is made by history alone without further investigation for mono-symptomatic enuresis (Tekgul et al. 2009).

ICCS guidelines, derived from "what evidence there is" (described as weak) and expert consensus, recommend the following:

- Urinalysis to evaluate glycosuria and/or proteinuria
- No renal ultrasound
- A 2-day chart of urinary frequency/volume and fluid volume consumed
- A 1-week chart of enuresis, daytime incontinence, and bowel movements (Neveus et al. 2010).

Treatment

Behavioral Interventions (Random Awakening, Fluid Restrictions, Rewards)

Cochrane review of RCTs reported wakening not triggered by a wetting episode was not effective therapy for enuresis.

Cochrane review of behavioral and educational interventions for enuresis, including wakening not triggered by a wetting episode, as well as night-time fluid restriction and reward systems, analyzed 18 trials involving 1,174 children. Behavioral interventions alone were not as effective as alarms alone or alarms plus behavioral therapy, with RR for failure or relapse with behavioral intervention versus alarm plus intervention 2.81 (95 % CI 1.80–4.38) (Glazener et al. 2008).

Alarm Conditioning

Cochrane review reported alarm use for 2–22 weeks resulted in 14 consecutive dry nights in 50–75 % of children. Approximately 50 % of children remained dry after active treatment.

A more rapid response may be achieved using medication, but overall effectiveness during therapy was considered similar by Cochrane review.

Relapse rates were less after alarm therapy versus medication.

Cochrane review of 56 RCTs involved 3,257 children, 2,412 of whom used an alarm. Duration of treatment varied but ranged from 2 to 8 weeks in 16 trials, up to more than 12 weeks in 22 trials. Only 29/56 (52 %) studies provided follow-up data to determine relapse rates. Here is a summary of key findings:

- Alarm versus no treatment: About two-thirds of patients using alarms became dry (RR for failure 0.38 [95 % CI 0.33–0.45]), and about half failed or relapsed after alarm conditioning, while nearly all controls remained wet.

- Alarm versus placebo: Alarms were better than placebo for fewer wet nights during and after treatment.
- Alarm versus desmopressin: Desmopressin may achieve dryness faster than alarm, although there appear to be no differences during an entire treatment course, RR 0.85 (95 % CI 0.53–1.37). In two small trials, relapse was less after alarm therapy (26/57 [46 %] vs. 40/62 [65 %]).
- Alarm versus tricyclics: There was no difference in response during treatment, RR 0.59 (95 % CI 0.32–1.09), but alarms had lower relapse rates after treatment, RR 0.58 (95 % CI 0.36–0.94).
- Alarm plus desmopressin: there was no difference in treatment success in alarm versus alarm plus desmopressin trials.

There were no clear-cut differences noted in types of alarms (body vs. pad), although two small trials demonstrated fewer wet nights among alarms with immediate wakening versus time delay of 3 min (Glazener et al. 2009a).

Desmopressin

Cochrane meta-analysis reported that desmopressin achieved 14 consecutive dry nights in approximately 20 % of children versus 2 % of controls.

One trial increased desmopressin dosing at 2-week intervals, reporting progressively decreased wet nights with increasing dose to 0.6 mg, but only 8 % of treated children became dry.

Relapse after therapy is similar in children treated with desmopressin and those receiving no medication.

One RCT reported desmopressin plus tolterodine achieved >50 % reduction in wet nights during 1 month of therapy in patients with enuresis failing desmopressin alone.

Cochrane review included 47 RCTs involving 3,448 children, with 2,210 receiving desmopressin. All but 10 of these studies involved the intranasal route (no longer available), with the remaining using oral tablets. Sample sizes of these studies ranged from 10 to 182 patients (mean 73) and were conducted for various lengths of time at varying dosing regimens. Key summarized findings included the following:

- Desmopressin versus placebo: At an intranasal dose of 20 μg, pooled data demonstrated a mean of 1.34 fewer wet nights per week (95 % CI 1.11–1.57). Doses of 40 μg and 60 μg decreased the number of wet nights per week by 1.33 and 1.50 nights/week, respectively (95 % CI 1.67–0.99 and 1.92–1.08). Nineteen percent of treated children became dry versus 2 % of controls. Four trials suggested results were not sustained after treatment ended.
- Desmopressin versus tricyclics: More children in two trials became dry with desmopressin during treatment, RR for failure to achieve 14 consecutive dry nights 0.44 (95 % CI 0.27–0.73), but there were no data regarding relapse after therapy.
- Desmopressin versus alarms: See section above.
- Adverse Events: All reported events were minor and did not result in stopping treatment. There is a risk for water intoxication, which is minimized by fluid restriction before bedtime (Glazener and Evans 2009).

In one multicenter dose-escalation study, 148 children (ages 6–16 years, 73 % males, average 10–11 wet nights per 2 weeks) were assigned to placebo or desmopressin beginning at 0.2 mg at bedtime for 2 weeks, and then increased every 2 weeks at 0.2-mg increments until either dry or receiving a maximum 0.6 mg. There was a significant linear decrease in wet nights from baseline a mean of 10, 27, 30, and 40 % for placebo, 0.2, 0.4, and 0.6 mg desmopressin. A 50 % reduction in wetting from baseline occurred in 28 % of patients at 0.2 mg, 16 % at 0.4 mg, and 9 % at 0.6 mg. However, only 11/141 (8 %) desmopressin patients became dry versus 0/47 receiving placebo (Schulman et al. 2001).

One RCT enrolled 34 nonresponders or partial responders to desmopressin with mono-symptomatic enuresis (mean age 10.5 years, 70 % males) to desmopressin plus 4 mg tolterodine versus desmopressin plus placebo for 1 month. Treatment outcomes were described as either success (>50 % reduction in wet nights) or no success. Success was achieved significantly more with desmopressin plus tolterodine, 8/18 (44 %) versus desmopressin plus placebo 5/16 (31 %) (Austin et al. 2008).

FDA Adverse Events Reporting

Desmopressin in combination with excessive fluid intake can result in hyponatremia, which can lead to brain swelling, seizure, and, rarely, death. However, no RCTs involving its use for bedwetting reported these events during the study period. In 2007, the FDA indicated post-marketing reports of 61 seizures among users of desmopressin nasal spray to treat various medical conditions. Thirty-one of these patients had other concomitant medicines/diseases associated with hyponatremia and/or seizures. Nevertheless, the FDA recommended against intranasal administration for the treatment of primary nocturnal enuresis in children.

Imipramine

Cochrane review found that imipramine was more effective than placebo for enuresis, with approximately 20–33 % achieving 14 consecutive dry nights during therapy.

Relapse occurred in approximately 66 % of patients when treatment stopped at 3 months.

Cochrane review included 58 RCTs involving 3,721 children. Results were pooled for the various tricyclics, which was primarily imipramine but also included desipramine, amitriptyline, nortriptyline, viloxazine, trimipramine, mianserin, and clomipramine. Study sample sizes were generally small. Various dosing regimens and lengths of treatment were used. Key findings included the following:

- Tricyclics versus placebo: There were fewer wet nights for patients receiving tricylics versus controls. Meta-analysis was possible using data from only three trials, finding an average of one fewer wet night per week, –0.92 (95 % CI –1.38 to –0.46). Eleven trials found 21 % of treated children achieved 14 consecutive dry nights, versus 5 % on placebo, RR for failure 0.77 (95 % CI 0.72–0.83). After stopping therapy, only 4 % who took imipramine versus 3 % who took placebo remained dry.
- Dose-related efficacy: Two trials compared higher versus lower dose imipramine, with one reporting there was no difference (but not providing data), while the other showed one fewer wet night per week at 25 mg compared to 10 mg.
- Tricyclics versus desmopressin: See section above.
- Tricyclics versus alarm: See above.

Adverse Events

Twenty-nine trials provided some information regarding side effects, but no major adverse events, specifically arrhythmia or heart block, occurred (Glazener et al. 2009b).

Oxybutynin

Oxybutynin monotherapy is no more effective than placebo for enuresis.

NICE guidelines pooled results demonstrated no difference in patients receiving oxybutynin versus placebo to achieve either >90 % (6/16 [37.5 %] vs. 5/23 [21.7 %], RR 1.73 [95 % CI 0.63–4.69]), or 50–90 % dry nights (6/15 [37.5 %] vs. 8/23 [4.8 %] RR 1.08 [5 % CI 0.46–2.51]) (NICE 2010).

A crossover double-blinded RCT of 30 children (mean age 10 years, 83 % boys, some previously treated with imipramine) with primary nocturnal enuresis assigned to placebo versus oxybutinin 5 mg nightly for 4 weeks demonstrated no difference in the number of dry nights. There was a mean decrease in wetting of 1.9 nights/week (Lovering et al. 1988).

Alternative Therapies: Acupuncture, Hypnosis, Psychotherapy, Chiropractor Adjustment, Homeopathy

No alternative therapy listed here has been found effective for enuresis treatment.

A 2011 update regarding complementary and miscellaneous interventions for enuresis was performed by the Cochrane Incontinence Group. Several small, poor-quality trials provide weak evidence in support of hyponosis, psychotherapy, acupuncture, chiropractic, and medicinal herbs (Huang et al. 2011).

Order of Therapy

Synthesizing outcomes data and cost analysis, NICE guidelines recommended, in descending order, the following:

- Alarm as first-line therapy
- Alarm plus desmopressin or desmopressin alone if alarm is ineffective
- Desmopressin plus anticholinergic
- Imipramine

Impact of Therapy on Self-Esteem

One study of enuretics versus matched controls using non-validated instruments to determine personality attributes and behavioral problems reported that parent and therapist assessment, but not that by teachers, improved with successful alarm therapy.

Subsequent trials using validated instruments found parent-rated behavior improved in patients regardless of treatment outcomes.

Two trials concluded that successful treatment of enuresis did not impact psychological health of the child, although another reported significant improvement in self-concept. One trial using imipramine found improved behavior that correlated with decreased wetting, but could not determine if the changes were secondary to therapeutic success versus euphoric effects of the medication.

A study of 30 enuretic children and 60 gender- and age-matched controls assessed personality characteristics and behavioral problems. Median age was 8 years (6–12), 20 boys, and enuresis occurred nightly in "more than half." Of the 30 with bedwetting, 10 were treated with alarms, 10 with scheduled night wakening, and 10 were not treated. Parents completed (non-validated) rating scales to assess personality attributes (confidence, anxiety) and behavioral problems (such as tantrums, thumb-sucking) before and "several weeks" after treatment. Their teachers used a different rating scale modified for the study and filled out just before treatment, 10 weeks later (end of treatment), and another 3 months later. The enuretic children and 30 of the controls were also tested by a psychologist using a novel "self-image questionnaire" created for the study and a "neurotic inventory" previously reported in another study of enuretics. There was no difference in patients versus controls on any pretreatment test. Parent ratings after treatment were significantly better in patients who stopped wetting. Teacher scores did not change regardless of response to therapy. Therapist ratings were improved in patients who stopped wetting, significantly different than the "improvement" during the same time in controls. No children who stopped wetting had worsening in adjustment symptoms, but rather were reported to be happier and less anxious (Baker 1969).

A subsequent study used similar methods but included more patients, used validated assessment instruments, and had longer follow-up to 1 year after treatment. There were 83 enuretic children (male to female ratio 3:1) who had been referred at median age 9 years to a child guidance center because of their bedwetting who were treated either with alarm ($n=64$), psychotherapy/counseling ($n=10$), or no treatment ($n=9$), and of these 51, 2, and 2, respectively, had success (13 consecutive dry nights). Mothers completed a behavioral questionnaire, the children a personality assessment, and their teachers a different behavioral rating before and 1, 6, and 12 months after treatment. There was no difference in the three groups in pretreatment or at 1 month posttreatment ratings. All three showed a decrease in mother-reported behavioral problems at 1 month post treatment, which the authors concluded represented either placebo effect (change in parental perception because of clinic contacts) or the result of repeat testing, but was not due specifically to enuresis therapy. Similarly, 6- and 12-month data showed patients successfully treated continued to have decreased mother-reported ratings, but so did those not achieving "cure." Consequently, there was no evidence that enuresis treatment impacted psychological health (Sacks et al. 1974).

A RCT enrolled children with enuresis and allocated them to alarm ($n=66$) or no treatment ($n=55$, "waiting list"). Treatment continued until patients had 14 consecutive dry nights, and then "overlearning" was done, having them drink additional fluids at bedtime with alarm use continued until there was another 14 consecutive dry nights. Validated self-concept and behavioral questionnaires were rated by children and parents at baseline and after treatment. Parent-rated behavior improved in both groups without difference. Significant self-concept improvement occurred in the treated patients (Moffatt et al. 1987).

Another trial recruited subjects from local pediatric clinics and by advertisements that attracted 148 children, from which a total of 40 were enrolled on the basis of several inclusion criteria. These were randomized to alarm, imipramine, or no treatment ("waiting list"), with treatment continued until the child was dry for 14 consecutive nights or for 14 weeks. Behavioral health and emotional health were determined by child and parent ratings on validated instruments before and after treatment. There were no significant behavioral or emotional effects from treatment. Despite different success rates, there was no difference in post-treatment psychological assessments in patients using alarms versus imipramine (Wagner et al. 1982).

While imipramine is used to stop enuresis, the fact that most enuretics have no psychiatric defect raised questions regarding effects of an antidepressant medication in psychologically normal children. A double-blinded, placebo-controlled crossover study was designed using 50 mg imipramine for 3 weeks in boys recruited by a newspaper story. There were 21 completers. Imipramine effects included significant but small increases in resting heart rate (placebo 82 vs. 98) and diastolic blood pressure (placebo 65 vs. 73). There was nonsignificant improvement in cognitive performance on imipramine. A low but significant correlation was found between changes in wetting and behavior, but it was not possible to determine if this was due to decreased wetting or any euphoric effect of imipramine. The authors concluded imipramine has similar psychotropic effects to stimulants, such as those used for hyperactivity (Werry et al. 1975).

References

Alexopoulos EI, Kostadima E, Pagonari I, Zintzaras E, Gourgoulianis K, Kaditis AG. Association between primary nocturnal enuresis and habitual snoring in children. Urology. 2006;68(2):406–9.

Austin PF, Ferguson G, Yan Y, Campigotto MJ, Royer ME, Coplen DE. Combination therapy with desmopressin and an anticholinergic medication for nonresponders to desmopressin for monosymptomatic nocturnal enuresis: a randomized, double-blind, placebo-controlled trial. Pediatrics. 2008;122(5):1027–32.

Baeyens D, Roeyers H, Demeyere I, Verte S, Hoebeke P, Vande WJ. Attention-deficit/hyperactivity disorder (ADHD) as a risk factor for persistent nocturnal enuresis in children: a two-year follow-up study. Acta Paediatr. 2005;94(11):1619–25.

Baker BL. Symptom treatment and symptom substitution in enuresis. J Abnorm Psychol. 1969;74(1):42–9.

Bakwin H. Enuresis in twins. Am J Dis Child. 1971;121(3): 222–5.

Barone JG, Hanson C, DaJusta DG, Gioia K, England SJ, Schneider D. Nocturnal enuresis and overweight are associated with obstructive sleep apnea. Pediatrics. 2009;124(1):e53–9.

Butler RJ, Golding J, Northstone K. Nocturnal enuresis at 7.5 years old: prevalence and analysis of clinical signs. BJU Int. 2005;96(3):404–10.

Butler R, Heron J. An exploration of children's views of bed-wetting at 9 years. Child Care Health Dev. 2007;34(1):65–70.

Butler RJ, Heron J. The prevalence of infrequent bedwetting and nocturnal enuresis in childhood. A large British cohort. Scand J Urol Nephrol. 2008;42(3): 257–64.

Capdevila OS, Kheirandish-Gozal L, Dayyat E, Gozal D. Pediatric obstructive sleep apnea: complications, management, and long-term outcomes. Proc Am Thorac Soc. 2008;5(2):274–82.

Carotenuto M, Esposito M, Pascotto A. Facial patterns and primary nocturnal enuresis in children. Sleep Breath. 2011;15(2):221–7.

Elia J, Takeda T, Deberardinis R, Burke J, Accardo J, Ambrosini PJ, et al. Nocturnal enuresis: a suggestive endophenotype marker for a subgroup of inattentive attention-deficit/hyperactivity disorder. J Pediatr. 2009;155(2):239–44. e5.

Ersu R, Arman AR, Save D, Karadag B, Karakoc F, Berkem M, et al. Prevalence of snoring and symptoms of sleep-disordered breathing in primary school children in istanbul. Chest. 2004;126(1):19–24.

Fergusson DM, Horwood LJ, Shannon FT. Factors related to the age of attainment of nocturnal bladder control: an 8-year longitudinal study. Pediatrics. 1986;78(5): 884–90.

Fergusson DM, Horwood LJ, Shannon FT. Secondary enuresis in a birth cohort of New Zealand children. Paediatr Perinat Epidemiol. 1990;4(1):53–63.

Forsythe WI, Redmond A. Enuresis and spontaneous cure rate. Study of 1129 enuretis. Arch Dis Child. 1974;49(4): 259–63.

Glazener C, Evans J, Peto RE. Complex behavioural and educational interventions for bedwetting (nocturnal enuresis) in children. Cochrane Database Syst Rev. 2008. Art. No.: CD004668. doi: 10.1002/14651858. CD004668.

Glazener C, Evans J, Peto RE. Alarm interventions for nocturnal enuresis in children. Cochrane Database Syst Rev. 2009. Art No. CD002911. doi: 10.1002/14651858. CD002911.

Glazener C, Evans J, Peto RE. Tricyclic and related drugs for nocturnal enuresis in children. Cochrane Database Syst Rev. 2009b. Art No. CD002117. doi: 10.1002/14651858. CD002117.

Glazener CM, Evans JH. Desmopressin for nocturnal enuresis in children. Cochrane Database Syst Rev. 2009. Art No. CD002112. doi: 10.1002/14651858. CD002112.

Hodges SJ, Anthony EY. Occult megarectum–a commonly unrecognized cause of enuresis. Urology. 2012;79(2):421–4.

Huang T, Shu X, Huang YS, Cheuk DK. Complementary and miscellaneous interventions for nocturnal enuresis in children. Cochrane Database Syst Rev. 2011;(12): CD005230.

Hublin C, Kaprio J, Partinen M, Koskenvuo M. Nocturnal enuresis in a nationwide twin cohort. Sleep. 1998;21(6): 579–85.

Inan M, Aydiner CY, Tokuc B, Aksu B, Ayvaz S, Ayhan S, et al. Factors associated with childhood constipation. J Paediatr Child Health. 2007;43(10):700–6.

Jarvelin MR, Vikevainen-Tervonen L, Moilanen I, Huttunen NP. Enuresis in seven-year-old children. Acta Paediatr Scand. 1988;77(1):148–53.

Jeyakumar A, Rahman SI, Armbrecht ES, Mitchell R. The association between sleep-disordered breathing and enuresis in children. Laryngoscope. 2012;122(8): 1873–7.

Joinson C, Heron J, Emond A, Butler R. Psychological problems in children with bedwetting and combined (day and night) wetting: a UK population-based study. J Pediatr Psychol. 2007;32(5):605–16.

Kajiwara M, Inoue K, Kato M, Usui A, Kurihara M, Usui T. Nocturnal enuresis and overactive bladder in children: an epidemiological study. Int J Urol. 2006; 13(1):36–41.

Lovering JS, Tallett SE, McKendry JB. Oxybutynin efficacy in the treatment of primary enuresis. Pediatrics. 1988;82(1):104–6.

Moffatt ME, Kato C, Pless IB. Improvements in self-concept after treatment of nocturnal enuresis: randomized controlled trial. J Pediatr. 1987;110(4):647–52.

Neveus T, Eggert P, Evans J, Macedo A, Rittig S, Tekgul S, et al. Evaluation of and treatment for monosymptomatic enuresis: a standardization document from the International Children's Continence Society. J Urol. 2010;183(2):441–7.

NICE (National Institute for Clinical Excellence). Nocturnal enuresis—the management of bedwetting in children and young people. Clinical guidelines, CG111. Issued: October 2010.

Robson WL, Leung AK, Van Howe R. Primary and secondary nocturnal enuresis: similarities in presentation. Pediatrics. 2005;115(4):956–9.

Sacks S, De Leon G, Blackman S. Psychological changes associated with conditioning functional enuresis. J Clin Psychol. 1974;30(3):271–6.

Schulman SL, Stokes A, Salzman PM. The efficacy and safety of oral desmopressin in children with primary nocturnal enuresis. J Urol. 2001;166(6):2427–31.

Shreeram S, He JP, Kalaydjian A, Brothers S, Merikangas KR. Prevalence of enuresis and its association with attention-deficit/hyperactivity disorder among U.S. children: results from a nationally representative study. J Am Acad Child Adolesc Psychiatry. 2009;48(1): 35–41.

Sureshkumar P, Jones M, Cumming R, Craig J. A population based study of 2,856 school-age children with urinary incontinence. J Urol. 2009;181(2):808–15. discussion 15–6.

Tekgul S, Riedmiller H, Gerharz E, Hoebeke P, Kokvara R, Nijman R, et al. Monosymptomatic enuresis. Guidelines on pediatric urology. Arnhem, The Netherlands: European Association of Urology; 2009. p. 29–31.

von Gontard A, Hollmann E, Eiberg H, Benden B, Rittig S, Lehmkuhl G. Clinical enuresis phenotypes in familial nocturnal enuresis. Scand J Urol Nephrol. 1996;183: 11–6.

von Gontard A, Heron J, Joinson C. Family history of nocturnal enuresis and urinary incontinence: results from a large epidemiological study. J Urol. 2011a;185(6):2303–6.

von Gontard A, Moritz AM, Thome-Granz S, Freitag C. Association of attention deficit and elimination disorders at school entry: a population based study. J Urol. 2011b;186(5):2027–32.

Wagner W, Johnson SB, Walker D, Carter R, Wittner J. A controlled comparison of two treatments for nocturnal enuresis. J Pediatr. 1982;101(2):302–7.

Werry JS, Dowrick PW, Lampen EL, Vamos MJ. Imipramine in enuresis–psychological and physiological effects. J Child Psychol Psychiatry. 1975;16(4): 289–99.

Yeung CK, Sreedhar B, Sihoe JD, Sit FK, Lau J. Differences in characteristics of nocturnal enuresis between children and adolescents: a critical appraisal from a large epidemiological study. BJU Int. 2006;97(5):1069–73.

Undescended Testes

5

Warren T. Snodgrass

Primary aims in diagnosis and treatment of undescended testes (UDT):

1. **Improve fertility.**
2. **Preserve testosterone production.**
3. **Reduce cancer risk.**

Secondary aims:

1. **Repositioning the testis into the dependent scrotum without atrophy**
2. **Normal scrotal appearance**
3. **Distinction between UDT versus retractile testes**

Summary of evidence for these goals:

- **Limited available data suggest paternity rates in men with former unilateral UDT are similar to those of normal men, whereas paternity rates are diminished with formerly bilateral UDT.**
- **One RCT reported preoperative intranasal GNRH improved the fertility index (adult spermatogonia/tubule) over patients undergoing orchiopexy alone.**
- **The overall risk that an operated UDT will develop cancer is <0.5 %; risk for nonoperated UDT is unknown.**
- **While cancer risk doubles if orchiopexy is done after age 13 versus before, 69 patients have to be operated before that age to prevent one tumor in males between ages 13 and 55 years.**
- **Surgical reports on orchiopexy rarely state final testicular position or objectively assess testicular size. Based on "intra-scrotal" position, a RCT reported 94 % success with both traditional inguinal and scrotal orchiopexy for palpable UDT.**
- **Meta-analysis found no difference between open versus laparoscopic orchiopexy for nonpalpable testis.**
- **A systematic review found a 5 % benefit to two-stage versus single-stage Fowler-Stephens orchiopexy, but cautioned data quality was poor.**
- **Our review found a single study using a parent questionnaire that reported no difference in satisfaction between inguinal versus scrotal orchiopexy.**
- **Surgeons perform approximately two times more orchiopexies than the rate of UDT, suggesting confusion between UDT versus retractile testes.**

UDT is the most common congenital anomaly affecting boys. Three percent of newborns have an undescended testis, but most subsequently descend within the first few months of life, resulting in a prevalence of approximately 0.8 %.

W.T. Snodgrass, M.D. (✉)
Department of Pediatric Urology, University of Texas Southwestern Medical Center and Children's Medical Center Dallas, 1935 Medical District Drive, MS F4.04, Dallas, TX 75235, USA
e-mail: warren.snodgrass@childrens.com

W.T. Snodgrass (ed.), *Pediatric Urology: Evidence for Optimal Patient Management*, DOI 10.1007/978-1-4614-6910-0_5, © Springer Science+Business Media New York 2013

Prevalence at Birth and Natural History

Of term males, 1.5–3 % have UDT.

Presumably stimulated by the postnatal testosterone surge 50 % or more will descend by 3 months, with greater likelihood for descent in bilateral versus unilateral cases.

Scorer reported observations in 3,222 term males, noting 90 (3 %) had UDT. Descent was specifically defined as mid-testicular position greater than 4 cm from the superior border of the pubic bone with downward traction on the testicle. Of these 90, 45 spontaneously descended during the first month of life into the dependent scrotum 7–8 cm from the pubic bone, and another 22 descended between 6 and 12 weeks of life to 5–6 cm from the pubic bone. The others remained undescended (i.e., <4 cm below the pubic bone), comprising 0.7 % of the total study group (Scorer 1964).

A report from 10,000 consecutive army recruits in the 1940s stated 80 (0.8 %) either had prior surgery for UDT or had one on physical examination (Baumrucker 1946).

A prospective study of 7,032 consecutive males examined at birth and again at 3 months using the same measurements as Scorer reported a total of 270 (3.8 %) had UDT, 179 unilateral and 91 bilateral cases. At 3 months, 59 % of unilateral and 72.5 % of bilateral UDT had descended into the dependent scrotum, $p = 0.0004$, leaving a 1.4 % prevalence of UDT. The authors were uncertain why their rates were higher than those of Scorer earlier, but believed they indicated a true increased prevalence of UDT (John Radcliffe Hospital Cryptorchidism Study Group 1992).

However, another prospective study involving 6,360 term males also using Scorer examinations did not find this apparent increased prevalence, but instead reported very similar results as had Scorer, with 2.2 % of newborns and 0.9 % of 3-month-old males having UDT (Berkowitz et al. 1993).

Finally, another prospective trial examined 6,246 newborn males >34 weeks gestation using Scorer methodology, reporting 95 (1.5 %) had UDT, unilateral in 83 (87 %) and bilateral in 12 (13 %). Repeat examination at 3 months found descent to have occurred in 44 %, leaving unilateral UDT in 94 % and bilateral UDT in 6 %, $p = 0.03$; four considered to descend by 3 months were noted to be reascended at 12 months (Wagner-Mahler et al. 2011).

UDT Prevalence

Unilateral Versus Bilateral

Bilateral UDT occurs in <20 % of cases.

The prospective study of 7,032 consecutive males described above (John Radcliffe Hospital Cryptorchidism Study Group) reported 99 testes remained undescended at 3 months of age, of which 83 (84 %) were unilateral and 16 (16 %) were bilateral.

Similarly, the prospective trial of 6,246 males reported 52 cases with persistent UDT at 3 months of age, unilateral in 94 % and bilateral in 6 % (Wagner-Mahler et al. 2011).

Prospective evaluation of boys referred to surgical specialists for nonscrotal testis reported UDT were unilateral in 90 % and bilateral in 10 % (Snodgrass et al. 2011).

Palpable Versus Nonpalpable

Approximately 75 % of UDT are palpable. Of the remaining nonpalpable testes, the condition is unilateral in 90 % and bilateral in 10 %.

Retrospective review of a clinical series of 1,866 patients operated for UDT reported 447 (24 %) had a nonpalpable testis, unilateral in 89 % and bilateral in 11 % (Kirsch et al. 1998).

Location of the Undescended Testis

Palpable

Most palpable testes are below the external ring, while a minority are between the internal and external rings in the inguinal canal.

A retrospective analysis reported surgical location of 488 palpable UDT: 324 (66 %) were distal to the external ring while 164 (34 %) were canalicular (Cendron et al. 1993).

In a surgical series of 120 consecutive palpable UDT, only 12 (10 %) were within the inguinal canal, while all others were in various positions below the external ring (Bianchi and Squire 1989).

Differences in these two reports likely relate to the surgical approach used to expose the testis. Manipulation of the cord structures through an inguinal incision may pull a testis proximally through the external ring, whereas dissection from below in the scrotum could move a testis distally through the external ring.

Unilateral Nonpalpable

Of *unilateral* nonpalpable testes (comprising 90 % of cases with nonpalpable testes), prenatal testicular loss has occurred in two-thirds. Nearly all of these are represented by a scrotal nubbin.

Of the other third having a viable testis, approximately half are located in the abdomen and the other half are extra-abdominal within the inguinal canal.

Although nonpalpable testes found to be nubbins traditionally have been included in series of UDT, the underlying pathophysiology is different in these cases, as they are presumed to represent intrauterine torsion or other vascular compromise of the testis before or during descent.

Combining two prospective series of consecutive boys with unilateral nonpalpable testes, a total of 83 nonpalpable testes were evaluated. Of these, 53 (64 %) had evidence of prenatal testicular loss, with scrotal nubbins ($n=48$), canalicular nubbins ($n=2$), or intra-abdominal vanished testis without extra-abdominal nubbin ($n=3$). The other 30 (36 %) had a viable testis that was extra-abdominal (despite examination under anesthesia) in 11 (13 %), and intra-abdominal in 19 (23 %) (Snodgrass et al. 2004, 2007).

One-hundred four consecutive males with nonpalpable testes, unilateral in 102 and bilateral in 2, underwent laparoscopy. Testicular loss was diagnosed in 63/104 (60.5 %), an intra-abdominal testis in 23 (22 %), and an inguinal testis in 18 (17 %) (Diamond and Caldamone 1992).

A prospective observational study included 75 patients with unilateral nonpalpable testes who underwent initial laparoscopy, with final diagnosis of testicular loss in 44 (59 %), intra-abdominal testis in 13 (17 %), and extra-abdominal testis in 18 (24 %) (Moore et al. 1994).

Bilateral Nonpalpable

***Bilateral* nonpalpable testes are most often both viable, with approximately half located intra-abdominally and half extra-abdominally.**

Anorchia is found in 5–25 % of patients.

The only prospective study regarding nonpalpable testes that distinguishes unilateral from bilateral cases reported findings in 44 bilateral nonpalpable testes in 22 patients. A viable testis was found in 40/44 testes (91 %), equally likely in the abdomen (20, 48 %) or inguinal canal (19, 45 %). The others sustained prenatal loss. The difference in findings in unilateral (mentioned above) versus bilateral cases was statistically significant (Moore et al. 1994).

Reported findings from surgical series for non-intersex patients with bilateral nonpalpable testes are potentially influenced by preoperative hormonal assessment, which can obviate need for surgical exploration. Anorchia was diagnosed in 5 and 25 % of cases in two series of consecutive patients (Moore et al. 1994; Tennenbaum et al. 1994).

Diagnosis

History and Physical Examination

A positive birth history for UDT greatly increases the likelihood that a boy referred for evaluation has UDT rather than a retractile testis.

Since most UDT are unilateral, visual inspection should precede palpation to detect scrotal asymmetry.

Assessment of the prepubertal boy with unilateral nonpalpable testis should include measurement of the contralateral descended testis for compensatory hypertrophy, which correlates with prenatal testicular loss. Testis length

≥1.8 cm measured with a ruler has a positive predictive value of 90 % that the nonpalpable testis is not viable.

A prospective study of 118 consecutive referrals reported only 50 % had UDT. Boys younger than 1 year of age and those older than 10 years old in puberty were more likely to have a correct diagnosis by PCPs, versus those 1–10 years of age, who were more likely to have retractile testes. UDT was predicted by the following:

- A positive birth history for UDT, OR 21.4 (95 % CI 3.8–120.8).
- Scrotal asymmetry (visual inspection before palpation), OR 121.3 (95 % CI 14.3 to >999).

Only 6 % of referred boys with a negative birth history and visual scrotal symmetry had UDT (Snodgrass et al. 2011).

In patients 7 months to 11 years with unilateral nonpalpable testis, a scrotal testis measuring 1.8 cm or greater in length positively predicts monorchidism in nearly 90 % of cases. One study of 60 boys with unilateral nonpalpable testis reported 14/15 1.8 to 2 cm and 14/16 > 2 cm had monorchidism (Hurwitz and Kaptein 2001).

Another prospective study of boys median age 23 months found 26/30 (87 %) had monorchidism for scrotal testis ≥1.8 cm, versus 8/10 (80 %) having a viable testis when the scrotal testis was <1.8 cm (Snodgrass et al. 2007).

Both performed office measurements using rulers, which may differ from ultrasound measurements of testicular length. There are no published data regarding ultrasound-determined compensatory hypertrophy.

UDT Versus Retractile Testis

Orchiopexy rates are approximately two times the prevalence of UDT.

A regional policy was adopted in a British health trust stating that boys in whom there was any doubt as to normal scrotal position of both testes at 8 months of age were to be referred to surgical specialists for evaluation. When this policy was implemented, the number of orchiopexies decreased by 50 %, with most reduction occurring in school-age boys, when testicular retraction is most common (Brown et al. 2004).

A review of a New York Department of Health database for the years 1984–2002 considered orchiopexy rates determined by the number of operations versus live male births. While surgical rates were stable throughout the study period, the average of 1.4 % operations consistently exceeded the expected 0.8 % prevalence of UDT (Capello et al. 2006).

The John Radcliffe Hospital Cryptorchidism Study Group calculated the orchiopexy rate from the earlier Scorer report and noted surgery was done twice as often as the UDT rate (1.9 % vs. 0.9 %). Their own evaluation of newborns and infants using Scorer's technique found a higher rate of UDT of 1.4 %, but their orchiopexy rate was also higher, at 2.9 % (John Radcliffe Hospital Cryptorchidism Study Group 1960).

Ascending Testes

Secondary ascent of a previously normally descended testis has been proposed to explain higher orchiopexy rates than UDT prevalence.

One prospective study using trained nurses reported testicular ascent in 4 % at 12 months of age. Another prospective study with a single pediatrician performing all examinations reported no testicular ascent at 12 months.

Two studies reported ascending testes were bilateral in over 30 % of cases, versus UDT, which is bilateral in <20 % (see above).

Spontaneous re-descent of ascended testes by mid-puberty was reported by two studies in approximately 60 % of cases.

A prospective study performed by five "trained research nurses" within the Cambridge Baby Growth Study involved longitudinal examinations in newborn males for testicular position. UDT were noted in 6 % at birth, declining to 2 % at age 3 months, but rising to 6.7 % at 12 months from 4 % ascending. Continued exams showed additional new cases of ascending testes, which by 24 months reached 7 % (Acerini et al. 2009).

However, another prospective study involving 6,246 newborns >34 weeks gestation, with examinations by the same pediatrician at birth, 3, and 12 months using Scorer methodology, assigned two controls to each case with UDT. None of 170 controls developed an ascended testis at 12 months (Wagner-Mahler et al. 2011).

Based on a policy of not operating on boys presenting with possible UDT if a normal newborn examination was documented, two studies prospectively evaluated patients diagnosed with ascending testes observed without surgery into puberty.

One reported findings in 557 consecutive patients referred for possible UDT at mean age of 7.4 years (0.3–16.5). Of these, 415 (479 testes) were considered from examination to have UDT, congenital in 116 (129 testes) and acquired (ascending) in 299 (350 testes); 108/350 (31 %) ascended testes were bilateral. There was completed follow-up in 139 patients (164 testes), with spontaneous descent in 98 (60 %) testes; 70 at Tanner stage G2, 26 at Tanner G3-4, and 2 at Tanner 5. Another 32 testes were confirmed to be undescended at ≥Tanner G3 and underwent surgery, while 14 were lost to follow-up and 21 had surgery elsewhere (Sijstermans et al. 2006).

A similar study followed 107 boys (133 testes) with ascended testes. Of these testes, bilateral involvement was diagnosed in 50 (38 %); 75 (57 %) of the testes descended; 3 before puberty, 40 at G2, and 32 at G3-4 (Eijsbouts et al. 2007).

Imaging

Genital US is sometimes used by PCPs to confirm suspicions of UDT before referral to surgical specialists, even though the test does not reliably distinguish between UDT and retractile testes.

Meta-analysis of US for nonpalpable testes reported detection in 97 % extra-abdominal versus 38 % intra-abdominal testes.

MRI was reported by three studies as having 60–85 % accuracy for nonpalpable UDT, with false-negative rates of 8 and 14 %.

Ultrasound

Meta-analysis of 12 studies involving 591 testes reported sensitivity/specificity for US to locate a nonpalpable testis to be 45 % (95 % CI 29–61) and 78 % (95 % CI 43–94), respectively. US detected 97 % of extra-abdominal and 38 % of intra-abdominal viable testes (Tasian and Copp 2011).

Thirty of 118 (25 %) consecutive boys referred in one prospective study had scrotal US ordered by their primary care physician; nonscrotal testes was reported in 29. Physical exam found 15 patients had UDT, while 14 had descended testes (Snodgrass et al. 2011).

MRI for Nonpalpable Testis

MRI was used preoperatively in the evaluation of 47 nonpalpable testes in boys ages 1–12 years, and found to be accurate in 39 (85 %), with a false-negative rate of 4/28 (14 %) and false-positive rate of 4/19 (21 %). All false positives were lymph nodes, and all false-negative testes were found in the inguinal canal at operation. The 24 MRI-identified testes were found "in the inguinal canal or just proximal to the internal ring" (n=19), in the abdomen (n=2), or in the scrotum (n=3) (Kanemoto et al. 2005).

MRI and diffusion-weighted MRI were performed in 36 boys and 38 testes, in which laparoscopy found 19 extra-abdominal, 11 low, and 4 high intra-abdominal testes (<3 cm vs. >3 cm from internal ring), and 4 nubbins. Results were presented from two radiologists, with the combination of the two methods giving overall accuracy in 92 and 86 %. Considering the observer with 92 % accuracy, there were no false positives and 3 (8 %) false-negative assessments, which were not further explained except that one was an intra-abdominal "atrophic" testis (Kantarci et al. 2010).

In a retrospective study in 26 boys with 29 nonpalpable testes, MRI correctly identified 10/12 intra-abdominal testes, 4/6 canalicular testes, 4/10 nubbins, and 0/1 scrotal testis, for an overall accuracy of 62 % (Desireddi et al. 2008).

Diagnosis of Anorchia

Basal LH and FSH levels >3× normal are considered diagnostic for anorchia.

MIS was reported in one study to have 92 %/98 % sensitivity/specificity for anorchia.

Twenty-eight prepubertal boys <11 years of age with bilateral nonpalpable testes had hCG therapy (3,000 u/m^2 BSA injection daily for 5 days, then 2x weekly for 5 weeks); 21 had an "adequate" rise in testosterone, and all had viable testes at exploration, versus 7 with no rise in testosterone, of which 6 had surgery, with none having a viable testis. Six of seven with no testosterone response had baseline LH and FSH >3x normal (Jarow et al. 1986).

Nine patients ranging from 10 months to >12 years with surgically confirmed anorchia had endocrine evaluation preoperatively, including LHRH stimulation in five and hCG stimulation in seven using varied protocols. There was no testosterone response to stimulation. FSH was ≥3x normal in 5/9 (56 %), with variation based on age (Lustig et al. 1987).

One series of 107 consecutive patients with nonpalpable testes reported none of 12 with bilateral nonpalpable testes met their criteria of elevated baseline gonadotrophin levels with negative hCG stimulation testing, although 3 were confirmed surgically to have anorchism (Tennenbaum et al. 1994).

One report compared assays for testosterone secretion versus MIS in 17 boys with anorchia. Diagnostic sensitivity and specificity for MIS was 92 and 98 %, versus 69 and 83 % for testosterone. Mean serum concentration of MIS was 0.8 ± 0.6 ng/mL in boys with anorchia, which was significantly less than the concentration of 48.2 ± 42.1 ng/mL in boys with testes (Lee et al. 1997).

Management

Hormonal Monotherapy

Hormone monotherapy results in complete testicular descent in ≤14 % of UDT.

A meta-analysis was performed using Cochrane Collaboration methodology to determine efficacy of hormonal therapy for UDT:

- Intramuscular hCG versus intranasal GnRH: Data from two RCTs comprising 201 patients reported complete testicular descent was 25 % versus 18 %, absolute risk reduction 7 % (95 % CI 0.012–0.170).
- Intranasal LHRH versus placebo: Nine RCTs with 1,049 boys reported complete testicular descent in 19 % versus 5 %, OR 3.59 (95 % CI 2.52–5.12).

Age of patients at treatment was not stated (Henna et al. 2004).

Adjunctive Hormonal Therapy

One RCT reported that preoperative intranasal GNRH improved the fertility index over orchiopexy alone.

A RCT randomized 42 boys (63 inguinal testes, 21 unilateral and 21 bilateral UDT) with mean age 33.5 months (11–100) to 1.2 mg/day intranasal GNRH for 4 weeks then orchiopexy versus orchiopexy alone. Intraoperative testis biopsies were obtained from UDT, with fertility index calculated by counting the number of adult spermatagonia per tubule in at least 80 tubules. Treated patients had a significantly higher mean fertility index of 1.05 ± 0.71 (0.27–3.33) spermatagonia/tubule versus nontreated with 0.51 ± 0.39 (0–1.17), $p = 0.007$. Considering only the 21 with bilateral UDT, the 9 treated had a mean fertility index of 0.96 ± 0.47 versus 12 untreated with 0.56 ± 0.38 (0–1.12), $p = 0.005$ (Schwentner et al. 2005).

The possibility that hormonal therapy may harm the testis has been proposed. One retrospective study involved patients managed for UDT over a 5-year period, 1985–1990, during which time 19 were given intranasal GHRH then orchiopexy; 8, IM hCG and orchiopexy; and 45, operated without preoperative hormones. Median fertility indexes were 0.07 (0–0.31), 0.06 (0.0025–0.21) and 0.14 (0–0.86), reported as a significant difference between hormonally treated versus only surgery groups. However, the numbers of patients lacking any germ cells was the same in all groups (Cortes et al. 2000). Reasons for hormonal stimulation in some patients and not in others were not stated, nor was the time at which surgery was done after stimulation.

An analysis of testis biopsies taken from the UDT and the descended scrotal testis in 73 patients compared apoptosis of spermatagonia in 43 with preoperative hCG (2 injections/week × 2 weeks, dose per injection: 250 IU if <12 months of age,

500 IU for 1–7 years of age, 1,000 IU if >7 years of age) versus 30 without injection. Effects of hCG were considered for three treated groups, those operated <1 month, at 1–3 months, and at 3–14 months after last injection. Apoptosis was increased in both the scrotal and UDT in treated patients at <1 months, but was similar to untreated patients by >1 month (Heiskanen et al. 1996).

Orchiopexy Timing

Orchiopexy is recommended between ages 6 and 12 months.

One RCT reported UDT had volume less than 50 % of descended testes at 6 months of age, with subsequent growth in those operated versus those not operated.

Current recommendations for surgery between 6 and 12 months are based on the observation that spontaneous descent that occurs after birth does so before 6 months, while decrease in germ cell counts can be diagnosed by 1 year of age (AAP 1996).

A RCT randomized boys with unilateral palpable UDT to orchiopexy at age 9 months versus 3 years, following them with periodic US performed at age <1, 6, 12, and 24 months. From birth to 6 months, scrotal testes increased in volume by 89 % without further increase through age 2 years. UDT also grew from birth through 6 months, but by a significantly less 50 %. Initial and 6-month US demonstrated significantly less volume in UDT versus scrotal testes (median volume at 6 months UDT 0.36 mL vs. scrotal 0.53 mL, $p<0.001$). However, further significant growth of the operated UDT was observed by 2 years (0.36–0.47 mL, $p<0.001$); this was not seen in the non-operated UDT (Kollin et al. 2007).

Palpable Testes

Traditional orchiopexy includes an inguinal incision to mobilize the testis and ligate an associated patent processus vaginalis and a separate scrotal incision for testis placement.

Observations that up to 90 % of palpable testes have exited the external ring support single-incision orchiopexy through the scrotum as an alternative. Additional inguinal incision to obtain greater spermatic cord length is reported in 0–4 % of cases.

Single upper scrotal incision was used in 104 consecutive boys aged 2–12 years with 120 palpable UDT. Scrotal orchiopexy resulted in a mid- to lower scrotal position in 111 testes, and a testis in the mid- to upper scrotum in 4. The other 5 required an additional inguinal incision to gain sufficient vascular length for orchiopexy. All testes were described as viable, without specific mention of atrophy with follow-up at 6 months to 3 years (mean not stated) (Bianchi and Squire 1989).

A prospective study analyzed single scrotal incision orchiopexy in 114 consecutive patients with 148 palpable UDT, accomplished in all cases without need for additional inguinal incision. With mean follow-up of 10 months (3–22), all were described as palpable within the scrotum, without specific mention of either atrophy or low versus high scrotal position (Callewaert et al. 2010).

A RCT assigned 292 children mean age 40 ±10 months with 398 palpable UDT to either scrotal or inguinal orchiopexy between 2007 and 2010. Surgical success at 12 months was defined as "intrascrotal testis." With follow-up in 107 children (146 testes) after scrotal orchiopexy and 105 children (141 testes) after inguinal orchiopexy, there was no difference in overall success: 135/146 (92 %) versus 136/141 (96 %). Nine of 201 (4 %) scrotal orchiopexies additionally required inguinal incision (Na et al. 2011).

Nonpalpable Testes

Since exploration for nonpalpable testes can find nubbins, extra-abdominal viable testes, or intra-abdominal viable testes, several management options are available, and approach can be tailored by likely findings in specific cases (Fig. 5.1):

1. **Unilateral nonpalpable testes with a contralateral scrotal testis measuring ≥1.8 cm have a 90 % probability of prenatal testis**

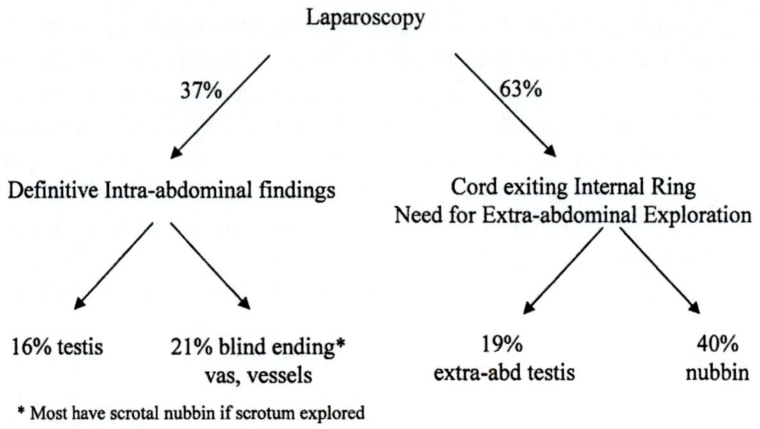

Fig. 5.1 Unilateral non-palpable testis. Findings if laparoscopy performed first. Created with data from (Moore et al. 1994; Diamond and Caldamone 1992)

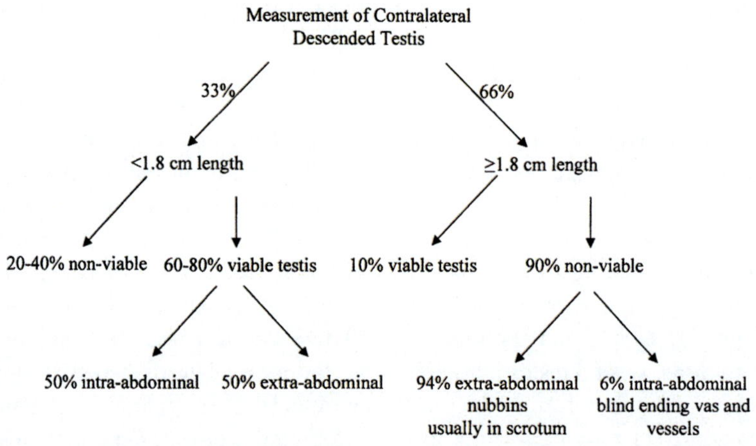

Fig. 5.2 Unilateral non-palpable testis. Findings are based on the length of the descended testis. Data from (Hurwitz and Kaptein 2001; Snodgrass et al. 2007)

loss, with a nubbin found in the scrotum in nearly all cases. Therefore, a scrotal incision can be made initially, reserving laparoscopy for the few without a nubbin (or testis) in the scrotum or inguinal canal (Fig. 5.2).

As discussed above, testicular length ≥1.8 cm in the contralateral descended testis has a 90 % predictive value that prenatal testicular loss has occurred. Patients with nubbins had contralateral testicular length a mean of 2.0±0.56 cm, which was significantly longer than those with a viable testis, whose contralateral testicular length was 1.69±0.09 cm (Hurwitz and Kaptein 2001; Snodgrass et al. 2007).

A prospective observational study in which consecutive patients with unilateral nonpalpable UDT underwent scrotal exploration first followed by laparoscopy reported testicular absence in 23 boys having a scrotal nubbin in 22 and blind ending vas and vessels at the internal ring without a nubbin in the other. Of the 22 scrotal nubbins, six had blind ending vas and vessels at or above the internal ring at laparoscopy, indicating that this finding more often represents the proximal extension of torsion after the testis reaches the scrotum rather than an intra-abdominal event (Snodgrass et al. 2004).

2. **Unilateral nonpalpable testes with a contralateral scrotal testis measuring <1.8 cm most often have a viable testis with an equal likelihood to be found extra- versus intra-abdominally.**

Preoperative ultrasound can detect the extra-abdominal testes, which are then approached either by inguinal or scrotal incision, as with palpable testes. Without preoperative imaging, scrotal or inguinal incision versus laparoscopy is an option.

Bilateral nonpalpable testes most often are found to have two viable testes. Preoperative ultrasound can be used to detect those that are extra-abdominal, or inguinal incision versus laparoscopy can be done.

Inguinal incision provides exposure to identify scrotal nubbins and extra-abdominal testes, and after opening the internal ring and peritoneum allows intra-abdominal inspection and orchiopexy. A retrospective series of 447 nonpalpable testes reported 181 (40 %) were nubbins or vanished, 175 (40 %) were extra-abdominal, and only 91 (20 %) intra-abdominal. All were managed inguinally, with 33 standard, 38 one-stage Fowler-Stephens, and 4 two-stage orchiopexies. Postoperative follow-up in 76 of the 91 intra-abdominal cases found 55 (72 %) described as having a "good sized" testis in the mid- to low scrotum versus 9 (12 %) in the upper scrotum and another 12 (16 %) with atrophy, including 26 % of those with Fowler-Stephens orchiopexy (Kirsch et al. 1998).

A prospective analysis of initial laparoscopy in 104 boys with 126 nonpalpable testes reported only 33 (26 %) intra-abdominal testes and 8 (5 %) blind ending vas and vessels. Others had vas and vessels exiting the internal ring associated with a patent processus vaginalis in 26 of 75 cases, comprising 19/38 (50 %) with an extra-abdominal testis (meaning the others had a closed internal ring with an extra-abdominal testis) and 7/37 (19 %) with an extra-abdominal nubbin. In 75 cases, there were vas and vessels exiting the internal ring, leading to an extra-abdominal testis in 38. The authors stated that "in most cases" those without a viable extra-abdominal testis had "attenuated" vas and vessels (Moore et al. 1994).

Retrospective review was done for results of laparoscopy in 111 boys with 124 nonpalpable testes, reporting that status of the internal ring correlated with findings of viable testis versus nubbin in those without an intra-abdominal testis. In this series, there were 38 intra-abdominal testes, 7 extra-abdominal testes, and 77 absent/vanished testes. Six extra-abdominal testes had a widely patent processus vaginalis that allowed them to be manipulated back into the abdomen for laparoscopic orchiopexy, whereas in one, "no hernia was visualized" but at inguinal exploration a viable testis with "a small patent processus vaginalis" was encountered (Elder 1994).

From these data, if neither an intra-abdominal testis nor blind ending vas and vessels were found on laparoscopy, extra-abdominal exploration would be mandated, since neither examination under anesthesia nor presence or absence of a patent processus vaginalis (open vs. closed internal ring) predicted whether or not a testis would be found. The possible exception would be those with "attenuated" vessels who might not need further extra-abdominal exploration, but our review did not find objective criteria for this determination.

No RCT evaluates inguinal exploration versus laparoscopy. The primary disadvantage of laparoscopy arises when neither a testis nor blind ending structures are encountered, as extra-abdominal exploration is still needed. Considering all patients undergoing initial laparoscopy in the prospective trial by Moore et al., only 32.5 % had either an intra-abdominal testis or blind ending vas and vessels, meaning the remainder needed extra-abdominal assessment. Whether or not a hernia sac extended through the internal ring did not predict whether an extra-abdominal viable testis or nubbin would be found, as 50 % of the testes had a closed internal ring, while 20 % of the nubbins had an open sac (Moore et al. 1994).

Extra-abdominal exploration after laparoscopy traditionally is done using an inguinal incision, followed by a scrotal incision if a testis is found. Alternatively, a scrotal incision can be used to remove a nubbin or to perform orchiopexy, without an inguinal incision.

Intra-abdominal Orchiopexy

Best management when there is insufficient vascular length to deliver the intra-abdominal testis into the scrotum—staged ochiopexy preserving the spermatic cord vessels versus one- or two-stage Fowler-Stephens orchiopexy—cannot be determined from available data.

A summary of reported orchiopexies included 248 intra-abdominal testes treated with two-stage orchiopexy preserving the spermatic cord vessels, of which 73 % were considered by the various authors to be successful. Success for one-stage Fowler-Stephens orchiopexy was reported as 63 % versus success for two-stage Fowler-Stephens of 77 %. This difference was not considered statistically significant (Docimo 1995).

To date no RCT compares one-stage versus two-stage orchiopexy with spermatic cord division.

No data were found regarding simultaneous bilateral one- or two-stage Fowler-Stephens orchiopexy.

Outcomes

Surgical Success

Surgical success is usually defined as "scrotal position without atrophy," with few articles reporting actual scrotal position (high, mid, low) or objective measurement of testicular size.

One review of series published before 1995 reported surgical success of 89 % for extra-abdominal and 74.5 % for intra-abdominal testes. Fowler-Stephens orchiopexy success was 67 %, while staged orchiopexy without vessel division was 72.5 %.

No RCT compares intra-abdominal orchiopexy with versus without vessel division, or one-stage versus two-stage Fowler-Stephens procedures.

Review of published literature identified 64 articles with 8,425 UDT with data that could be evaluated to determine surgical success, defined as "scrotal position and absence of atrophy." Of patients with postoperative evaluations ≥6 months, 420/564 (74.5 %) intra-abdominal testes and 1,000/1,126 (89 %) extra-abdominal testes had surgical success. Fowler-Stephens orchiopexy had overall surgical success in 214/321(67 %), with no difference reportedly found in staged (43/56 [77 %]) versus single-stage (data not shown) procedures. Two-stage orchiopexy without vessel division had surgical success in 180/248 (72.5 %) (Docimo 1995).

The RCT by Na et al. described above comparing inguinal versus scrotal orchiopexy for palpable UDT reported success as an intrascrotal testis achieved in 271/287 (94 %) testes, with no difference by technique used.

Meta-analysis compared open versus laparoscopic abdominal orchiopexy using data obtained from two RCTs and five case series totaling 263 and 176 cases, reporting no differences in:

- Testicular retraction, OR 0.6 (95 % CI 0.13–2.72).
- Viable testis, OR 1.61 (95 % CI 0.30–8.52).
- Testicular atrophy, OR 1.70 (95 % CI 0.49–5.98) (Guo et al. 2011).

A systematic review was done comparing single- versus two-stage Fowler-Stephens orchiopexy, with nine articles for single-stage, 36 for two-stage, and 16 including both. Pooled estimated success rates were 80 % (95 % CI 75–86) for single-stage versus 85 % (95 % CI 81–90) for two-stage orchiopexy, with no differences as to whether orchiopexy was laparoscopic or open. Despite the apparent increased success for two-stage orchiopexy, quality of the data from which the observations were made was low (Elyas et al. 2010).

Cosmetic Results

One study reported parents equally satisfied with cosmetic results of inguinal versus scrotal orchiopexy.

The RCT by Na et al. described above comparing inguinal versus scrotal orchiopexy included a parent questionnaire with response options of "satisfied," "not fully satisfied," or "not satisfied" (questionnaire not shown) regarding cosmetic results. No parent was "not satisfied," and only 3 % were "not fully satisfied," with no difference in response based on surgical procedure.

Reoperative Orchiopexy

Two retrospective studies reported outcomes of reoperative orchiopexy via scrotal incision for testicular retraction after prior orchiopexy or hernia repair. Only one (3 %) boy had second testicular retraction, and there was no atrophy.

A retrospective review of operated patients from 2005 to 2009 reported 17/687 (2.5 %) UDT reascended after orchiopexy, of which eight found distal to the external ring were included for study. In another two cases, a testis ascended following inguinal hernia/hydrocele repairs. Three additional patients failed orchiopexy elsewhere, and three had ascent of a testis after hernia surgery elsewhere, giving a total of 16 reoperative orchiopexies all for testes distal to the external ring and approached by scrotal incision. One required additional inguinal incision and "wide preperitoneal" dissection to gain adequate cord length. At mean follow-up of 12 months (3–36), all were reported to have normal scrotal position and no atrophy on physical exam (Karaman et al. 2010).

Retrospective review reported 24 patients mean age 6 years (1–16) undergoing 27 orchiopexies after prior hernia ($n=13$) or orchiopexy ($n=6$). Scrotal incision was used if it "could be manipulated near or over the testis," comprising 24/27 (89 %). At mean follow-up of 12 months in 20 of the 21 patients with scrotal surgery, one testis was high and none were atrophic (Dudley et al. 2011).

One retrospective study reported outcomes in 32 reoperations for UDT (15 high scrotum, eight at external ring, and nine in the inguinal canal). Two inguinal testicles were only able to be brought down into the high scrotum, and one patient underwent orchidectomy. Overall, after a mean follow-up period of four (1–7) years following the second operation, 29 (93.5 %) testes were scrotal without evidence of atrophy (Ziylan et al. 2004).

Another retrospective study reported outcomes in 35 patients with recurrent UDT after failed inguinal orchiopexy. Ten inguinal testes were treated directly with open inguinal redo orchidopexy. Laparoscopy-assisted orchiopexy was attempted in the remaining 25 based on an impalpable testis or need for additional vascular length. In two (8 %) of these cases, scarring was present between the cord and the inguinal canal, impeding the laparoscopy approach. After a mean follow-up of 22 months (6–32), all 33 testicles were within the scrotum. Atrophy (not defined) was reported in four (11 %) patients (two with laparoscopy, two after the inguinal procedure) (Tong et al. 2009).

Cancer Risk

The overall risk that a previously operated UDT will develop a germ cell tumor is less than 0.5 %.

Nonoperated UDT are more likely to develop seminoma, whereas tumors developing after orchiopexy are more likely nonseminomas.

It is unclear if orchiopexy performed before puberty is protective against cancer development.

There is a theoretic risk for cancer to develop in nubbins, since germ cells are found in ≤10 %, but no case has been reported.

The overall risk for a germ cell tumor associated with UDT was characterized by a study of 16,983 men surgically treated for UDT and then followed for a mean of 12±7 years (209,984 man-years), during which time only 56 (0.3 %) developed a germ cell tumor (Pettersson et al. 2007).

Meta-analysis of seven reported series found seminomas developed in 74 % of 121 nonoperated UDTs that developed germ cell tumors versus 37 % of 247 previously UDTs repositioned into the scrotum that developed tumors; the others were nonseminomas (Wood and Elder 2009).

Two studies conclude orchiopexy performed before puberty is protective against tumor development:

- In 56 cases of testis cancer in former UDTs, the relative risk was 2.23 (95 % CI: 1.58–3.06) when surgery was performed before age 13 years, versus 5.40 (95 % CI: 3.20–8.53) when surgery was done after 13 years. Sixty-nine patients had to undergo orchiopexy before age 13 to prevent one malignancy between ages 13 and 55 years (Pettersson et al. 2007).

- The other report was a meta-analysis of five studies with 80 germ cell malignancies associated with UDTs. Although the authors stated prepubertal orchiopexy was protective, their finding that surgery after approximately age 11 years was three times more likely to be associated with cancer than when surgery was performed earlier was not statistically significant (OR 3.4 95 % CI 0.7–17.7) (Walsh et al. 2007).

Nubbins are found to have germ cell elements in <10 % of cases. A single case found intratubular germ cell neoplasia (Rozanski et al. 1996), but no overt malignancies have been reported arising from a nubbin.

Fertility

Paternity rates for men with previously operated unilateral UDT are considered similar to those of men born with normal testes.

Paternity rates in those with formerly bilateral UDTs are less than in normal men.

Two articles report successful sperm retrieval in >60 % men with prior UDT, similar in one to infertile men without prior UDT.

Paternity data was obtained in 40 men who underwent orchiopexy with testis biopsy between 1950 and 1960. Of 20 men with prior unilateral orchiopexy who attempted to have children, 87 % reported success, versus 33 % of nine men with prior bilateral orchiopexy. Sperm counts were obtained in 16 men, with 75 % having $<20 \times 10^6$ sperm; findings did not predict reported paternity (Cendron et al. 1989).

Questionnaires were distributed to patients (numbers not stated) undergoing orchiopexy or other minor surgery (controls) between 1955 and 1969 at Children's Hospital of Pittsburg, reporting responses from 363 men with former UDTs (313 unilateral and 50 bilateral) and 336 controls. There was no difference in paternity reported by patients formerly with unilateral UDT versus controls (90.2 and 93.1 %, respectively), but there was significantly less paternity after bilateral orchiopexy (64.5 %) (Lee et al. 1995).

Several publications emphasize histological appearance of seminiferous tubules obtained by biopsy during orchiopexy. While a detailed discussion of potential fertility is beyond the scope of this review, it may be noteworthy that two recent reports concern sperm retrieval in men previously undergoing orchiopexy, with successful results in over 60 % of cases despite azoospermia on semen specimens (Wiser et al. 2009); (Haimov-Kochman et al. 2010). Prior orchiopexy at age <10 years versus later did not impact results (Wiser et al. 2009). Success in men after orchiopexy was the same as in other men undergoing sperm retrieval without a history of UDT (Haimov-Kochman et al. 2010).

References

AAP. Timing of elective surgery on the genitalia of male children with particular reference to the risks, benefits, and psychological effects of surgery and anesthesia. Pediatrics. 1996;97(4):590–4.

Acerini CL, Miles HL, Dunger DB, Ong KK, Hughes IA. The descriptive epidemiology of congenital and acquired cryptorchidism in a UK infant cohort. Arch Dis Child. 2009;94(11):868–72.

Baumrucker GO. Incidence of testicular pathology. Bull U S Army Med Dep. 1946;5:312–4.

Berkowitz GS, Lapinski RH, Dolgin SE, Gazella JG, Bodian CA, Holzman IR. Prevalence and natural history of cryptorchidism. Pediatrics. 1993;92(1):44–9.

Bianchi A, Squire BR. Transscrotal orchidopexy: orchidopexy revised. Pediatr Surg Int. 1989;4:189–92.

Brown JJ, Wacogne I, Fleckney S, Jones L, Ni Bhrolchain C. Achieving early surgery for undescended testes: quality improvement through a multifaceted approach to guideline implementation. Child Care Health Dev. 2004;30(2):97–102.

Callewaert PR, Rahnama'i MS, Biallosterski BT, van Kerrebroeck PE. Scrotal approach to both palpable and impalpable undescended testes: should it become our first choice? Urology. 2010;76(1):73–6.

Capello SA, Giorgi Jr LJ, Kogan BA. Orchiopexy practice patterns in New York State from 1984 to 2002. J Urol. 2006;176(3):1180–3.

Cendron M, Keating MA, Huff DS, Koop CE, Snyder 3rd HM, Duckett JW. Cryptorchidism, orchiopexy and infertility: a critical long-term retrospective analysis. J Urol. 1989;142(2 Pt 2):559–62. discussion 72.

Cendron M, Huff DS, Keating MA, Snyder 3rd HM, Duckett JW. Anatomical, morphological and volumetric analysis: a review of 759 cases of testicular maldescent. J Urol. 1993;149(3):570–3.

Cortes D, Thorup J, Visfeldt J. Hormonal treatment may harm the germ cells in 1 to 3-year-old boys with cryptorchidism. J Urol. 2000;163(4):1290–2.

John Radcliffe Hospital Cryptorchidism Study Group. Cryptorchidism: a prospective study of 7500 consecutive male births, 1984–8. Arch Dis Child. 1992;67(7):892–9.

Desireddi NV, Liu DB, Maizels M, Rigsby C, Casey JT, Cheng EY. Magnetic resonance arteriography/venography is not accurate to structure management of the impalpable testis. J Urol. 2008;180(4 Suppl):1805–8. discussion 8–9.

Diamond DA, Caldamone AA. The value of laparoscopy for 106 impalpable testes relative to clinical presentation. J Urol. 1992;148(2 Pt 2):632–4.

Docimo SG. The results of surgical therapy for cryptorchidism: a literature review and analysis. J Urol. 1995;154(3):1148–52.

Dudley AG, Sweeney DD, Docimo SG. Orchiopexy after prior inguinal surgery: a distal approach. J Urol. 2011;185(6):2340–3.

Eijsbouts SW, de Muinck Keizer-Schrama SM, Hazebroek FW. Further evidence for spontaneous descent of acquired undescended testes. J Urol. 2007;178(4 Pt 2):1726–9.

Elder JS. Laparoscopy for impalpable testes: significance of the patent processus vaginalis. J Urol. 1994;152(2 Pt 2):776–8.

Elyas R, Guerra LA, Pike J, DeCarli C, Betolli M, Bass J, et al. Is staging beneficial for Fowler-Stephens orchiopexy? A systematic review. J Urol. 2010;183(5): 2012–8.

Guo J, Liang Z, Zhang H, Yang C, Pu J, Mei H, et al. Laparoscopic versus open orchiopexy for non-palpable undescended testes in children: a systemic review and meta-analysis. Pediatr Surg Int. 2011;27(9):943–52.

Heiskanen P, Billig H, Toppari J, Kaleva M, Arsalo A, Rapola J, et al. Apoptotic cell death in the normal and cryptorchid human testis: the effect of human chorionic gonadotropin on testicular cell survival. Pediatr Res. 1996;40(2):351–6.

Haimov-Kochman R, Prus D, Farchat M, Bdolah Y, Hurwitz A. Reproductive outcome of men with azoospermia due to cryptorchidism using assisted techniques. Int J Androl. 2010, 33(1):e139–43.

Henna MR, Del Nero RG, Sampaio CZ, Atallah AN, Schettini ST, Castro AA, et al. Hormonal cryptorchidism therapy: systematic review with metanalysis of randomized clinical trials. Pediatr Surg Int. 2004;20(5): 357–9.

Hurwitz RS, Kaptein JS. How well does contralateral testis hypertrophy predict the absence of the nonpalpable testis? J Urol. 2001;165(2):588–92.

Jarow JP, Berkovitz GD, Migeon CJ, Gearhart JP, Walsh PC. Elevation of serum gonadotropins establishes the diagnosis of anorchism in prepubertal boys with bilateral cryptorchidism. J Urol. 1986;136(1 Pt 2):277–9.

John Radcliffe Hospital Cryptorchidism Study Group. Cryptorchidism: an apparent substantial increase since 1960. Br Med J (Clinical research ed.) 1986;293(6559):1401–4.

Kanemoto K, Hayashi Y, Kojima Y, Maruyama T, Ito M, Kohri K. Accuracy of ultrasonography and magnetic resonance imaging in the diagnosis of non-palpable testis. Int J Urol. 2005;12(7):668–72.

Kantarci M, Doganay S, Yalcin A, Aksoy Y, Yilmaz-Cankaya B, Salman B. Diagnostic performance of diffusion-weighted MRI in the detection of nonpalpable undescended testes: comparison with conventional MRI and surgical findings. AJR Am J Roentgenol. 2010;195(4):W268–73.

Karaman I, Karaman A, Erdogan D, Cavusoglu YH. The transscrotal approach for recurrent and iatrogenic undescended testes. Eur J Pediatr Surg. 2010;20(4):267–9.

Kirsch AJ, Escala J, Duckett JW, Smith GH, Zderic SA, Canning DA, et al. Surgical management of the nonpalpable testis: the Children's Hospital of Philadelphia experience. J Urol. 1998;159(4):1340–3.

Kollin C, Karpe B, Hesser U, Granholm T, Ritzen EM. Surgical treatment of unilaterally undescended testes: testicular growth after randomization to orchiopexy at age 9 months or 3 years. J Urol. 2007;178(4 Pt 2):1589–93. discussion 93.

Lee PA, O'Leary LA, Songer NJ, Bellinger MF, LaPorte RE. Paternity after cryptorchidism: lack of correlation with age at orchidopexy. Br J Urol. 1995;75(6):704–7.

Lee MM, Donahoe PK, Silverman BL, Hasegawa T, Hasegawa Y, Gustafson ML, et al. Measurements of serum mullerian inhibiting substance in the evaluation of children with nonpalpable gonads. N Engl J Med. 1997;336(21):1480–6.

Lustig RH, Conte FA, Kogan BA, Grumbach MM. Ontogeny of gonadotropin secretion in congenital anorchism: sexual dimorphism versus syndrome of gonadal dysgenesis and diagnostic considerations. J Urol. 1987;138(3):587–91.

Moore RG, Peters CA, Bauer SB, Mandell J, Retik AB. Laparoscopic evaluation of the nonpalpable tests: a prospective assessment of accuracy. J Urol. 1994; 151(3):728–31.

Na SW, Kim SO, Hwang EC, Oh KJ, Jeong SI, Kang TW, et al. Single scrotal incision orchiopexy for children with palpable low-lying undescended testis: early outcome of a prospective randomized controlled study. Korean J Urol. 2011;52(9):637–41.

Pettersson A, Richiardi L, Nordenskjold A, Kaijser M, Akre O. Age at surgery for undescended testis and risk of testicular cancer. N Engl J Med. 2007;356(18): 1835–41.

Rozanski TA, Wojno KJ, Bloom DA. The remnant orchiectomy. J Urol. 1996;155(2):712–3. discussion 4.

Schwentner C, Oswald J, Kreczy A, Lunacek A, Bartsch G, Deibl M, et al. Neoadjuvant gonadotropin-releasing hormone therapy before surgery may improve the fertility index in undescended testes: a prospective randomized trial. J Urol. 2005;173(3):974–7.

Scorer CG. The descent of the testis. Arch Dis Child. 1964;39:605–9.

Sijstermans K, Hack WW, van der Voort-Doedens LM, Meijer RW, Haasnoot K. Puberty stage and spontaneous descent of acquired undescended testis: implications for therapy? Int J Androl. 2006;29(6):597–602.

Snodgrass W, Chen K, Harrison C. Initial scrotal incision for unilateral nonpalpable testis. J Urol. 2004;172(4 Pt 2):1742–5. discussion 5.

Snodgrass WT, Yucel S, Ziada A. Scrotal exploration for unilateral nonpalpable testis. J Urol. 2007;178(4 Pt 2): 1718–21.

Snodgrass W, Bush N, Holzer M, Zhang S. Current referral patterns and means to improve accuracy in diagnosis of undescended testis. Pediatrics. 2011;127(2):e382–8.

Tasian GE, Copp HL. Diagnostic performance of ultrasound in nonpalpable cryptorchidism: a systematic review and meta-analysis. Pediatrics. 2011;127(1): 119–28.

Tasian GE, Copp HL, Baskin LS. Diagnostic imaging in cryptorchidism: utility, indications, and effectiveness. J Pediatr Surg. 2011;46(12):2406–13.

Tennenbaum SY, Lerner SE, McAleer IM, Packer MG, Scherz HC, Kaplan GW. Preoperative laparoscopic localization of the nonpalpable testis: a critical analysis of a 10-year experience. J Urol. 1994;151(3): 732–4.

Tong Q, Zheng L, Tang S, Mao Y, Wang Y, Liu Y, et al. Laparoscopy-assisted orchiopexy for recurrent undescended testes in children. J Pediatr Surg. 2009;44(4): 806–10.

Wagner-Mahler K, Kurzenne JY, Delattre I, Berard E, Mas JC, Bornebush L, et al. Prospective study on the prevalence and associated risk factors of cryptorchidism in 6246 newborn boys from Nice area, France. Int J Androl. 2011;34(5 Pt 2):e499–510.

Walsh TJ, Dall'Era MA, Croughan MS, Carroll PR, Turek PJ. Prepubertal orchiopexy for cryptorchidism may be associated with lower risk of testicular cancer. J Urol. 2007;178(4 Pt 1):1440–6. discussion 6.

Wiser A, Raviv G, Weissenberg R, Elizur SE, Levron J, Machtinger R, et al. Does age at orchidopexy impact on the results of testicular sperm extraction? Reprod Biomed Online. 2009;19(6):778–83.

Wood HM, Elder JS. Cryptorchidism and testicular cancer: separating fact from fiction. J Urol. 2009;181(2):452–61.

Ziylan O, Oktar T, Korgali E, Nane I, Ander H. Failed orchiopexy. Urol Int. 2004;73(4):313–5.

Hernias and Hydroceles

6

Micah A. Jacobs

The primary reason to operate on hernias is to prevent bowel incarceration.

Secondary aims of surgery:

1. **Avoid recurrent hernia.**
2. **Decrease metachronous hernia.**
3. **Treat bother associated with the hernia.**

Summary of evidence for these aims:

- **Incarceration was reported by one case series in 12 % of patients, decreasing with age from 39 % in preterm neonates to 6 % in teenagers.**
- **Bowel resection for necrosis is rare, occurring in <1 % of incarcerated hernias.**
- **One prospective longitudinal study reported 84 % of newborn communicating hydroceles resolved by 18 months of age.**
- **Two studies reported 0 and 5 % of communicating hydroceles observed in children <2 years of age developed hernias, none with incarceration.**
- **Recurrent hernia occurs in ≤4 %, with meta-analysis finding no difference in open versus laparoscopic repair.**
- **Meta-analysis of unilateral open repair found metachronous hernia in 7 %, not predicted by age <2 years versus older, or gender, although left hernias had higher risk.**
- **Meta-analysis of laparoscopic versus open repair reported significant reduction in metachronous hernia with laparoscopic surgery.**
- **Our review found no data regarding bother of untreated hydroceles or hernias in children.**

M.A. Jacobs, M.D., M.P.H. (✉)
Department of Pediatric Urology, University of Texas Southwestern Medical Center and Children's Medical Center Dallas, 1935 Medical District Drive, MS F4.04, Dallas, TX 75235, USA
e-mail: micah.jacobs@childrens.com

Definitions

Hydrocele: Fluid distending the tunica vaginalis.

Communicating hydrocele: A patent processus vaginalis allows fluid to intermittently distend the tunica vaginalis.

Hernia: Intestinal contents (bowel, omentum, bladder) enter a patent processus vaginalis.

Incarcerated hernia: Intestinal contents become entrapped within the processus vaginalis.

Prevalence

One analysis of consecutive newborn males undergoing circumcision reported hydrocele in 6 %, with approximately half communicating.

Similar data were not found for prevalence of hernia in newborns; review articles cite ≤5 % in full-term and ≤10 % in preterm newborns.

No data were found for prevalence of hydrocele/hernia in older children.

W.T. Snodgrass (ed.), *Pediatric Urology: Evidence for Optimal Patient Management*,
DOI 10.1007/978-1-4614-6910-0_6, © Springer Science+Business Media New York 2013

A prospective determination of the prevalence of communicating hydrocele was made during 2002 and 2006 among 2,715 consecutive neonates, mean age 8 ± 4 days, presenting to a university hospital in Nigeria for circumcision. Of these, 158 (6 %) had 190 hydroceles. Repair was done in 25 patients and 27 hydroceles due to "parental anxiety"; the remaining 163 hydroceles were further characterized as communicating in 75 (46 %) and non-communicating in 88 (54 %). These 163 hydroceles were bilateral in 69 %, right in 12 %, and left in 19 %. Of the patients, 28 % were preterm (Osifo and Osaigbovo 2008).

Our review found no cross-sectional analysis of consecutive premature and full- term newborns to determine prevalence of hernia. Review articles quote 3.5–5 % prevalence in full-term newborns and 9–11 % in preterm infants (Grosfeld 1989).

No data were found for hydrocele/hernia prevalence in older children.

Natural History

Hydroceles

Most newborn hydroceles, communicating or not, close spontaneously by 18–24 months, with 0 to <5 % developing a hernia (two studies).

There are no data regarding observation for communicating hydroceles in patients >2 years of age.

In the prospective study of newborn males undergoing circumcision mentioned above, one pediatric urologist performed monthly examinations and took photographs of those diagnosed with hydrocele for 2 years. Spontaneous resolution occurred in 135 (83 %), with most resolving by 6 months and none after 18 months. There was no difference in resolution among preterm versus term boys, or communicating versus non-communicating hydroceles (63/75 [84 %] communicating hydroceles resolved). Of the 27 persisting at 2 years (1 lost to follow-up) progressive enlargement was documented in 13, while the other 14 remained stable. No patient developed a clinical hernia, although two "found to have a hernia" were excluded from analysis (Osifo and Osaigbovo 2008).

A retrospective review of 110 infants presenting with communicating hydrocele at <18 months of age and initially observed reported 69 (63 %) resolved spontaneously in a mean of 9 (2–55) months. Only six developed a hernia during observation, none with incarceration, and of those that apparently resolved, only two recurred. The remainder underwent surgery after mean observation of 9 months and at a mean age of 14 months for hernia, persistent communicating hydrocele after age 1 year and/or for increasing size of the hydrocele. Age at presentation and history of prematurity <37 weeks did not influence likelihood for resolution. Based on findings, the authors changed their practice to include observation until ≥2 years of age before surgical intervention (Koski et al. 2010).

Another retrospective review concerned 302 boys >1 year of age (mean 4, median 3, range 1–18) presenting as outpatients with new-onset hydrocele from 1994 to 2002. Of these, 35 % were non-communicating, 59 % communicating, and 6 % cord hydroceles. Repair was done in all but five (3 %) of the communicating hydroceles, and three of these resolved; surgery was done in 35 % of non-communicating hydroceles either at diagnosis or after a median of 8.5 months observation. Of the remaining 70 non-communicating hydroceles, 19 were lost to follow-up and 51 were observed, with resolution reported by phone ($n = 41$) or follow-up exam ($n = 8$) in 39/49 (80 %) at a mean of 6 months. Of 17 cord hydroceles, 5 were observed and 3 resolved (interval not stated) (Christensen et al. 2006).

Hernias

There are no long-term observational studies of hernias.

The overall incidence of incarceration in hernias is ≤12 %, and is greater in premies and infants than in older children or teens.

Bowel resection in patients with incarceration was reported in two case series in ≤0.2 %.

The long-term clinical course of non-operated hernias is unknown, since no longitudinal observation studies have been reported.

A retrospective analysis of 6,361 children with hernias operated by a single surgeon over a 35-year period ending in 2004 reported incarceration occurred overall in 12 %. Incidence was 39 % of 191 premies <36 weeks and 6 % in 143 teens aged 13–18 years. Of a total of 743 incarcerated hernias, only 8 % could not be reduced preoperatively, only 0.1 % presented with bowel obstruction, and only two patients needed simultaneous bowel resection (Ein et al. 2006).

Another retrospective review specifically comprised premature infants (gestational age <37 weeks) undergoing hernia repair during a 2-year period from 2006 to 2008. There were 172 patients, 81 % males, with mean gestational age 30.7 ± 3.9 weeks and birth weight 1,428 ± 713 g. Of these, 80 (47 %) were diagnosed in the NICU; 45 were repaired before discharge and 35 electively after discharge at the discretion of the surgeon, while the remainder were diagnosed and operated after NICU discharge. Duration of observation between diagnosis and surgery for those discharged from NICU with a known hernia or diagnosed after discharge was not stated. In the entire series, incarceration occurred in only eight (5 %), with all successfully reduced without sedation and none progressing to bowel infarction. Of these eight, five occurred before discharge from NICU and the other three had incarceration at initial presentation (Lee et al. 2011).

A retrospective study reviewed a Canadian Institute of Health database to compare risk for incarceration based on waiting time from diagnosis of hernia to elective surgery during the year 2002–2003. The overall rate of incarceration was 12 % in 1,065 patients during a median wait time of 35 days (interquartile range 17–77 days). Those operated within a median 14 days had a significantly lower incarceration rate of 5 % versus 10 % for median wait time of ≤35 days ($p < 0.001$). Additionally, patients <1 year of age had RR 1.75 (95 % CI 1.04–2.93) for incarceration versus those 1–2 years of age, as did girls versus boys, RR 2.07 (95 % CI 1.32–3.23) (Zamakhshary et al. 2008).

Testicular Atrophy, Vasal Injury

Testicular atrophy and/or vasal injury is reported in <1 % of cases, without association to preterm versus full-term birth, age at surgery, or incarceration.

A prospective study used testicular ultrasound preoperatively and then at <48 h and 6 months following laparoscopic hernia repair to assess volume and blood flow (resistive index) in 100 boys mean age 4 years with 125 hernias. Of these, five presented with incarceration and were reduced with elective repair after 2 days. All testes showed consistent blood flow, and there was no difference in mean testicular volume between preoperative and last postoperative scan (Parelkar et al. 2011).

A retrospective review of hernias in children <2 years of age during a 3-year period included 269 patients, of which 98 (37 %) were premature. Of repairs, 39 (15 %) were emergent (defined as not electively scheduled), and all surgeries were open repairs performed by five surgeons. Testicular atrophy occurred in one patient, while injuries to the vas were documented in three; preterm versus full-term birth, age at surgery, or emergent versus elective repair did not predict these occurrences (Baird et al. 2011).

The retrospective review by Ein et al. (2006) reported 0.3 % testicular atrophy and 0.06 % transection/avulsion of the vas. Of the 16 cases of testicular atrophy, 8 (1 %) were associated with an incarcerated hernia.

Ventriculoperitoneal Shunt

A matched cohort study found that ventriculoperitoneal (VP) shunts in children 0–5 years of age increased risk for hernia development during the initial 2 years after placement (HR 20 and 11 at years 1 and 2), but thereafter risk was equivalent to that of children without shunts.

A nationwide database covering >99 % of the Taiwanese population was accessed to identify more than 1.5 million children born between 1996 and 2000, from which a study group of 675 less than 5 years of age who underwent VP shunt were compared over an 8-year follow-up period to a sex- and age-matched cohort of 6,704 children without VP shunt. A total of 353 children underwent inguinal hernia surgery, 12 % of those with a VP shunt at a mean time interval of 2 years versus 4 % of the control group. The adjusted HR was 19.67 (95 % CI 9.89–39.12) during the first year after VP shunt placement, and 11.36 (95 % CI 4.22–30.54) during the second year, but subsequently was no different than controls (Chen et al. 2011).

Indirect Versus Direct Hernias

The retrospective study by Ein et al. (2006) described above stated that 64/6,361 (0.1 %) were direct.

Surgical Management

Open Versus Laparoscopic Repair

Meta-analysis and two prospective studies comparing laparoscopic to open repair report no differences in hernia recurrence rates (≤4 %).

Unilateral laparoscopic surgery (with sac division and ligation) is associated with longer operative times, and there are variable results regarding differences in postoperative pain versus open repair.

Laparoscopic hernia repair can be done using intracorporeal instruments or by percutaneous sac ligation, with no difference in recurrences.

Open repair (OHR): The retrospective review by Ein et al. (2006) mentioned earlier using high sac division and ligation with mean follow-up of 6 months reported recurrent hernia in 84 (1 %), with 54 % detected within 1 year, 96 % by 5 years, and 100 % by 10 years after surgery.

Laparoscopic repair (LHR): This technique can be done either transperitoneally or preperitoneally with transperitoneal scope placement. The technique has included division of the sac at the internal ring with suture closure, or suture closure of an intact sac. It can be accomplished using working ports or by percutaneous suture ligation without additional ports.

Three-Instrument Laparoscopic Repair

A prospective series of 161 patients, mean age 5.2 years (1 month-16 years), undergoing a minimally invasive repair (number of alternative repairs was not mentioned), used a transperitoneal laparoscopic technique with two working trocars to divide and ligate the sac just distal to the internal ring. Follow-up in 146 patients >1 year after surgery, mean 3 years, found four (2 %) recurrences (Tsai et al. 2011).

A retrospective review using a similar laparoscopic technique in 315 patients, of whom 50 were under 1 year of age at repair were analyzed. There were no conversions to open surgery and with follow-up greater than 1 year in all patients, recurrence was noted in one (2 %) (Esposito et al. 2010).

A single surgeon analyzed repair in 542 consecutive children, median age 1.6 years (4 days-14 years), ligating (without dividing) the sac (4–0 permanent monofilament) using two laparoscopic transperitoneal needle holders. At median follow-up of 39 months (1–84), recurrence occurred in 20 (4 %) (Schier 2006).

Two randomized single-blinded trials compared OHR to LHR with two working trocars. One performed LHR with sac ligation ($n=47$) versus OHR ($n=42$) in children with median age of 6 years (0.65–16) and a unilateral hernia undergoing day surgery. Follow-up was >6 months in 98 % and >2 years in 84 %. Recurrent hernia occurred in three—two LHR and one OHR. The primary study outcome was time to resume normal activity, which was 2.5 days in both cohorts. Secondary outcomes included operative time and postoperative pain before and after discharge. Operative time in minutes (mean 33 [15–59] LHR vs. mean 15 [8–35] OHR) and time (minutes) in the day surgical unit before discharge (mean 300 [185–635] LHR vs. mean 230 [145–432] OHR) were greater after LHR. LHR was associated with significantly greater postoperative pain, which required rescue fentanyl analgesia before discharge and ibuprofen on postoperative day 2 (Koivusalo et al. 2009).

The other series used the same laparoscopic technique and randomized consecutive patients to outpatient LHR ($n=41$) versus OHR ($n=42$). The primary outcome was postoperative pain requiring acetaminophen, which was less with LHR than OHR. Operative time for unilateral repair was significantly less with OHR (18 min ± 5.7) than

LHR (23 min ± 6.3), whereas time for bilateral surgeries was the same (Chan et al. 2005).

A meta-analysis of LHR versus OHR involving 10 studies (2 RCTs, 1 nonrandomized trial, 7 observational comparative studies) with 2,699 patients reported the following:

- No differences in hernia recurrences: OR 1.81 (95 % CI 0.89–3.67).
- Longer operative time for unilateral LR: WMD 10.23 (95 % CI 8.82–11.64).
- Reduction in metachronous hernias after LR: OR 0.37 (95 % CI 0.20–0.67).

There were insufficient data to analyze postoperative pain differences (Alzahem 2011).

One-Instrument Percutaneous Sac Ligation with Laparoscopy

Subcutaneous endoscopically assisted ligation (SEAL) used a single endoscope with percutaneous sac ligation with either Maxon absorbable or Ticron nonabsorbable suture (size used not stated) through a stab incision over the internal ring. A retrospective series reported 204 patients mean age 2 years (3 days–16 years) with mean follow-up of approximately 8 months. During the study period, another 68 patients underwent OHR for incarcerated hernia that could not be reduced, difficult laparoscopic visualization, hemodynamic instability during insufflation, an "extraordinarily large" hernia, and parent or surgeon preference (numbers for each indication not stated). Of the laparoscopic cases, eight were incarcerated. Complications occurred in 28/204 (14 %), comprising 12 (6 %) hernia recurrences, 10 suture abscesses or granulomas, 3 wound infections, 2 umbilical hernias, and 1 femoral nerve injury. Recurrences were not associated with suture type (absorbable vs. nonabsorbable) (Ozgediz et al. 2007).

A retrospective review compared laparoscopy using two working ports and suture ligation with 3–0 silk to percutaneous (SEAL) laparoscopy with suture ligation using 1–0 polyglactin in repair of 67 and 146 hernias, respectively. Median age was 5 years (1–14). One percutaneous ligation converted to open surgery. Recurrence was noted in 2/67 (3 %) versus 7/146 (5 %), $p = 0.49$. SEAL recurrences were greater with single purse-string ligation versus double ligation (5/35 vs. 2/77, $p = 0.02$) (Bharathi et al. 2008).

Another retrospective study reported SEAL in 221 consecutive children (144 males) at mean age 3 years (9 days–21 years) with mean body weight 14 kg (2–77). Nonabsorbable suture was used (size, type not stated). The technique could not be performed in two infants (13 and 80 days of age). Duration of follow-up was not stated; two (1 %) developed recurrences at 43 and 161 days (Chang et al. 2011).

Consecutive patients (1,107) with a pediatric inguinal hernia underwent SEAL and were analyzed retrospectively. Contralateral patent processus vaginalis (not defined) was found in 20 % of patients and repaired. Mean follow-up was 36 months (range 9–74 months); six recurrences were seen (0.54 %) within 2–6 months. All occurred in boys with hernia ring defects larger than 2.5 cm, and were reoperated using the same laparoscopic technique successfully. Other complications were noted in seven cases—one puncture of the iliac artery (which stopped with external pressure), four umbilical hernias, and two suture-site abscesses or granulomas) (Li et al. 2012).

Contralateral Exploration for Unilateral Hernia

Meta-analysis reports approximately 7 % of unilateral herniorraphies will have a metachronous contralateral hernia.

Risk is not influenced by age at initial repair or gender.

Left-sided hernias are more likely than right-sided ones to develop metachronous hernia.

One study found contralateral laparoscopic appearance of the ring (open vs. closed) through the ipsilateral sac did not predict metachronous hernia.

One study reported that eight contralateral explorations would be needed to avoid one hernia.

Most metachronous hernias occur within 1 year after initial repair.

Metachronous hernia occurs significantly less often after laparoscopic versus open surgery.

A meta-analysis of unilateral hernia repairs published from 1941 to 1996 that included 35 studies with 15,310 children reported 7 % (95 % CI 0.68–0.72) developed a metachronous contralateral hernia. Analysis of potential risk factors found the following:

- Age <2 years did not increase risk: OR 1.34 (95 % CI 0.91–1.97).
- Male gender did not increase risk: OR 1.15 (95 % CI 0.87–1.53).
- Left hernia increased risk: OR 1.49 (95 % CI 1.23–1.81).

Most new contralateral hernias occurred within 5 years, with only 1 % presenting with incarceration (Miltenburg et al. 1997).

A subsequent prospective study limited contralateral exploration to premature babies less than post-conceptual age 56 weeks in a series of 264 infants and children undergoing unilateral repair. During follow-up from 36 to 72 months, only 14 (5 %) developed a metachronous hernia. These were statistically more likely to occur with initially left-sided hernias, but there was no significant association by gender (although none occurred in females), age <2 years versus older, or presentation with incarceration. If contralateral exploration had been done to those with unilateral left hernias, 84 procedures would have been done to prevent 11 metachronous hernias. Eighty-five percent of metachronous hernias presented within 1 year of initial surgery. Overall, unilateral exploration in this series avoided 153 unneeded contralateral procedures (Manoharan et al. 2005).

Another prospective study evaluated the role of laparoscopy (70° or 110° lens) through the hernia sac in unilateral operations to assess the contralateral internal ring. Bilateral surgery was only done if this visualization resulted in a bulge and/or crepitance in the groin. There were 299 cases, with 13 (4 %) undergoing bilateral surgery. Of the remaining 286, laparoscopy showed a closed ring in 127 (44 %) and an open ring in 115 (40 %), and was not technically feasible in the remaining 44 (15 %) due to a small ipsilateral sac. With follow-up to 53 months (clinical examination at 1 month, annual phone calls thereafter) in 222 patients, metachronous hernia developed in 15 (7 %). Of the 115 with an open internal ring at laparoscopy, follow-up in 88 found a metachronous hernia in 9 (10 %). Of the 127 apparently closed internal rings, follow-up in 97 included a metachronous hernia in 4 (4 %), $p = 0.149$ (Maddox and Smith 2008).

Meta-analysis of eight articles reporting contralateral patent processus vaginalis and metachronous hernia found the contralateral processus was patent in 21–47 % at laparoscopy. There was a significant reduction in metachronous hernia associated with laparoscopy (14/1,571, 0.9 %) versus unilateral open surgery (72/1,144, 6 %), OR 0.4 (95 % CI 0.2–0.7). Number needed to treat is 19 LHR to prevent one metachronous hernia by OHR (Alzahem 2011).

Sutured Versus Skin Adhesive Wound Closure

Inguinal incisions can be closed using either subcuticular sutures or skin adhesives, with equivalent functional and cosmetic outcomes.

One RCT compared 70 subcuticular suture approximations (5–0 Monocryl) to 64 adhesive skin (2-octylcyanoacrylate) closures in children of mean age 3.7 years and mean weight 16 ± 0.8 kg. Outcomes were assessed at 6 weeks by the operating surgeon using a validated visual analog scale and an ordinate scale, and by an independent surgeon using photographs. There were no cosmetic differences, and no clinical wound complications for either group (Brown et al. 2009).

References

Alzahem A. Laparoscopic versus open inguinal herniotomy in infants and children: a meta-analysis. Pediatr Surg Int. 2011;27(6):605–12.

Baird R, Gholoum S, Laberge JM, Puligandla P. Prematurity, not age at operation or incarceration, impacts complication rates of inguinal hernia repair. J Pediatr Surg. 2011;46(5):908–11.

Bharathi RS, Dabas AK, Arora M, Baskaran V. Laparoscopic ligation of internal ring-three ports versus single-port technique: are working ports necessary? J Laparoendosc Adv Surg Tech A. 2008;18(6):891–4.

Brown JK, Campbell BT, Drongowski RA, Alderman AK, Geiger JD, Teitelbaum DH, et al. A prospective, randomized comparison of skin adhesive and subcuticular suture for closure of pediatric hernia incisions: cost and cosmetic considerations. J Pediatr Surg. 2009;44(7):1418–22.

Chan KL, Hui WC, Tam PK. Prospective randomized single-center, single-blind comparison of laparoscopic vs open repair of pediatric inguinal hernia. Surg Endosc. 2005;19(7):927–32.

Chang YT, Lee JY, Tsai CJ, Chiu WC, Chiou CS. Preliminary experience of one-trocar laparoscopic herniorrhaphy in infants and children. J Laparoendosc Adv Surg Tech A. 2011;21(3):277–82.

Chen YC, Wu JC, Liu L, Chen TJ, Huang WC, Cheng H. Correlation between ventriculoperitoneal shunts and inguinal hernias in children: an 8-year follow-up. Pediatrics. 2011;128(1):e121–6.

Christensen T, Cartwright PC, Devries C, Snow BW. New onset of hydroceles in boys over 1 year of age. Int J Urol. 2006;13(11):1425–7.

Ein SH, Njere I, Ein A. Six thousand three hundred sixty-one pediatric inguinal hernias: a 35-year review. J Pediatr Surg. 2006;41(5):980–6.

Esposito C, Montinaro L, Alicchio F, Savanelli A, Armenise T, Settimi A. Laparoscopic treatment of inguinal hernia in the first year of life. J Laparoendosc Adv Surg Tech A. 2010;20(5):473–6.

Grosfeld JL. Current concepts in inguinal hernia in infants and children. World J Surg. 1989;13(5):506–15.

Koivusalo AI, Korpela R, Wirtavuori K, Piiparinen S, Rintala RJ, Pakarinen MP. A single-blinded, randomized comparison of laparoscopic versus open hernia repair in children. Pediatrics. 2009;123(1):332–7.

Koski ME, Makari JH, Adams MC, Thomas JC, Clark PE, Pope JC, et al. Infant communicating hydroceles–do they need immediate repair or might some clinically resolve? J Pediatr Surg. 2010;45(3):590–3.

Lee SL, Gleason JM, Sydorak RM. A critical review of premature infants with inguinal hernias: optimal timing of repair, incarceration risk, and postoperative apnea. J Pediatr Surg. 2011;46(1):217–20.

Li B, Nie X, Xie H, Gong D. Modified single-port laparoscopic herniorrhaphy for pediatric inguinal hernias: based on 1,107 cases in China. Surg Endosc. 2012;26(12):3663–8.

Maddox MM, Smith DP. A long-term prospective analysis of pediatric unilateral inguinal hernias: should laparoscopy or anything else influence the management of the contralateral side? J Pediatr Urol. 2008;4(2):141–5.

Manoharan S, Samarakkody U, Kulkarni M, Blakelock R, Brown S. Evidence-based change of practice in the management of unilateral inguinal hernia. J Pediatr Surg. 2005;40(7):1163–6.

Miltenburg DM, Nuchtern JG, Jaksic T, Kozinetz CA, Brandt ML. Meta-analysis of the risk of metachronous hernia in infants and children. Am J Surg. 1997;174(6):741–4.

Osifo OD, Osaigbovo EO. Congenital hydrocele: prevalence and outcome among male children who underwent neonatal circumcision in Benin City, Nigeria. J Pediatr Urol. 2008;4(3):178–82.

Ozgediz D, Roayaie K, Lee H, Nobuhara KK, Farmer DL, Bratton B, et al. Subcutaneous endoscopically assisted ligation (SEAL) of the internal ring for repair of inguinal hernias in children: report of a new technique and early results. Surg Endosc. 2007;21(8):1327–31.

Parelkar SV, Oak S, Bachani MK, Sanghvi B, Prakash A, Patil R, et al. Laparoscopic repair of pediatric inguinal hernia–is vascularity of the testis at risk? A study of 125 testes. J Pediatr Surg. 2011;46(9):1813–6.

Schier F. Laparoscopic inguinal hernia repair-a prospective personal series of 542 children. J Pediatr Surg. 2006;41(6):1081–4.

Tsai YC, Wu CC, Ho CH, Tai HC, Yang SS. Minilaparoscopic herniorrhaphy in pediatric inguinal hernia: a durable alternative treatment tostandard herniotomy. J Pediatr Surg. 2011;46(4):708–12.

Zamakhshary M, To T, Guan J, Langer JC. Risk of incarceration of inguinal hernia among infants and young children awaiting elective surgery. CMAJ. 2008;179(10):1001–5.

Testicular Torsion

7

Warren T. Snodgrass, Linda A. Baker, and Nicol C. Bush

Two primary goals in diagnosis and management of testicular torsion:

1. **Preserve the ipsilateral testis, when it remains viable.**
2. **Prevent contralateral torsion.**

Secondary goals include the following:

1. **Avoidance of risk factors for infertility.**
2. **Maintain a normal scrotal appearance.**

Evidence for these aims—perinatal torsion:

- **Most case series report no ipsilateral testis salvage from neonatal surgery. One reported 2 of 30 explored testes had normal size at follow-up.**
- **Risk for contralateral postnatal torsion is not well defined, but case series report neonatal ultrasound to be unreliable to exclude vascular compromise.**
- **Our review found no data regarding fertility or psychologic impact of asymmetric scrotal appearance after perinatal torsion.**

Evidence for these aims—torsion in children and teenagers:

- **Few objective criteria are described to guide orchiopexy versus orchiectomy, and there is no agreed-upon definition for atrophy after orchiopexy.**
- **Two retrospective studies that defined atrophy as ≥15 % or >50 % volume loss reported 27 and 13 % occurrence.**
- **We found one case of simultaneous bilateral torsion, and none of asynchronous torsion, after the neonatal period. Contralateral orchiopexy is done based on potential risks.**
- **One retrospective review reported recurrent torsion in 4 % of patients after orchiopexy.**
- **There are few data regarding fertility in men after torsion. Semen analyses most often are normal, with oligospermia in 0–35 %. Antisperm antibodies reported in three studies were positive in only 2/80 patients.**
- **Our review found no article regarding psychologic impact of orchiectomy or testicular atrophy after orchiopexy for torsion.**

Prenatal and Perinatal Torsion

Most prenatal torsion presents as unilateral nonpalpable testis and is managed as a potential undescended testis (*see* Chap. 5). Our review found no report of contralateral postnatal torsion in these patients.

Newborns with evidence of recent prenatal torsion (firm, discolored testis), or neonates who develop unilateral torsion postnatally, do have risk for contralateral torsion. Bilateral torsion is either suspected on preoperative assessment or encountered despite a lack of preoperative findings in most cases. Asynchronous torsion less commonly occurs.

W.T. Snodgrass, M.D. (✉) • L.A. Baker, M.D.
N.C. Bush, M.D., M.S.C.S.
Department of Pediatric Urology, University of Texas Southwestern Medical Center and Children's Medical Center Dallas, 1935 Medical District Drive, MS F4.04, Dallas, TX 75235, USA
e-mail: warren.snodgrass@childrens.com; linda.baker@childrens.com; nicol.bush@childrens.com

W.T. Snodgrass (ed.), *Pediatric Urology: Evidence for Optimal Patient Management*,
DOI 10.1007/978-1-4614-6910-0_7, © Springer Science+Business Media New York 2013

Preoperative color Doppler ultrasound erroneously reported blood flow to contralateral clinically normal testes in several reported cases that were found, at exploration, to have ischemic necrosis.

A systematic literature review reported salvage (not defined) in 9 % of published cases, increasing to 22 % with "urgent exploration." Larger case series (16–27 patients) together comprising 108 cases report three testes with normal volume after orchiopexy and another two with partial atrophy.

No study reported perioperative anesthesia-related morbidity from surgery in newborns.

No study reported testis tumor mimicking torsion. Scrotal incision is an option, especially since extravaginal torsion can be identified before the tunica vaginalis is opened, with extravaginal dissection to the internal ring or conversion to an inguinal incision if torsion is not found.

A systematic review of published literature identified 18 case series reporting ≥5 newborns with perinatal torsion, comprising a total of 284 patients, of which 268 were operated. All but four patients were full-term. Testicular salvage was described in 24 (9 %). Three of these 24 were diagnosed within 2 h of birth and considered to be prenatal events, while 10 were diagnosed between 12 and 36 h and the remainder up to 72 h after birth. There were 19 cases with bilateral torsion reported, 6 synchronous; in 7 cases, a preoperative diagnosis of unilateral torsion was found to have bilateral torsion. The authors concluded from their review that only one case of asynchronous torsion was clearly reported. One-hundred six cases were described as emergent operations, with salvage (i.e., detorsion) reported in 23 (22 %) (Nandi and Murphy 2011). Subsequent outcomes from detorsion, specifically atrophy, were not discussed.

A retrospective series found 23 cases, all ≥37 weeks of gestational age and all stated to have abnormal testicular examination at birth. Nineteen were operated urgently upon arrival (4 needed NICU stabilization), with 14 undergoing surgery at age 6–12 h. No viable testis was found, and no testicular salvage occurred. Two had bilateral torsion and resultant anorchia. Despite an obvious necrotic appearance, six testes were maintained, and all six atrophied. In eight (35 %) cases, contralateral exploration/fixation was not done and none had abnormal exams at follow-up (Brandt et al. 1992).

Another retrospective series reviewed 27 neonates and 30 testes operated between 2 h and 2 months of age, with orchiectomy performed in 19 due to obvious necrosis. Orchiopexy was done in 11/30 testes, with follow-up physical examination in 10. Of these 10, 4 were atrophic, 2 were symmetric to the contralateral side, and 4 had partial atrophy. Therefore, salvage was achieved in 6/30 (20 %) testes, of which 2/30 (7 %) were considered on palpation to be normal (Pinto et al. 1997).

A third retrospective review found 18 cases of neonatal torsion, with all having a normal contralateral testis on examination. Each underwent urgent exploration (two delayed by transfer from another facility). No ipsilateral testis was salvaged; 4 (22 %) had asymptomatic contralateral torsion encountered during surgery, each of which atrophied postoperatively. In two of these four cases, the contralateral testis was imaged preoperatively by US (color Doppler vs. other methods not stated) and reported to have "good flow" (Yerkes et al. 2005).

A retrospective review included 24 neonates, 2 with clinically bilateral torsion, of which 21 had exploration. Time interval from diagnosis to operation was not stated. No testis was salvaged. In one case described in detail, a unilateral abnormal testis first noted on routine exam on "day 1" prompted US, which reported normal bilateral blood flow. At exploration on day 3, both testes were necrotic (John et al. 2008).

Still another retrospective review reported 16 neonatal torsions, 13 (2 bilateral) considered to have occurred prenatally and the other 3 postnatally. All prenatally torsed testes were necrotic, and two that were preserved were atrophied at 3-month assessment. One postnatally detected testis was salvaged despite absent blood flow on color Doppler US, and at 3-month follow-up remained normal (method of postoperative assessment not stated). Timing of surgery after diagnosis was not mentioned (Kaye et al. 2008a).

A case report described a newborn with bilateral hard testes within an enlarged, indurated scrotum. Color Doppler US showed no flow on the left, but central flow on the right. At exploration, the left was necrotic and was removed; the right was blue and was preserved, with follow-up US at 5 months reporting a normal testis (Zinn et al. 1998).

Torsion in Children and Adolescents

Acute Scrotum: Incidence of Testicular Torsion Versus Torsed Appendage or Epididymitis

Several retrospective series report findings from "universal" exploration for patients presenting with "acute scrotum." Generally, torsed appendage testis was the most common diagnosis, found in 32–57 %. Testicular torsion was found in 21–33 % and epididymitis in 8–18 %.

A retrospective review of universal exploration for "acute scrotum" (not defined) between 1977 and 1995 included 388 consecutive boys <17 years of age. Findings included testicular torsion in 100 (26 %), torsed appendage in 174 (45 %), and epididymitis in 38 (10 %). Testicular torsion occurred most often in the first year of life and at ages 13–16 years, torsed appendages between 9 and12 years, and epididymitis within the first year of life. Urine cultures were positive in 10/21 boys less than 1 year of age, and fever was present in 6, diagnosed with epididymitis (Makela et al. 2007).

Another retrospective review reported 100 consecutive males, mean age 13.6 years (3 months to 37 years), with acute scrotal pain managed by exploration without routine imaging. Testis torsion occurred in 33 at mean age 15.7 years, torsed appendage in 32 at mean age 11.6 years, and epididymitis in 18 at mean age 14.8 years (Hegarty et al. 2001).

A third unit with a policy for universal exploration for acute scrotal pain or swelling did retrospective review of 121 boys mean age 11 years (1–14). Of these, 113 had surgery and 8 were observed, 2 with positive urinalyses and US diagnosis of epididymitis, 3 with clinical signs of a torsed appendage, and 3 with normal US. Of the 113 operated cases, testis torsion was found in 31 (27 %), 9 (29 %) of which were removed. A torsed appendage occurred in 64 (57 %) and epididymitis in 12 (11 %) (Murphy et al. 2006).

Review of 135 patients 1–16 years of age presenting with acute scrotal pain over a 5-year period beginning in 2003 who all underwent exploration, found 89 (66 %) with torsed appendage, 41 (30 %) with testicular torsion, and 2 (1 %) with epididymitis (Soccorso et al. 2010).

Another retrospective study used color Doppler US to assess the acute scrotum, but performed surgical exploration in all cases with suspected testicular torsion regardless of US findings. In 298 males, mean age 11±4 years, 62 (21 %) had testicular torsion, 168 (56 %) had torsed appendage, and 24 (8 %) epididymitis (Waldert et al. 2010).

If all these five centers identified similar patients with similar ages and categorized "acute scrotum" the same, and if all those testes that were detorsed were subsequently healthy (all unlikely suppositions), then universal surgery would result in five scrotal explorations for each testis salvaged.

Clinical Parameters to Predict Testicular Torsion

The main differential diagnosis for testicular torsion is a torsed appendage.

Patients with torsion tend to be older than those with a torsed appendage. Three studies have reported mean ages >12 versus <12 years, respectively.

When present, nausea/vomiting increases likelihood for testicular torsion.

Two studies reported abdominal pain correlated with testis torsion, while another did not.

Studies found pain duration <24 h at presentation predicted testis torsion.

Three studies report an elevated ("high-riding") testicle most often indicates testicular torsion.

Five studies report that absent cremasteric reflex most often predicts testicular torsion.

Scrotal edema and scrotal erythema do not reliably distinguish between testicular torsion, torsed appendage, and epididymitis.

Patient Age

A retrospective study of 179 patients who underwent scrotal exploration for suspected torsion at median age 14 years (0–92), reported there was a significant difference in the median age of those with torsed appendage versus those with testicular torsion or epididymitis (11 vs. 15 vs. 21.5 years). A cutoff of 12 years of age gave a positive predictive value for torsed appendage of 52 % (95 % CI 0.66–0.91), whereas patients >12 years were unlikely to have this diagnosis (Molokwu et al. 2011).

Another retrospective study reviewed cases undergoing exploration during a 10-year period beginning in 1986 (number of patients with acute scrotum not operated during this period was not stated). Of 115 patients, 83 had testicular torsion, 27 a torsed appendage, and 5 epididymitis. Mean age of those with a torsed appendage was 9 years, versus 14 years in those with testicular torsion or epididymitis (Jefferson et al. 1997).

A study of 135 consecutive boys with acute scrotum who all underwent surgery reported that the median age of those with torsed appendage was 9 years (7–11) versus those with testicular torsion, whose median age was 14 years (3–16) (Soccorso et al. 2010).

Nausea and Vomiting

A review of records in a pediatric emergency department from 2005 to 2007 found 492 children with mean age 10.75 ± 5 years evaluated for an acute scrotum. In this series, the majority (169, 32 %) had no diagnosis, with testis torsion in only 17 (3 %). Compared to all other etiologies, nausea/vomiting increased the likelihood for testicular torsion (OR 8.87 [95 % CI 2.6–30.1]) (Beni-Israel et al. 2010).

The study by Jefferson et al. (1997) mentioned above found that nausea/vomiting was present in 69 % of patients found to have testicular torsion, versus 8 and 0 % in those with a torsed appendage or epididymitis, OR 30.80 (95 % CI 6.8–139.5).

The Waldert study (2010) found nausea or vomiting in 32 % of torsion cases, versus 3 % for torsed appendage and 12.5 % for epididymitis, OR 22.98 (95 % CI 8.76–60.2).

A retrospective review of 138 boys with a diagnosis of acute scrotum found nausea and vomiting in 47.4 % of torsion cases, 3.3 % of torsed appendage, and none with epididymitis, OR 21.6 (95 % CI 4.9–93.4) (Boettcher et al. 2012).

A prospective 5-month study of 79 boys with acute scrotum, 8 with torsion, performed multivariable analysis of predictive clinical factors and reported nausea/vomiting was significantly associated with testicular torsion versus all other diagnoses (data not shown) (Srinivasan et al. 2011).

In contrast, the review by Makela et al. (2007) described above, which reviewed 388 boys with an acute scrotum, found nausea/vomiting reported in 5/100 with torsion versus 3/174 (2 %) and 1/38 (3 %) with torsed appendage or epididymitis.

Abdominal Pain

The Beni-Israel et al. (2010) retrospective review of children with acute scrotum demonstrated an increased likelihood of torsion diagnosis when abdominal pain was present, OR 3.19 (95 % CI 1.15–8.89).

Similarly, the Waldert et al. (2010) retrospective review of boys with an acute scrotum who also underwent scrotal US showed an increased presence of abdominal pain in torsion cases, OR 4.33 (95 % CI 2.13–8.84).

In contrast, the Makela et al. (2007) retrospective review of acute scrotum cases did not show this relationship, with only 7 % of torsion cases with abdominal pain versus 7 % of appendiceal torsion and 8 % of epididymitis, OR 1.01(95 % CI 0.39–2.51).

Pain Duration >24 h

The Beni-Israel et al. (2010) study demonstrated that boys who presented with pain with duration of less than 24 h were more likely to have testis torsion, OR 6.66 (95 % CI 1.54–33.33).

Boettcher et al. (2012) similarly found shorter pain duration in the torsion group (mean 17.2 h) versus the non-torsion group (mean duration of pain not reported), OR 4.2 (95 % CI 1.3–13.4).

Soccorso et al. (2010) also reported that pain duration less than 24 h was more frequent with testis torsion (69 %) versus non-torsion (37 %), OR 3.63 (95 % CI 1.66–7.92).

High Testicular Position

The analysis of 17 patients with testicular torsion by Beni-Israel et al. (2010) discussed above calculated OR 58.8 (95 % CI 19.2–166.6) for torsion versus other diagnoses when the testicle was observed in a high position.

A retrospective review of 160 patients with acute scrotum at mean age 12 years (8 months to 15 years) between 1970 and 2000 reported an elevated testicular position had 83 % sensitivity and 90 % specificity for testicular torsion (Ciftci et al. 2004).

The report by Murphy et al. (2006) discussed above with the policy of universal exploration stated that a high testicular position was found in 16/31 (52 %) patients with testicular torsion, versus 7/64 (11 %) and 1/12 (8 %) with epididymitis, OR 9.07 (95 % CI 3.28–25.21).

Cremasteric Reflex

An absent cremasteric reflex was identified in the multivariable analysis by Srinivasan et al. mentioned above (2011) to predict testicular torsion versus other causes for acute scrotum.

Absence of the cremasteric reflex was reported to have 92 % sensitivity and 98 % specificity for testicular torsion in the retrospective review by Ciftci et al. (2004).

The study by Waldert et al. (2010) described above that included exploration in all acute scrotum cases reported absent cremasteric reflex in 43/62 (70 %) with testicular torsion versus 24/192 (12.5 %) with torsed appendage or epididymitis, $p<0.001$.

Another retrospective review from 1997 to 2002 identified 177 boys, mean 9 years (0–18), with an acute scrotum, of which testicular torsion was diagnosed in 41 (23 %). Absent cremasteric reflex was noted in 28/31 (90 %) patients in whom it was recorded, versus 30/122 (25 %) of those with a torsed appendage or epididymitis, $p<0.001$ (Karmazyn et al. 2005).

The previously described study of emergency department records by Beni-Israel et al. (2010) calculated from 17 patients with testicular torsion versus 475 with other or no diagnoses that abnormal (absent/ "reduced") cremasteric reflex had OR 27.77 (95 % CI 7.5–100) for testicular torsion.

Scrotal Reaction

A retrospective review of 90 patients <18 years diagnosed with testicular torsion, torsed appendage, or epididymitis reported that scrotal erythema/ edema was present in 1/13 (8 %) with testicular torsion versus 45/77 (58 %) without testicular torsion, $p<0.007$ (Kadish and Bolte 1998).

The retrospective study by Karmazyn et al. (2005) previously mentioned reported scrotal erythema in 15/40 (37.5 %) boys with testicular torsion versus 93/127 (73 %) with torsed appendage or epididymitis, $p<0.001$. However, scrotal swelling was similar between those with versus those without testicular torsion: 31/30 (77.5 %) and 104/131 (79 %), $p=0.6$.

Similarly, the review by Makela et al. (2007) described above reported scrotal erythema in 16/100 (16 %) boys <17 years with testicular torsion versus 69/211 (32 %), $p<0.002$, with torsed appendage or epididymitis, but scrotal swelling did not vary between these etiologies and was recorded in <20 % of cases of each.

The retrospective review by Beni-Israel et al. (2010) stated univariable analysis found scrotal erythema did not distinguish between those with testicular torsion versus other diagnoses [OR 1.37 (95 % CI 0.47–3.95)] (Beni-Israel et al. 2010).

The retrospective study by Waldert et al. described above, in which all patients with acute scrotum underwent surgery, reported scrotal swelling in 47/62 (75 %) testicular torsions versus

81/192 (42 %) in those with torsed appendage or epididymitis, $p=0.001$.

Another retrospective review in which all patients had exploration found scrotal swelling in 40/41 (98 %) with testicular torsion versus 63/92 (68 %) with torsed appendage or epididymitis, $p=0.001$, OR 58.4 (95 % CI 7.83–435). However, erythema was present in 15/41(37 %) with testicular torsion versus 46/92 (50 %) with torsed appendage or epididymitis, $p=0.2$, OR 0.58 (95 % CI 0.27–1.22) (Soccorso et al. 2010).

Although scrotal edema and erythema potentially indicate a subacute presentation, neither duration of symptoms at presentation nor findings at surgery (viable versus necrotic testis) in testicular torsion with versus without scrotal reaction were stated in any of these reports.

Clinical Algorithms

Three groups reported algorithms to predict testicular torsion versus other diagnoses based on clinical parameters. The largest prospective study was conducted in Brazil over a 2-year period identifying 282 patients with a mean age of 12.1 years (41 with torsion). A 5 variable scoring system including scrotal swelling (2 points), hard testicular mass (2 points), high-riding testis (1 point), and absent cremasteric reflex (1 point) could stratify patients into low (0–2 points), intermediate (3–4 points), and high risk of torsion (5–7). They validated their system on a retrospective cohort of 116 patients and found that the high- and low-risk categories could predict the presence and absence of torsion in all cases (Barbosa et al. 2012).

The study by Boettcher et al. (2012) identified four factors that were highly predictive of testicular torsion: pain <24 h, nausea or vomiting, high position of testis, and abnormal cremasteric reflex. They reported that presence of two or more of those findings included 100 % of torsion cases at exploration ($n=19$), but did not validate this score on any other sample.

Similarly, Srinivasan et al. (2011) found that the presence of three factors, namely, absence of cremasteric reflex, nausea/vomiting, and scrotal skin changes, could predict all cases of testicular torsion ($n=8/79$) and that absence of all three factors could rule out torsion. This was not validated in other samples.

Testicular Ultrasonography to Diagnose Torsion

A multi-institutional study reported high-resolution US to detect spermatic cord twist correctly identified 96 % of testicular torsions, versus 76 % diagnosis by color Doppler of intra-parenchymal vascular loss.

Several retrospective analyses of color Doppler US report sensitivity/specificity for testicular torsion ranging from 89 to 100 % and 98 to 100 %.

A multicenter European study compared color Doppler to high-resolution US for the diagnosis of testicular torsion in 919 boys, mean age 9 years (1 day to 18 years) with acute scrotum who underwent both examinations. The final diagnosis was testicular torsion in 208 (23 %). Of these, color Doppler stated intra-parenchymal vascularization was absent in 158 (76 %), but was reported normal to increased in the other 50 (24 %). Color Doppler findings in the patients without testicular torsion were not stated. High-resolution scanning detected cord twisting in 199 (96 %), while in the remaining 9 cases it was not seen due to high position in 5 and confused with epididymitis in 4. In the other 711 patients without testicular torsion, high-resolution US reported no cord twisting in 705 (99 %) and was falsely positive in the other 6 with various findings at surgery (Kalfa et al. 2007).

A retrospective study compared color Doppler US findings to surgical exploration in 298 boys, mean age 11 ± 4 years, with acute scrotum. All patients had US followed by surgery regardless of radiologic findings. Of these, 62 had surgically proven testicular torsion, with color Doppler US correctly predicting the diagnosis in 60 (97 %) and falsely negative in 2 (3 %). Therefore, sensitivity/specificity for US to detect testicular torsion was 97 % and 98 % (Waldert et al. 2010).

A retrospective study considered the use of B-mode US, and color Doppler for those with low vascular flow, in patients with acute scrotum who were not considered to have clinical findings of testicular torsion sufficient to warrant immediate exploration (number undergoing surgery without imaging was not stated). Of 130 patients <23 years of age, 17 had US evidence for torsion, prompting surgery, with 1 false-negative. Of 110 patients in which US reported no testicular torsion, 2/85 (2 %) with follow-up had atrophy indicating missed torsion. Sensitivity/specificity for color Doppler US was 89 and 99 % (Baker et al. 2000).

Another retrospective study reviewed 61 boys, mean age 8 years (1 day to 17 years), with acute scrotum evaluated by color Doppler US. Fourteen had decreased or absent intraparenchymal perfusion leading to surgical exploration with torsion confirmed in all cases. Another 12 were operated for pain, despite normal to increased perfusion, and none had testicular torsion. Thirty-three with normal to increased perfusion were not operated, and at follow-up in 32 "up to 2 years" none had atrophy. In this series, sensitivity and specificity of color Doppler US were both 100 % (Gunther et al. 2006).

Investigational Tools to Diagnose Torsion

Trans-scrotal near-infrared spectroscopy (NIRS) was evaluated in 16 males, mean age 18 years, with acute scrotum; non-torsion cases ($n=5$) had mean testicular oxygen saturations of 61 % in both the affected and non-affected testis. Testis torsion cases ($n=11$) showed a significant difference with the mean testicular oxygen saturation with the affected testis measuring 40 % compared to 64 % in the non-affected testis. A cutoff value of −11.5 units difference between affected and non-affected testes could distinguish between torsion and non-torsion cases (100 % sensitivity and 100 % specificity) (Baker 2011).

Factors Predicting Testicular Viability

There is no emergency to operate on a dead testicle. Preoperative factors predicting testicular viability include the duration of symptoms at presentation and the echogenic pattern on US.

Retrospective reviews report that detorsion within a mean of 4–8 h of symptom onset is significantly more likely to result in testicular salvage than is later presentation.

Our review found one article that reported scrotal erythema associated with a nonviable testis.

Two retrospective studies report that normal parenchymal echogenecity by US predicts a viable testis at surgery, versus hypoechogenicity and heterogenous parenchyma, which predict a nonviable testis.

Duration of Symptoms

A retrospective review of 186 operations for testicular torsion in boys, median age 14 years (18 month to 20 years), reported median pain duration of 5 h (0.5 h to 6 days) in those treated by orchiopexy, versus 2.2 days (2.5 h to 2 weeks) for those with orchiectomy. Of 116 orchiopexies, there was follow-up in 90, with 34/116 (29 %) having median follow-up at 8 months (1–39). Volume loss of ≥15 % compared to the contralateral testis was seen in 11/90 (12 %) (Sessions et al. 2003).

Another retrospective study of 86 boys, mean age 14 years, undergoing surgery for torsion found that mean pain duration in the 51 (61 %) with orchiopexy was 4 h (40 min to 12 h) versus 58 h (20 h to 5 days) in the 32 with orchiectomy. Of the 51 orchiopexies, there was follow-up in 37 at 1 month, with 2 (5 %) "mildly atrophic" (Jefferson et al. 1997).

Review of 100 testicular torsions in boys <17 years of age reported that all 35 operated at ≤6 h from onset of pain had salvage, versus 8/16 operated between 6–12 h and 2/51 operated at >12 h (Makela et al. 2007).

A retrospective analysis of 97 boys with surgery for testicular torsion found mean pain duration was 8 versus 56 h for those undergoing orchiopexy versus orchiectomy, and that all with pain for more than 36 h had orchiectomy (Bayne et al. 2010).

Another review of 63 testis torsions in patients mean age 18 years (11–45) reported no testicular loss (either orchiectomy or atrophy >50 % at 3 months) in the 24 operated at <4 h, versus 8/27 (30 %) explored at 4–24 h and 10/12 (83 %) at >24 h after symptom onset (Al-Hunayan et al. 2004).

Scrotal Reaction

Although testicular salvage rates potentially are different in patients with no scrotal reaction versus those with erythema and edema, our review found only one report of viability correlated with these findings on physical examination:

One prospective study of 19 pubertal patients with testicular torsion (median 14 years, range 12–16) reported that 13/13 patients with non-salvageable testes (necrotic appearance with no active bleeding with incision of tunica albuginea) had scrotal erythema versus 0/6 patients with salvageable testes. Median time to presentation in the non-salvageable versus salvageable groups was 96 h (12–168) versus 6 (4–48) (Bush and Bagrodia 2012).

Preoperative US

A retrospective analysis was done of color Doppler US done preoperatively in 55 of 79 boys, aged 1–17 years, with torsion. Parenchymal heterogeneity was found in 37/55 (67 %), and all had orchiectomy; homogeneity was found in 18, of which 16 had orchiopexy without atrophy (not defined) 4 months later (Kaye et al. 2008b).

Another retrospective study reviewed findings on color Doppler US before exploration for testicular torsion in 16 patients aged 14–40 years. Of these, seven had orchiectomy, and all were diffusely or focally hypoechoic or had parenchymal heterogeneity. The other nine had normal echogenicity and homogenous parenchyma and were salvaged, with none "who returned for follow-up" demonstrating subsequent atrophy (not defined) (Middleton et al. 1997).

Manual Detorsion

Manual untwisting can be performed to restore blood flow while awaiting surgery. Most torsion occurs inwardly, so initial derotation is from medial to lateral.

One retrospective series reported persistent torsion in 32 %.

A retrospective review included 61 patients with clinical diagnosis of testicular torsion, of which 44 underwent immediate surgery, and 17, with mean age of 15 years (13–28), had attempted manual detorsion, based on the preference of the attending urologist. Initial attempt was to derotate outwards, but if pain increased or there was resistance to lateral rotation, turning was done inwardly. The goal was immediate pain relief, which could not be achieved in three who then had surgery. The other 14 had elective orchiopexy at mean 12 h (2 h to 3 months), and all testes were reported as normal without atrophy (not defined) at either exploration or during follow-up at mean 22 months (9–72) (Cornel and Karthaus 1999).

Another retrospective review of 186 operations for testicular torsion reported information on the direction and number of turns in 162 cases. Inward twisting occurred in 67 %, and outward twisting occurred in 33 %; turns ranged from one-half to three. In 56 cases, manual detorsion was done, followed by immediate surgery; 18/56 (32 %) had persistent twisting a mean of 360° (180–720) (Sessions et al. 2003).

Intraoperative Tests to Determine Testis Viability

Two prospective studies of young children with testicular torsion (mean ages <12 years) used a similar protocol of incision through the tunica albuginea ± into parenchyma, followed by observation for arterial bleeding within 10 min. Orchiopexy was done in those with bleeding, with subsequent atrophy in 17–22 %.

A prospective study involved 19 children mean age 9 years (0–13) with testicular torsion in which the tunica albuginea and testicular parenchyma were incised deeply for biopsy and warm sponges applied. The surgeon observed for fresh arterial bleeding for up to 10 min, pexing those with flow ($n = 12$) and removing those without. Follow-up was done using color Doppler US at 15 days and 1 year in all undergoing orchiopexy. Atrophy (not defined) was diagnosed in 2/12 (17 %) "after a month of follow-up" (Arda and Ozyaylali 2001).

Another prospective study reported 15 boys, median age 8 years (6–12), with testicular torsion who were operated, each having the tunica albuginea incised followed by observation for arterial bleeding for 10 min. Flow noted within 10 min resulted in orchiopexy in nine; using color Doppler US at follow-up a median of 2.6 years (0.8–4), atrophy defined as volume loss of 50 % on the contralateral side occurred in two (22 %) (Cimador et al. 2007).

A retrospective review was done in 59 boys, aged 1–17 years, who underwent surgical detorsion after a minimum of 6 h of symptoms, who had at least one postoperative follow-up. Following surgical detorsion, 31 (53 %) with mean symptom duration of 13 h had improved intraoperative "appearance and color" and underwent orchiopexy. In the other 28 testes with a grossly ischemic appearance following detorsion, a tunica albugineal incision was made along the entire length of the testis; if blood flow to the parenchyma was observed ($n = 11$, mean duration of symptoms 31 h), the defect was covered with a vascularized tunica vaginalis flap and the testis preserved. Nineteen underwent orchiectomy for no parenchymal blood flow (mean symptom duration 67.5 h). Salvage rates were defined as testicular volume of 50 % or greater compared with the normal contralateral testis and presence of flow on Doppler ultrasound. The testicular viability rates were 62.5 % for the orchiopexy group and 55 % of the tunica vaginalis flap group; there was no difference in duration of symptoms in the salvaged versus atrophied patients (Figueroa et al. 2012).

Testicular Salvage Rates with Detorsion and Orchiopexy

Our review found few reports with follow-up to determine if detorsion and orchiopexy resulted in salvage or atrophy.

All are retrospective, and criteria used to determine orchiopexy versus orchiectomy were not stated by any.

Only three defined atrophy, as volume loss ≥15 % or >50 % versus the contralateral testis.

Orchiopexy was done in 61–71 % of these cases, with atrophy reported in from 5 to 45 %.

A review of 186 operations for testicular torsion found 116 (62 %) had orchiopexy at median 5 h (0.5 h to 6 days) after onset of pain. During follow-up (time not clearly stated) in 90 after orchiopexy, atrophy ≥15 % contralateral testis volume, which was determined using an orchidometer, occurred in 11 (27 %) (Sessions et al. 2003).

Of 83 patients with testicular torsion identified on retrospective review, orchiopexy was done in 51 (61 %). Thirty-seven of 51 (73 %) had follow-up at 1 month, with 2 (5 %) demonstrating "mild atrophy" (not defined) (Jefferson et al. 1997).

In another review of 63 patients, mean age 18 years (11–45), with surgery for testis torsion, orchiopexy was done in 52 (82.5 %), of which 7 (13 %) developed atrophy (volume <50 % non-torsed testis measured by US) by 3 months (Al-Hunayan et al. 2004).

Thirty-one patients with torsion had mean pain duration of 6 h (1 h to 7 day), with orchiopexy done in 22 (71 %). At follow-up (not clearly stated for torsion patients) one (5 %) had atrophy (not defined) (Murphy et al. 2006).

In the study by Figueroa et al. (2012) described in the section above, atrophy occurred in approximately 40 % thought to have "good appearance and color" after detorsion or parenchymal blood flow after tunica albuginea incision.

A retrospective study identified 65 cases of torsion with varying durations of preoperative symptoms: mean 13 h in those with detorsion plus orchiopexy, 31 h for detorsion, tunica albuginea incision plus tunica vaginalis flap, and 67 h in those with detorsion and then orchiectomy. Decision-making was not defined. Of those with albuginea incision and grafting, "salvage" (not defined, postoperative US done "at least 4 weeks" postoperatively) occurred in 55 %. "Salvage" (determined without systematic postoperative US) in those with detorsion plus orchiopexy was 62.5 % (Figueroa et al. 2012).

Risk for Contralateral Torsion

Contralateral orchiopexy is done by most, though not all, surgeons during operations for testicular torsion.

Only one study we reviewed reported synchronous bilateral torsion in a single patient.

Our review found no report of asynchronous torsion after the neonatal period.

With unknown risk for contralateral asynchronous testicular torsion, contralateral orchiopexy is based on concern for the consequences of subsequent torsion, especially after unilateral orchiectomy, the reported high prevalence of contralateral bell clapper deformity, and the assumption that there is little risk from the procedure to testicular function.

One of 41 boys aged 1–16 years was found to have synchronous, asymptomatic torsion of 180° during routine contralateral exploration; it was treated by detorsion and orchiopexy (Soccorso et al. 2010).

Bell Clapper Deformity

Surgical anatomy was described in 25 patients, mean age 15 years (12–23), with unilateral testicular torsion and contralateral orchiopexy. Of all 50 testes, 40 (80 %) had bell clapper deformity, 8 (16 %) had a long mesorchium between the epididymis and testis, and 2 (4 %) had normal anatomy, both on the contralateral side (Favorito et al. 2004).

Testicular Prosthesis

One study reported successful testicular prosthesis placement at the time of orchiectomy for torsion.

One prospective study demonstrated no evidence of infection or extrusion in 12 consecutive adolescents who underwent placement of a saline-filled testicular prosthesis within the tunica vaginalis at the time of orchiectomy for torsion, despite scrotal reaction in all patients (Bush and Bagrodia 2012).

In the study typically referenced to justify delayed prosthesis placement, a survey study of 488 urologists who were asked to recall the number of complications they encountered after testicular prosthesis placement reported complications in 87 (16 %) of 527 patients who had prostheses secondary to testicular torsion. While the authors concluded this complication rate was greater in patients with torsion due to the underlying inflammatory process, these data are subject to recall bias (Marshall 1986).

Recurrent Torsion After Orchiopexy

Torsion despite orchiopexy has been reported in both detorsed and contralateral testes, after orchiopexy using either absorbable or nonabsorbable sutures.

A literature review reported 20 cases of recurrent torsion in patients with median age of 16 years (10–24) that occurred at a median of 15 months (4–72) after initial orchiopexy. Twelve of 20 developed in the contralateral pexed testis. Suture material used was stated in 17 case reports; 15 were absorbable (catgut, polyglactin), and the others were polypropylene and silk. Suture placement was only reported by five, ranging from a single stitch to four stitches (Sells et al. 2002).

A retrospective review of testis torsion cases operated between 1991 and 2003 identified 179 patients, mean age 18 years (neonates-45 years), of which 8 had recurrent torsion at mean age 18 years (12–30) and 6 months to 23 years after initial surgery. The method of orchiopexy changed during this time: the first three cases had fixation of tunica albuginea to dartos with two stitches medially and two stitches laterally using catgut; the next four cases used the same method, but substituted polyglactin; the final case occurred after three sutures of polypropylene (Mor et al. 2006).

A survey of pediatric surgeons in the UK elicited response from 83 %; a total of 95 completed the questionnaire. Fourteen (15 %) used sutureless fixation in a dartos pouch. The remainder used suture fixation alone ($n=51$, 54 %) or in combination with a dartos pouch or Jaboulay procedure ($n=30$, 32 %). Of the 51 using suture fixation alone, 30 used nonabsorbable and 21 absorbable suture. Four of 95 (4 %) did not pex the contralateral testis (Bolln et al. 2006).

Infertility After Torsion

Few studies report semen parameters in men after testicular torsion. Our review of four studies included 97 patients, with oligospermia reported in 0–35 %.

Antisperm antibodies were tested in 80 patients in three studies, with only 2.5 % positive results.

One study with 16 patients reported elevated baseline and stimulated LH and FSH levels in torsion patients, whereas another with 28 patients found elevated FSH only in 9 with torsion symptoms >24 h before surgery.

Biopsy of the contralateral testis reported for 51 patients in two studies was reported as abnormal in 47.

Semen Analysis/Sperm Antibodies

Fifty-one cases of prepubertal testis torsion with a "nonviable testis" replaced in the scrotum from 1960 to 1982 included 26 older than age 18 years at the time of study. Of these 26, 18 operated at a mean age 10 years (2–13) agreed to participate: 5 had proven fertility (married with children) and the remaining 13 were unmarried without reported fertility. Testicular volume on the affected side was 0–1 mL in all 18. Semen analysis (one sample following 3 days abstinence) found 3/13 (23 %) with oligospermia <20 million/mL, and no case with antisperm antibodies by IgG and IgA specific mixed agglutination reaction testing (Puri et al. 1985).

Thirty-five patients with testicular torsion between 1985 and 1990 were identified from chart review; 16 agreed to undergo fertility evaluation. Ten controls were randomly selected from a pool of semen donors with known fertility. A single semen analysis was obtained in 14/16 patients and all controls. Of patients, nine had detorsion with bilateral orchiopexy (with testicular atrophy to length <1 cm in 2), and seven had orchiectomy; mean age at surgery was 18 and 20 years for these two groups, and follow-up evaluation was done approximately 3 years later. Mean duration of torsion was 13 h in the detorsion group versus 69 h in the orchiectomy patients. Mean sperm density was 132 million/mL in controls, 117 million/mL in orchiopexy patients, and 29 million/mL following orchiectomy. One patient after orchiopexy had borderline density of 20 million/mL, versus three orchiectomy patients with <20 million/mL. There were no differences in motility or morphology among the three groups, and antisperm antibody testing done in 12/16 patients was negative (Anderson et al. 1992).

Of 48 potentially eligible patients treated for torsion and now with age >16 years, 24 agreed to further testing at age averaging 21–25 years, and were compared to a control group of 20 men for vasectomy (age not stated). One semen analysis was done after 2–4 days of abstinence. Nine patients had orchiopexy after mean 7 h ischemia, and 15 had orchiectomy with mean ischemia time of 48 h, $p=0.001$. Mean sperm density was similar in orchiopexy and orchiectomy patients and controls, although 3/9 and 3/15 patients had oligospermia. Mean motility was normal for patients and controls, while morphology was abnormal in both patients and controls. Antisperm antibodies were analyzed using Immunobead seminal assay with no significant differences in patients and controls (Arap et al. 2007).

Fifty-five patients out of a total of 123 with testicular torsion between 1971 and 1986 were contacted and agreed to the study. Mean age at torsion was 21.5 years (12–27), and management was detorsion in 44 and orchiectomy in 11. Duration of symptoms before surgery was <2 h in 11 and 2–6 h in 29 who all had detorsion, >6 h in 9, 4 with detorsion, and >12 h in 6 who all had orchiectomy. All 55 had two semen analyses 2–8 years later, reported only by WHO criteria as normal in 7, OAT (oligospermia, asthenospermia, and teratospermia) in 19, and apparently isolated decreased motility in 10 and increased abnormal forms in another 19. Serum from 36 patients was tested at the time of torsion for sperm antibody testing; 2 had positive results, with titers >1:1,064. Repeat testing 2–8 years later in these patients show no sperm antibodies in these two patients, but new evidence for antibodies in another two (Hagen et al. 1992).

Fifty-two men, mean age 23 years (17–46), with past history of testis torsion agreed to further evaluation 4–10 years later, which included semen analysis in 13 (selection for these not stated). Of these 13, the only 2 with abnormal results also had a history of surgery for undescended testis. Sperm density in the other 11 ranged from 27 to 150 million/mL (Daehlin et al. 1996).

Hormonal Assays

In the evaluation by Anderson et al. (1992) mentioned above, mean baseline and stimulated FSH levels were significantly different and highest in orchiectomy and intermediate in orchiopexy patients versus controls. Mean baseline and stimulated LH levels were significantly elevated in orchiectomy versus orchiopexy patients and controls. There was no difference in baseline or stimulated T levels between these three groups.

The report by Daehlin et al. (1996) above reported mean FSH levels significantly higher in the 9 patients with symptom duration >24 h (8.3 IU/l [5.9–10.4]) versus the 19 with symptoms <8 h (3.1 IU/l [2.4–3.6]). There were no differences in mean LH, T, or prolactin levels.

Contralateral Testis Biopsy

Contralateral testis biopsy was obtained in 34 of the 55 patients in the study by Hagen et al. (1992) mentioned above. Of these, 30/34 (88 %) were described as abnormal with "desquamated germinal epithelium and Leydig cell atrophy."

Seventeen patients, mean age 20 years (14–34), had contralateral testis biopsy during surgery for ipsilateral testis torsion after symptoms a mean of 4 ± 3 h (0.5–11). "Controls" comprised three men (age not stated) with biopsy for suspected infertility declared "in retrospect to be normal." Specimens were studied for apoptosis, found to be increased in all patients and especially impacting spermatocytes, spermatids, and Sertoli cells, but not spermatogonia and, less often, Leydig cells (Hadziselimovic et al. 1998).

Psychologic Impact of Unilateral Orchiectomy

Our review found no study concerning the psychological impact of orchiectomy in adolescents.

Intermittent Torsion

Three retrospective studies were reviewed that reported orchiopexy for acute, episodic testicular pain diagnosed as intermittent torsion. One study reported that 10 % developed acute torsion while waiting for surgery, but it did not state the interval.

Due to the retrospective nature of chart review identifying surgical patients, boys similarly diagnosed who did not undergo surgery were not included. Therefore, risk for torsion and the natural history of non-operated intermittent torsion are not known.

Two studies reported anatomy in at least some patients, with 85–100 % bell clapper deformity affecting the ipsilateral testis and 80–90 % affecting the contralateral testes.

Pain resolution was reported for nearly all patients with follow-up.

A retrospective review of 30 patients seen from 1973 to 1982 with episodic pain thought to be due to intermittent testicular torsion noted that 3 (10 %) developed acute torsion while awaiting elective orchiopexy (duration of waiting in these and the other 27 patients was not stated) (Creagh et al. 1988).

A retrospective review searched for patients with history of acute, episodic pain who had orchiopexy. During an 8-year period ending in 2003, there were 50 patients, mean age 12 years (4–17), with mean four episodes (1–30) before pexy. Nausea/vomiting occurred in 12 (24 %), and a horizontal testicular lie in 21 (42 %). Anatomy was described in 28 cases—24 with ipsilateral bell-clapper deformity that was bilateral in 22. Follow-up in 38 patients at a mean of

9 months (1–60) found persistent pain in 1 (3 %) (Eaton et al. 2005).

Another retrospective review of an 18-year period ending in 2006 found 17 patients, mean age 14 years, who were operated for acute testicular torsion and gave a history of a mean three prior pain episodes (51 with torsion but no prior pain episodes excluded), and another 30, mean age 12 years, with a mean of two pain episodes who had elective orchiopexy. Of the 30 with intermittent torsion, 18 were prepubertal and none had an apparent transverse testicular lie, while 6 of 12 pubertal adolescents were described as having this finding. Bell clapper deformity was reported in all torsed testes, 15/17 contralateral testes, all intermittently symptomatic testes, and 27/30 contralateral testes. Of the 17 needing emergent surgery, 6 had orchiectomy and 2 of the 12 with orchiopexy had subsequent atrophy versus no atrophy in the elective orchiopexy group. At mean follow-up at 4 months, no patient with intermittent torsion had recurrent pain (Hayn et al. 2008).

Surgery Versus Conservative Management of Torsed Appendages

Our review found no study regarding duration or intensity of pain comparing surgery to remove a torsed appendage versus nonoperative management.

References

Al-Hunayan AA, Hanafy AM, Kehinde EO, Al-Awadi KA, Ali YM, Al-Twheed AR, et al. Testicular torsion: a perspective from the Middle East. Med Princ Pract. 2004;13(5):255–9.

Anderson MJ, Dunn JK, Lipshultz LI, Coburn M. Semen quality and endocrine parameters after acute testicular torsion. J Urol. 1992;147(6):1545–50.

Arap MA, Vicentini FC, Cocuzza M, Hallak J, Athayde K, Lucon AM, et al. Late hormonal levels, semen parameters, and presence of antisperm antibodies in patients treated for testicular torsion. J Androl. 2007;28(4):528–32.

Arda IS, Ozyaylali I. Testicular tissue bleeding as an indicator of gonadal salvageability in testicular torsion surgery. BJU Int. 2001;87(1):89–92.

Baker LA, Sigman D, Mathews RI, Benson J, Docimo SG. An analysis of clinical outcomes using color Doppler testicular ultrasound for testicular torsion. Pediatrics. 2000;105(3 Pt 1):604–7.

Baker L. Feasibility of transscrotal near-infrared spectroscopy (NIRS) in the evaluation of acute scrotum: a pilot human study. American Urological Association Annual Meeting, Washington, DC, 2011.

Barbosa JA, Tiseo B, Barayan GA, Rosman BM, Torricelli F, Passerotti CC, et al. Development and initial validation of a scoring system for diagnosing testicular torsion in children. J Urol. 2012. http://dx.doi.org/10.1016/j.juro.2012.10.056.

Bayne AP, Madden-Fuentes RJ, Jones EA, Cisek LJ, Gonzales Jr ET, Reavis KM, et al. Factors associated with delayed treatment of acute testicular torsion-do demographics or interhospital transfer matter? J Urol. 2010;184 Suppl 4Suppl 4:1743–7.

Beni-Israel T, Goldman M, Bar Chaim S, Kozer E. Clinical predictors for testicular torsion as seen in the pediatric ED. Am J Emerg Med. 2010;28(7):786–9.

Boettcher M, Bergholz R, Krebs TF, Wenke K, Aronson DC. Clinical predictors of testicular torsion in children. Urology. 2012;79(3):670–4.

Bolln C, Driver CP, Youngson GG. Operative management of testicular torsion: current practice within the UK and Ireland. J Pediatr Urol. 2006;2(3):190–3.

Brandt MT, Sheldon CA, Wacksman J, Matthews P. Prenatal testicular torsion: principles of management. J Urol. 1992;147(3):670–2.

Bush N, Bagrodia A. Initial results for combined orchiectomy and prosthesis exchange for unsalvageable testicular torsion in adolescents: description of intravaginal prosthesis placement at orchiectomy. J Urol. 2012;188 Suppl 4Suppl 4:1424–8.

Ciftci AO, Senocak ME, Tanyel FC, Buyukpamukcu N. Clinical predictors for differential diagnosis of acute scrotum. Eur J Pediatr Surg. 2004;14(5):333–8.

Cimador M, DiPace MR, Castagnetti M, DeGrazia E. Predictors of testicular viability in testicular torsion. J Pediatr Urol. 2007;3(5):387–90.

Cornel EB, Karthaus HF. Manual derotation of the twisted spermatic cord. BJU Int. 1999;83(6):672–4.

Creagh TA, McDermott TE, McLean PA, Walsh A. Intermittent torsion of the testis. BMJ (Clin Res Ed). 1988;297(6647):525–6.

Daehlin L, Ulstein M, Thorsen T, Hoisaeter PA. Follow-up after torsion of the spermatic cord. Scand J Urol Nephrol. 1996;179:139–42.

Eaton SH, Cendron MA, Estrada CR, Bauer SB, Borer JG, Cilento BG, et al. Intermittent testicular torsion: diagnostic features and management outcomes. J Urol. 2005;174(4 Pt 2):1532–5. discussion 5.

Favorito LA, Cavalcante AG, Costa WS. Anatomic aspects of epididymis and tunica vaginalis in patients with testicular torsion. Int Braz J Urol. 2004;30(5):420–4.

Figueroa V, Pippi Salle JL, Braga LH, Romao R, Koyle MA, Bagli D, et al. Comparative analysis of detorsion alone versus detorsion and tunica albuginea

decompression (fasciotomy) with tunica vaginalis flap coverage in the surgical management of prolonged testicular ischemia. J Urol. 2012;188 Suppl 4Suppl 4:1417–23.
Gunther P, Schenk JP, Wunsch R, Holland-Cunz S, Kessler U, Troger J, et al. Acute testicular torsion in children: the role of sonography in the diagnostic workup. Eur Radiol. 2006;16(11):2527–32.
Hadziselimovic F, Geneto R, Emmons LR. Increased apoptosis in the contralateral testes of patients with testicular torsion as a factor for infertility. J Urol. 1998;160(3 Pt 2):1158–60.
Hagen P, Buchholz MM, Eigenmann J, Bandhauer K. Testicular dysplasia causing disturbance of spermiogenesis in patients with unilateral torsion of the testis. Urol Int. 1992;49(3):154–7.
Hayn MH, Herz DB, Bellinger MF, Schneck FX. Intermittent torsion of the spermatic cord portends an increased risk of acute testicular infarction. J Urol. 2008;180 Suppl 4Suppl 4:1729–32.
Hegarty PK, Walsh E, Corcoran MO. Exploration of the acute scrotum: a retrospective analysis of 100 consecutive cases. Ir J Med Sci. 2001;170(3):181–2.
Jefferson RH, Perez LM, Joseph DB. Critical analysis of the clinical presentation of acute scrotum: a 9-year experience at a single institution. J Urol. 1997;158(3 Pt 2):1198–200.
John CM, Kooner G, Mathew DE, Ahmed S, Kenny SE. Neonatal testicular torsion—a lost cause? Acta Paediatr. 2008;97(4):502–4.
Kadish HA, Bolte RG. A retrospective review of pediatric patients with epididymitis, testicular torsion, and torsion of testicular appendages. Pediatrics. 1998;102(1 Pt 1):73–6.
Kalfa N, Veyrac C, Lopez M, Lopez C, Maurel A, Kaselas C, et al. Multicenter assessment of ultrasound of the spermatic cord in children with acute scrotum. J Urol. 2007;177(1):297–301. discussion.
Karmazyn B, Steinberg R, Kornreich L, Freud E, Grozovski S, Schwarz M, et al. Clinical and sonographic criteria of acute scrotum in children: a retrospective study of 172 boys. Pediatr Radiol. 2005; 35(3):302–10.
Kaye JD, Levitt SB, Friedman SC, Franco I, Gitlin J, Palmer LS. Neonatal torsion: a 14-year experience and proposed algorithm for management. J Urol. 2008a;179(6):2377–83.
Kaye JD, Shapiro EY, Levitt SB, Friedman SC, Gitlin J, Freyle J, et al. Parenchymal echo texture predicts testicular salvage after torsion: potential impact on the need for emergent exploration. J Urol. 2008b;180 Suppl 4Suppl 4:1733–6.
Makela E, Lahdes-Vasama T, Rajakorpi H, Wikstrom S. A 19-year review of paediatric patients with acute scrotum. Scand J Surg. 2007;96(1):62–6.
Marshall S. Potential problems with testicular prostheses. Urology. 1986;28(5):388–90.
Middleton WD, Middleton MA, Dierks M, Keetch D, Dierks S. Sonographic prediction of viability in testicular torsion: preliminary observations. J Ultrasound Med. 1997;16(1):23–7. quiz 9–30.
Molokwu CN, Somani BK, Goodman CM. Outcomes of scrotal exploration for acute scrotal pain suspicious of testicular torsion: a consecutive case series of 173 patients. BJU Int. 2011;107(6):990–3.
Mor Y, Pinthus JH, Nadu A, Raviv G, Golomb J, Winkler H, et al. Testicular fixation following torsion of the spermatic cord—does it guarantee prevention of recurrent torsion events? J Urol. 2006;175(1):171–3. discussion 3–4.
Murphy FL, Fletcher L, Pease P. Early scrotal exploration in all cases is the investigation and intervention of choice in the acute paediatric scrotum. Pediatr Surg Int. 2006;22(5):413–6.
Nandi B, Murphy FL. Neonatal testicular torsion: a systematic literature review. Pediatr Surg Int. 2011; 27(10):1037–40.
Pinto KJ, Noe HN, Jerkins GR. Management of neonatal testicular torsion. J Urol. 1997;158(3 Pt 2):1196–7.
Puri P, Barton D, O'Donnell B. Prepubertal testicular torsion: subsequent fertility. J Pediatr Surg. 1985;20(6):598–601.
Sells H, Moretti KL, Burfield GD. Recurrent torsion after previous testicular fixation. ANZ J Surg. 2002; 72(1):46–8.
Sessions AE, Rabinowitz R, Hulbert WC, Goldstein MM, Mevorach RA. Testicular torsion: direction, degree, duration and disinformation. J Urol. 2003;169(2):663–5.
Soccorso G, Ninan GK, Rajimwale A, Nour S. Acute scrotum: is scrotal exploration the best management? Eur J Pediatr Surg. 2010;20(5):312–5.
Srinivasan A, Cinman N, Feber KM, Gitlin J, Palmer LS. History and physical examination findings predictive of testicular torsion: an attempt to promote clinical diagnosis by house staff. J Pediatr Urol. 2011;7(4):470–4.
Waldert M, Klatte T, Schmidbauer J, Remzi M, Lackner J, Marberger M. Color Doppler sonography reliably identifies testicular torsion in boys. Urology. 2010;75(5):1170–4.
Yerkes EB, Robertson FM, Gitlin J, Kaefer M, Cain MP, Rink RC. Management of perinatal torsion: today, tomorrow or never? J Urol. 2005;174(4 Pt 2):1579–82. discussion 82–3.
Zinn HL, Cohen HL, Horowitz M. Testicular torsion in neonates: importance of power Doppler imaging. J Ultrasound Med. 1998;17(6):385–8.

8 Varicocele

Micah A. Jacobs

The primary reason to diagnose and treat varicoceles in adolescents is to prevent future infertility.

Secondary reasons:

1. **Relieve testicular pain.**
2. **Correct the abnormal appearance of the left scrotum with grade 3 varicoceles.**

Evidence for these aims:

- **Evidence that treatment of varicoceles in adolescents reduces or prevents adult infertility is lacking.**
- **Treatment recommendations currently are based on semen parameters and/or left testicular volume loss, variously described as >2 mL, >10 %, or >20 %.**
- **Most adolescents with varicoceles do not have decreased testicular volume compared to controls. Up to 50 % of those with decreased left testicular volume on initial assessment have been reported to have spontaneous improvement within 1–2 years of observation. Up to 33 % of those with initial volume differences <20 % are reported to develop volume discrepancy >20 % within 1–2 years.**
- **Relationship between any extent of volume difference between the left and right testis with impaired semen parameters is poorly established in both adolescents and adults with varicoceles.**
- **Use of >10 % or >20 % volume discrepancy as an indication for surgery is not based on known infertility risks.**
- **There are limited semen analysis data in adolescents with varicoceles, with two studies reporting normal sperm densities but decreased motility and normal morphology, and one reporting decreased sperm density but normal motility and morphology.**
- **Our review found only a single study involving 33 adolescents with preoperative and postoperative semen analysis that indicated improved sperm density and motility.**
- **Three retrospective studies reported pain relief from varicocelectomy in from 68 to 97 %.**
- **One retrospective study stated that 87 % of teens had resolution of the scrotal mass with varicocelectomy.**

Prevalence

Population based studies report varicocele occurs in <1 % of boys <10 years of age vs. 8–19 % of those aged 11–19 years.

Approximately 90 % are unilateral, and three studies found grade 3 to comprise ≤25 % of these.

A prospective, population based cross-sectional study on growth and development examined 6,200 white Bulgarian boys equally distributed into

M.A. Jacobs, M.D., M.P.H. (✉)
Department of Pediatric Urology, University of Texas Southwestern Medical Center and Children's Medical Center Dallas, 1935 Medical District Drive, MS F4.04, Dallas, TX 75235, USA
e-mail: micah.jacobs@childrens.com

W.T. Snodgrass (ed.), *Pediatric Urology: Evidence for Optimal Patient Management*, DOI 10.1007/978-1-4614-6910-0_8,

20 age groups from <1 year to 19 years. All were healthy and were examined by a single physician. Diagnosis of varicocele was made by palpation, and Tanner stage was recorded. Prevalence of varicocele was 4 % overall, 0.2 % in boys <10 years, and 8 % in those >10 years. Prevalence significantly increased between Tanner stages until stage 3 and then remained constant. All were left-sided (grade not stated) (Kumanov et al. 2008).

Another prospective, population-based cross-sectional study involved examination for varicocele by two urologists in 1,938 Korean boys aged 13–16 years. A varicocele was diagnosed in 320 (16.5 %), left-sided in 303 (95 %), and bilateral in 17. Unilateral left varicoceles were grade 1 in 51 %, grade 2 in 27 %, and grade 3 in 25 %. The right varicocele in boys with bilateral findings was grade 1 or 2 in all cases (Baek et al. 2011).

In another prospective population-based study, 4,052 Turkish boys aged 2–19 years were examined by two urologists who reported varicocele in 293 (7 %), <1 % in boys <10 years of age, and 14 % in those ages 15–19. Of these, 1 was only on the right, while 30 were bilateral. All varicoceles in boys <10 years were grades 1 and 2, as were all bilateral varicoceles; in 249 boys >10 years with unilateral varicocele, grades were 1 in 92 (35 %), grade 2 in 112 (45 %), and grade 3 in 45 (18 %) (Akbay et al. 2000).

Examination in 3,186 Italian boys, mean age 13 ± 1.6 years, a varicocele was diagnosed in 609 (19 %), which were grade 1 in 332 (54.5 %), grade 2 in 143 (23 %), and grade 3 in 134 (22 %) (Zampieri and Cervellione 2008).

Assessing Testicular Size

Animal and human studies directly determining testicular volume after orchiectomy indicate that US using Lambert's formula ($L \times W \times H \times 0.71$) best correlates with true volume.

One clinical study found no difference in volume determined by orchidometry vs. US, while two others reported that orchidometry overestimates testicular volume.

A prospective study evaluated 159 consecutive men presenting for infertility using both an orchidometer and US (Lambert's formula). Mean right testicular volume was 18 ± 6 cc by orchidometer vs. 18 ± 9 cc by US, $p = 0.5$; mean left testicular volume was 17 ± 6 cc and 17 ± 8 cc, $p = 0.8$ (Schiff et al. 2004).

Testicular volume was also determined using Prader orchidometers vs. US (5 and 7.5-MHz transducers and Lambert's formula) in 469 men with infertility. Orchidometry overestimated US volumes by approximately 5 ± 3.7 cc, corresponding to a mean percent difference of 46 % ± 40 % and 54 % ± 45 % for the right and left testes. However, differences decreased as US-measured volume increased, such that there was a strong correlation between orchidometry and US ($r = 0.7$ on right and $r = 0.746$ on the left) (Sakamoto et al. 2007a).

Another study compared the Prader and Rochester orchidometers and US to determine volume discrepancies of 10, 15, 20, and 25 % in 65 males aged 7–24 years old. Considering US volume to be most accurate, orchidometry overestimated volume a significant 6 cc. Still considering US to be most accurate, neither orchidometers correlated well to define volume discrepancies (Diamond et al. 2000).

Testicular volume was determined in nine dogs using Prader and Rochester orchidometers and US using two transducers (6–13 MHz and 5–10 MHz). Three formulas to calculate volume from US measurements were compared (formula for an ellipsoid, for a prolate spheroid, and Lambert's formula). Bilateral orchiectomy was done, and the testes were weighed. In this study, true volume was considered weight/density, with density approximately 1.04 g/mL derived from prior studies in humans and dogs. Regression analysis showed US had a stronger linear relationship to true volume than either orchidometers, both of which overestimated volume. Lambert's formula ($L \times W \times H \times 0.71$) best approximated true volume with both US transducers, although there was no significant difference between the three formulas tested (Paltiel et al. 2002).

These methods were then used in a study of human adult testes removed for androgen ablation with true volume determined by water displacement. Again, US volumes calculated by any of the three formulas were more accurate than either of the orchidometers, and Lambert's formula best approximated true volume (Sakamoto et al. 2007b).

Prevalence of Testicular Volume Discrepancy

Two population-based studies reported that most adolescents with varicoceles do not have a left testicular volume discrepancy, defined as >2 mL and/or >10 % difference compared to the right testis.

One reported volume difference by varicocele grade: 4 % without varicocele, 12 % with grade 1, 27.5 % with grade 2, and 37.5 % with grade 3.

Two population-based studies compared testicular volume in varicocele patients vs. boys without varicoceles. One found no differences for either mean left or right testis volume. The other reported that boys with varicoceles had normal mean right testicular volume but decreased left mean volume beginning at age 14 and persisting through age 19 years (end of study period).

The prospective cross-sectional examination of 6,200 Bulgarian boys aged 0–19 years mentioned above measured testicular size using Prader orchidometers. All varicoceles were left-sided, and mean left testicular volume was decreased compared to normal boys beginning at age 14 and remaining less through age 19 years (end of study). Mean right testicular volume was the same in teens with varicocele vs. non-varicocele teens (Kumanov et al. 2008).

The prospective cross-sectional examination of 1,938 Korean boys described above also used Prader orchidometers but found no significant differences in either mean left or right testicular volumes between 486 (which would be ≥13 % in their data), the left testicle was smaller in 4 % without varicocele, 12 % with grade 1, 27.5 % with grade 2, and 37.5 % with grade 3 varicoceles (OR 3, 7, and 9, respectively) (Baek et al. 2011).

The prospective evaluation of 4,052 Turkish boys referenced above found a total of 293 (7 %) had a varicocele. Examination was performed by two urologists, determined testicular volume using Prader orchidometers, with a volume discrepancy defined as >2 mL or >10 %. None of the 14 boys less than 10 years of age with a varicocele had testicular size discrepancy, whereas 24 (10 %) of 249 boys >10 years of age with unilateral varicocele did (Akbay et al. 2000).

Semen Analysis

There are few semen analysis data in adolescents with varicocele.

One study found decreased sperm density and motility, but mean values were still within WHO guidelines for fertility. Two studies reported no difference in sperm concentration, but decreased percent motility and normal morphology in varicocele patients vs. controls.

One matched cohort study reported mean left testicular volume significantly decreased vs. controls. Mean sperm density was similar, while percent motility and normal morphology were reduced in patients.

One retrospective review with 15 varicocele patients found decreased sperm density in half the boys with <10 % left testicular volume discrepancy and all those with volume discrepancy >20 %, but normal motility and morphology.

Our review found no other studies that correlated semen analysis with testicular volume.

As discussed below, correlation of infertility with testicular volume discrepancy of any extent is poorly established in adult males with varicoceles.

A prospective study included 360 adolescents, mean age 15.7 ± 0.8 years, of which there were 100 with grade 2 ($n = 72$) or grade 3 ($n = 28$) varicoceles. Tanner stage for the 360 was 5 in 66 % and 4 in 31 %. Testicular volume was determined by orchidometers, and semen samples (number not stated) were obtained in 227. Findings on semen analysis were as follows:

Mean sperm density was significantly less in those with grades 2 and 3 varicoceles:

- No/grade 1: 88 ± 76 million/mL
- Grade 2: 50 ± 52 million/mL,
- Grade 3: 37 ± 41 million/mL, $p = 0.003$

Percent motility was also reduced in grades 2 and 3 varicoceles, but values were still above WHO fertility standards.

Normal morphology was not reduced.

Testicular volume discrepancy was defined as >10 %, and diagnosed in 42 % with grade 2 and 52 % with grade 3 varicoceles vs. 11 % in those without varicocele. Semen analysis in those with grades 2 and 3 varicoceles, with and without 10 % testicular volume difference, was not reported (Mori et al. 2008).

A cross-sectional study of 2,100 boys aged 10–20 years old identified those with a varicocele and selected 38 boys aged 17–19 years and Tanner stage 5 with grades 2 or 3 left varicocele, comparing them to 36 similar boys without varicocele. Testicular volume was determined by US, and all provided two semen samples with the following results:

- Mean right testicular volume was similar between controls and patients (18.7 ± 5 cc vs. 17.4 ± 4.6 cc).
- Mean left testicular volume was significantly less in patients (18.3 ± 4.5 cc vs. 14.4 ± 4.3 cc, $p = 0.01$).
- Sperm density was similar in controls vs. patients (55.7 ± 36 million/mL vs. 52.9 ± 30.6 million/mL).
- Percent motility and normal morphology were less in patients (Paduch and Niedzielski 1996).

Another retrospective review compared semen analyses in 31 adolescents, 14–20 years old, with left varicocele grade 1 in 8 (26 %), grade 2 in 15 (48 %), and grade 3 in 8 (26 %) to semen analyses in control men, mean age 34 years, who fathered a child within 1 year and had no varicocele, and to infertile men, mean age 32 years, with left varicocele:

- Sperm concentration was not significantly different between groups; adolescents with varicoceles having mean 63 ± 60 million/mL.
- Both motility and normal morphology were reduced in adolescents with varicocele compared to controls.
- There were no differences in semen parameters between adolescents with varicocele and adults with varicocele and infertility (Andrade-Rocha 2007).

A retrospective review compared ten adolescents with left varicocele and no testicular volume discrepancy by US to five with volume difference >20 %. Mean age was similar at 15 years (12–17), and all had grade 2 or 3 varicoceles. Differential testicular volume was 7 % (0–17) in those defined as without asymmetry vs. 30 % (20–61) in the five with asymmetry. A single semen specimen was obtained in all patients. Mean concentration in boys with testicular volume difference <20 % was 26 million/mL vs. 3 million/mL in those with >20 %, $p = 0.04$, whereas mean percent forward motility and percent normal morphology were not significantly different. Furthermore, 5/10 with <20 % volume difference had semen parameters (density and forward motility) below normal WHO adult criteria, as did all those with >20 % testicular volume difference (Keene et al. 2012).

Natural History of Testicular Growth

Testicular volume changes during pubertal growth, and patients with varicoceles potentially can spontaneously resolve left volume discrepancy observed at initial evaluation, or develop volume discrepancy not initially present.

One prospective and two retrospective reviews reported 25–50 % of left testes with volume discrepancy >10–20 % had improvement to <10–20 % within 12–24 months.

Development of volume discrepancy >20 % occurred in 9 % of 559 boys at mean time of 29 months in one observational study. Several retrospective studies reported 0–33 % of patients with volume discrepancy <20 % progressed to >20 % during 12–24 months.

One retrospective study reported outcomes in 19 adolescents with grade 1 varicoceles, of which 8 developed >20 % volume discrepancy during 4 years follow-up despite stable varicocele grade in 6.

Spontaneous Resolution of Testicular Size Discrepancy

One prospective study allocated 27 adolescents, median age 14.5 years (7–16), with left varicocele and US-measured testicular volume discrepancy >20 % to observation for 12 months. Eight (30 %) resolved to <20 % (Spinelli et al. 2010).

One retrospective review of 543 varicocele patients managed between 1994 and 2008 identified 181 at median age 14 years (range not stated) who were observed after initial diagnosis and had at least one follow-up measurement of testicular volume (most the others apparently had surgery). Measurements were performed by US in 143 and orchidometer in 38. Median time between initial and final examination was 12 months (interquartile range 8–21).

At initial examination, 54 (30 %) had discrepancy <10 %, 61 (34 %) had asymmetry of 10–20 %, and 66 (36 %) had >20 % volume discrepancy. At final measurement, 59 (33 %) had less than 10 % volume difference, representing no change in 27, reduction from 10 to 20 % in 20, and improvement from >20 % in 12.

Therefore, at a median follow-up of 12 months, decrease in volume discrepancy from >10 to <10 % occurred in 32/127 (25 %). Of the 66 with initial volume discrepancy >20 %, 31 (47 %) had <20 % at median 12 months reexamination (Poon et al. 2010).

Another retrospective study identified 33 patients at median age 13 years (9–16) with a varicocele that was grade 1 in 1, grade 2 in 11, and grade 3 in 21. Of these, 14 had volume discrepancy >20 % by US at diagnosis, of which 7 (50 %) had improvement to <20 % asymmetry during observation a median of 2 years (0.5–5) (Preston et al. 2008).

Development of Size Discrepancy During Observation

A longitudinal observational study enrolled 609 patients found during school screening with varicocele, grade 1 in 332 (54.5 %), grade 2 in 143 (23 %), and grade 3 in 134 (22 %). Of these, 40 (7 %) had >20 % volume discrepancy at initial diagnosis and underwent surgery. Follow-up occurred in 559 observed for <20 % testicular asymmetry on initial measurement, with 52 (9 %) developing >20 % volume discrepancy at a mean of 29 ± 3 months, occurring only in those with grades 2 and 3 (Zampieri and Cervellione 2008).

The retrospective review by Poon et al. (2010) mentioned above performed a follow-up examination at a median 12 months after the initial assessment and found that progression to >20 % size discrepancy occurred in 37/115 (32 %), comprising 17 (31 %) of 54 with <10 % discrepancy originally and 20 (33 %) of 61 with initial asymmetry 10–20 %.

A retrospective chart review identified 117 patients with varicocele presenting at mean age 13 years (7–18). Testicular volume discrepancy was defined as ≥15 % difference with measurement using calipers, and was found initially in 10/33 (30 %) patients with grade 2 and 38/84 (45 %) with grade 3. Of the remaining 69, volume discrepancy developed in 12/50 (24 %) with follow-up at a mean of 14 months (5–22), occurring in 3/16 (19 %) patients with grade 2 and 9/34 (26 %) with grade 3 (Thomas and Elder 2002).

Another retrospective review analyzed 89 adolescents, mean age 14 ± 2.7 years, with grades 1–3 left varicocele and <15 % testicular volume discrepancy by US or orchidometry, who were observed for a median 27 months (range not stated). Fifty-two (58 %) remained with <15 % volume difference, and 37 progressed—13 (15 %) to difference of 15–19 % and 24 (27 %) to >20 % (Korets et al. 2011).

In another retrospective review, 11 of 33 patients with varicocele diagnosed at median age 13 years (9–16) had initial testicular volume difference <20 %. During follow-up, a median of 2 years (0.5–5), none progressed to >20 % (Preston et al. 2008).

A retrospective review identified 21 adolescents, mean age 12.5 ± 0.4 years, with grade 1 left varicocele who were observed 4.8 ± 0.3 years. Two of these had testicular volume discrepancy >10 % determined by orchidometry. Of these varicoceles, 4 (19 %) resolved, 13 (62 %) remained stable, and 4 (19 %) progressed to grade 2. Of the 19 initially symmetric testes, 8 (42 %) developed volume difference >10 %, 2 of the 4 with progression to grade 2 and 6 with stable grade 1 varicocele (Shiraishi et al. 2009).

Varicoceles and Fertility in Adults

According to the Centers for Disease Control, approximately one-third of men with male factor infertility have a varicocele.

Infertile men with varicocele have been reported to have decreased left testicular volume in some retrospective reviews but not in others.

A WHO study reported that mean left testicular volume was significantly less than mean right volume in men with varicoceles, but still one-third of men with varicoceles had normal semen analysis.

A retrospective report of 611 infertile men with unilateral varicocele found 50 % had left testicular hypotrophy >3 mL, but mean motile sperm density was normal at 80 million/mL.

One report indicated total testicular volume (right + left testicular volume) < 30 cc correlated with diminished sperm density in infertile men.

One study found significant postoperative increased left testicular volume in men at a mean age 26 years, which would indicate that "catch-up" growth may not be restricted to adolescents.

Cochrane review of eight RCTs involving varicocele intervention for subfertility reported no benefit.

One subsequent RCT found infertile varicocelectomy patients had improved postoperative semen parameters and significantly greater spontaneous pregnancy rates compared to non-operated infertile men with varicocele.

Varicocele Prevalence in Infertile Men

The Division of Reproductive Health of the Centers for Disease Control and Prevention analyzed data from the 2002 National Survey of Family Growth, in which 4,109 sexually active men were questioned using structured interviews regarding infertility. A total of 308 (7.5 %) reported at least one physician visit for infertility, of which 18 % (95 % CI 12.9–24.8) were diagnosed with a male factor problem. Of those with a diagnosis, 6 % (95 % CI 2.6–13) had a varicocele (Anderson et al. 2009).

Prevalence of Testicular Size Discrepancy

Nine-thousand thirty-eight men reporting infertility of at least 12 months' duration who presented to 34 centers worldwide underwent standardized evaluation that included testicular volume measurement using Prader orchidometers and two semen analyses:

- 3,468 men had a normal semen analysis, of which 396 (12 %) had a varicocele that was grade 2 in 174 and grade 3 in 80.
- 3,626 men had an abnormal semen analysis, of which 857 (24 %) had a varicocele that was grade 2 in 374 and grade 3 in 191.
- Men without varicocele had symmetric mean right and left testicular volumes (18.8 mL left and 19.0 mL right).
- Men with varicoceles had mean testicular volume significantly less than the right (18.5 mL left vs. 19.5 mL right, $p < 0.001$).

Total testicular volume was lower for each grade of varicocele, regardless of normal vs. abnormal semen analysis, and it was less in men with abnormal vs. normal semen analysis. However, of 1,253 men with varicoceles identified because of an infertility assessment, 32 % had normal semen analyses despite palpable/visible varicocele and decreased left testicular volume (WHO 1992).

Another study involved 43 men, mean age 26 years (17–40), with left varicocele (fertility status not stated) who had testicular measurements by US and semen analysis pre-and post-varicocelectomy at 1 year. There were 6 grade 1, 16 grade 2, and 21 grade 3 varicoceles, of which 2 were bilateral. The authors stated that "more than 60 %" had decreased left testicular volume compared to the right (data not shown), but there was a significant increase in mean left testicular volume post-varicocelectomy (13.4 ± 4.4 ccm [4–24] vs. 14 ± 4.5 ccm [4–25]). Similarly, sperm count significantly increased from 38 ± 33 million/mL (2–80) to 48 ± 34 million/mL (5–60) (Zucchi et al. 2006).

A retrospective review considered 79 fertile men with varicocele, 71 infertile men (>1 year duration) with varicoceles, and 217 fertile men without varicocele (unilateral vs. bilateral varicoceles, and varicocele grade were not stated). Both left and right mean testicular volumes were significantly less in infertile men with varicocele than in fertile men with or without varicocele (left testis infertile men 17.6±8.9 cc vs. fertile men with varicocele 21.6±7.8 cc and 23.4±8.3 cc without varicocele; right testis infertile men 18.7±8.3 cc vs. fertile men with varicocele 25.2±13 cc and 24.9±10.7 cc without varicocele). There was no significant difference in left or right testicular size in fertile men with vs. without a varicocele (Pasqualotto et al. 2005).

Another study compared 143 men with a left varicocele—123 with infertility vs. 20 that were fertile (means to select fertile men with varicocele were not stated). There was no significant difference in the prevalence of decreased left testicular volume at any reduction from 5 to 35 % (Sakamoto et al. 2008).

A retrospective study included 611 men, mean age 34 years (19–55), with infertility and unilateral varicocele. Left testicular hypotrophy was defined as volume discrepancy >3 mL by orchidometer, and was diagnosed in 305 (50 %). Semen analyses were "performed in the standard fashion" (number of studies per patient not stated). Mean total motile sperm counts were significantly less in patients with vs. without hypotrophy, but both were within normal range by WHO criteria, $80 \pm 5 \times 10^6$ in those with hypotrophy (Sigman and Jarow 1997).

A study determined testicular volume in 486 infertile Japanese males, median 33 years of age (23–51), using orchidometers and correlated global volume (right and left) with semen analysis (two samples collected after 3–7 days abstinence). Total testicular volume was categorized into ten groups ranging at 5-mL intervals from <10 mL to >50 mL. Median volume was 32 mL (5–60). Decreased sperm density occurred at volumes <30 mL, and decreased motility occurred at volumes <45 mL (Arai et al. 1998).

Fertility After Varicocele Surgery

A RCT randomized 145 married men with infertility for >1 year with palpable varicoceles and at least one abnormal semen parameter (concentration <20 million/mL, progressive motility <50 %, normal morphology <30 %) to either observation ($n=72$) or subinguinal microscopic varicocelectomy. Varicoceles were unilateral in 106 (73 %) and bilateral in 39, comprising grade 1 in approximately 40 %, grade 2 in 32 %, and grade 3 in 28 %. At follow-up of 12 months, spontaneous pregnancy occurred in 14 % observed vs. 33 % treated patients, OR 3.04 (95 % CI 1.33-6.95) with number needed to treat five patients (95 % CI 1.55–8.99). No changes in semen parameters from baseline were noted in observed patients, whereas the mean of all parameters improved significantly in operated patients (Abdel-Meguid et al. 2011).

Prior to this study, Cochrane review included eight RCTs, stating that one excluded men with sperm counts <5 million/mL and another at <2 million/mL, and three specifically concerned subclinical varicoceles. Pregnancy rates was the outcome, with pooled analysis demonstrating OR 1.10 (95 % CI 0.73–1.68), indicating varicocele treatment was no better than no treatment (Evers et al. 2009).

Varicocelectomy in Patients <18 Years of Age

Reported indications for varicocele therapy include testicular volume discrepancy, abnormal semen parameters, pain, and cosmesis.

One cohort study allocated adolescents with varicocele and testicular volume discrepancy >20 % to varicocelectomy vs. observation for 1 year, reporting left testicular growth to <20 % asymmetry in significantly more operated patients, 85 % vs. 30 %.

Retrograde sclerotherapy technically cannot be performed in from 10 to 20 % of cases due to the venous anatomy. Of those able to be sclerosed, varicocele resolution is reported in approximately 80–90 %. Scrotal pain, thought secondary to phlebitis from the sclerosing agent traveling distally to the pampiniform plexus, occurred in 7–15 % of treated patients. Recurrence was reported by two studies in 8 and 21 %.

Antegrade sclerotherapy **was described in three studies in adolescents, with only one patient in whom a vein could not be cannulated. Persistent varicocele was reported in 2 and 7 %.**

***Open* vs. *laparoscopic varicocelectomy* was reviewed by meta-analysis, finding a 5 % persistent varicocele rate and 9.5 % development of hydrocele that was not different between the two methods. Analysis reported that artery-sparing varicocelectomy had a greater risk for varicocele persistence than the Paloma technique, and that lymph-sparing reduced risk for hydroceles.**

Varicocelectomy vs. Observation

Fifty-four adolescents, median 14.5 years (7–16), with left varicocele and US-determined testicular volume discrepancy >20 % were divided into two cohorts with similar Tanner stage and age: varicocelectomy vs. observation for 12 months. "Catch-up growth" to <20 % volume difference occurred in 8/27 (30 %) observed patients vs. 23/27 (85 %) operated patients, $p<0.01$ (Spinelli et al. 2010).

Retrograde Sclerotherapy

A retrospective review identified 367 patients with 396 varicoceles and testicular size discrepancy (not defined) at mean age 13 years (4–25) who were all recommended for retrograde sclerotherapy. Vascular anomalies in 36 (10 %) and "technical problems" in 11 precluded this treatment, whereas open surgery was performed for other reasons in 42, leaving 251 patients (277 varicoceles) that had sclerotherapy. A single procedure was successful to resolve 220/277 (79 %) varicoceles. Painful scrotal swelling developed in 17/251 (7 %) patients; there was no mention of hydroceles (Mazzoni et al. 1999).

Another retrospective review identified 86 patients with left grades 2 or 3 varicoceles at mean age 13.8 years (11–16) who underwent venography; it was possible to perform retrograde sclerotherapy in 72 (84 %) but not in the remaining 14 owing to "unfavorable anatomic variants in the left spermatic vein." Of these 72, the initial attempt was successful in 64, and a second attempt was successful in 2 of 5 patients, for a total success rate of 66/86 (77 %). No sedation was used, and mean procedure time was 50 min (35–75). Pampiniform phlebitis occurred in 11/72 (15 %) injected patients, attributed to the sclerosing agent reaching the scrotal aspect of the varicocele and causing scrotal swelling and pain 12–24 h post procedure that lasted "a few days." At mean follow-up of 31 months, 5/66 (8 %) initially successful patients relapsed, 4 at 12 months and 1 at 24 months. Three of these had recanalization of the left internal spermatic vein and were re-sclerosed (Granata et al. 2008).

A retrospective review comprised 319 teen and adult patients with grades 2 and 3 left varicocele, treated for a variety of indications that included infertility with abnormal semen analysis in 9 %, left scrotal pain in 25 %, cosmetic in 33 %, and volume discrepancy >15 % in 31 %. Of these patients, retrograde sclerotherapy under local anesthesia was attempted in 126 (39 %) at median age 15.7 years (11–61), while others had laparoscopic varicocelectomy or antegrade sclerotherapy (selection for various therapies was not described). The procedure could not be performed in 25 (20 %) cases, due to venous spasm in 3, proximal collateral veins in 6, distal collateral veins (iliac/lumbar) in 3, and difficulty with cannulating and/or perforating the internal spermatic vein in 11. Median follow-up for the entire population was 69 months (6–122), with success defined as "disappearance" of the varicocele on physical examination first done postoperatively at 3–6 months. Outcomes for the 71 patients <19 years of age with retrograde sclerotherapy were separately reported: recurrence in 15 (21 %), hydrocele in 1, and "epididymoorchitis" (probably scrotal phlebitis) in 5 (7 %) (Beutner et al. 2007).

Antegrade Sclerotherapy

A prospective study evaluated antegrade sclerotherapy in 45 consecutive adolescents, median age 15 years (13–17), with left varicocele that was grade 1 in 4 (9 %), grade 2 in 18 (40 %), and grade 3 in 23 (51 %). No immediate complications from sclerotherapy were noted, and at follow-up at 6 and 12 months, 1 (2 %) had persistent varicocele (Ficarra et al. 2004).

A retrospective review involved 88 consecutive males, mean age 13 years (9–19), who underwent scrotal antegrade sclerotherapy, 46 for grade 2 and 42 for grade 3 varicocele. In one 10-year-old the procedure converted to Palomo varicocelectomy due to inability to isolate a suitable vein scrotally. Follow-up was available in 84 at mean of 11 months (3–60), and included US. Persistent varicocele was diagnosed in 6 (7 %), grade 2 in 4, and grade 3 in 2. No hydroceles developed (Zaupa et al. 2006).

Another retrospective study involved 38 adolescents at mean age 15 years (12–18) with grade 1 ($n=3$), grade 2 ($n=22$), and grade 3 ($n=13$) left varicoceles treated with antegrade sclerotherapy followed by physical exam and Doppler US at 3-month intervals for a mean of 11 months (9–15). The procedure apparently was not completed in one boy who was uncooperative, and one developed postoperative "epididymitis." Two persistent grade 1 varicoceles were detected in two patients with initial grade 3 varicoceles (Mottrie et al. 1995).

Open vs. Laparoscopic Varicocelectomy

One RCT enrolled 654 patients, 7 to 17 years of age, with grades 2 or 3 left varicoceles randomized to either laparoscopic ($n=434$) or open retroperitoneal varicocelectomy ($n=220$) (randomization method and reason for disparate groups was not stated). In all patients, 0.3 mL methylene blue was injected under the tunica albuginea to delineate the lymphatic vessels for sparing. Paloma procedure without artery sparing was done. After the first 32 laparoscopic procedures done with vessel clipping had an 8 % recurrence rate, the remaining cases had cord ligation using two silk ties and coagulation of the intervening vessels. Duration of follow-up, postoperative assessment, and primary and secondary outcomes were not described. There were no differences in recurrence rates (<2 %) or hydroceles (<2 %) (Podkamenev et al. 2002).

Meta-analysis was used to compare open vs. laparoscopic varicocelectomy in children and adolescents. From 37 publications, 11 published between 2000 and 2009 met inclusion criteria, comprising 4 RCTs, 5 multicenter studies, and 2 clinical studies. Together there were 1,443 patients, mean age 14.6 years (6–17). Overall, recurrence rate was 5 %, and hydroceles occurred in 9.5 %, with no significant differences between surgical methods. Analysis comparing the Ivanissevich procedure (artery sparing) vs. Paloma (vein and artery ligation) showed OR 4 (95 % CI 1.6–10.3), less likely for recurrence using Paloma. Lymphatic sparing had OR 0.08 (95 % CI 0.67 to −2.32), less risk for hydrocele (Borruto et al. 2010).

Artery-Sparing vs. Non-sparing Laparoscopic Varicocelectomy

A RCT randomized patients with left grades 2 and 3 varicoceles and testicular volume discrepancy >20 % to laparoscopic varicocelectomy with artery ligation ($n=63$) vs. artery sparing ($n=59$) at mean age 14.3 years (12–16). Semen analyses were obtained at age 18 years, with the primary outcome "normal" vs. "abnormal" spermiograms (sperm concentration, motility, and morphology) using WHO criteria, and the secondary outcome surgical complications. Semen analysis was obtained in 110 and was normal in 76 (69 %), with no difference between cohorts. There were no persistent or recurrent varicoceles, whereas at 6 months postoperatively, 7/63 (11 %) artery ligating cases vs. 1/59 (2 %) artery sparing developed a hydrocele, $p=0.01$ (Zampieri et al. 2007).

Lymph Vessel Sparing vs. Non-sparing Laparoscopic Paloma Varicocelectomy

A RCT randomized 50 patients to laparoscopic Paloma varicocelectomy, 25 with mean age 16.5 years (8–22) having lymph vessel sparing via identification using isosulfan blue dye subdartos injection (successful in 24 cases) vs. 25 with mean age 17.9 years (11–25) who did not have lymph sparing. The primary outcome was procedure complications. At mean follow-up of 24 months (14–36), five (20 %) of the lymph vessel non-sparing patients had hydroceles, with three undergoing surgery, vs. 0 in the lymph-sparing cohort, $p=0.025$. All hydroceles were identified on the 3-month postoperative examination. Persistence of varicocele was noted in one (4 %) patient in each cohort (Schwentner et al. 2006).

In a meta-analysis including six studies, 489 lymphatic-sparing cases were compared to 307 non-sparing cases. The hydrocele rate was lower in the lymphatic-sparing group (OR=0.19 [95 % CI 0.10–0.36]), while no difference was found in recurrence rates or catch-up growth (Liang et al. 2011).

A retrospective study compared non-lymph sparing (first 59) to lymph-sparing (next 132) laparoscopic Paloma varicocelectomy. No dye injection was done; lymph vessels were identified visually during dissection within the spermatic cord. The 191 patients were mean age 15 years (10–22), and varicoceles were considered bilateral in 71 (37 %). At mean follow-up of 26 months, persistence/recurrence was 4/88 (4.5 %) for non-sparing vs. 6/174 (3.4 %) for lymph sparing sides, $p=0.7$. Hydroceles developed in 10/88 (11 %) non-sparing vs. 6/174 (3.4 %) with lymph sparing, $p=0.025$ (Glassberg et al. 2008).

Surgical Outcomes

Our review found only one article describing preoperative and postoperative semen analysis in adolescents undergoing varicocelectomy, reporting a significant increase in sperm density and motility.

One trial randomized patients with similar testicular volume discrepancy to surgery vs. observation, reporting that at 1 year surgical patients had less volume discrepancy (3 %) than those observed (9 %).

Meta-analysis of studies reporting preoperative volume discrepancy >10 % or >20 % reported that after varicocelectomy, the number of patients with persistent volume difference significantly decreased. Catch-up growth was a mean of 76 % the volume difference.

Several series that reported that pain was an indication for varicocelectomy did not report results of intervention for relief of symptoms. Of retrospective studies that did report outcomes, pain was relieved in from 68 to 97 %.

Our review found no report concerning change in scrotal appearance after varicocelectomy, even though cosmetic concerns were listed by several as an indication for intervention. One study mentioned scrotal mass resolution in 87 %.

Change in Semen Parameters

Preoperative and postoperative semen analyses were obtained in 33 adolescents aged 15–19 years. These patients were part of a series of 100 patients aged 7–19 undergoing varicocelectomy for grades 2 or 3 varicoceles with hypotrophy (>2 mL or 10 % discrepancy), "soft testis," pain, or "large size." Selection of these 33 for additional analysis was not discussed. Mean sperm concentration increased from 21.8 ± 3.6 million/mL to 39.6 ± 5.7 million/mL, $p=0.007$, and mean percent motility from 33.6 ± 3.8 to 48.5 ± 3.9 postoperatively, $p=0.001$ (Cayan et al. 2005). Neither Tanner stages nor time ("at least 1 year postoperatively") when semen analyses were obtained was stated.

Effect on Testicular Size Discrepancy

A meta-analysis concerning impact of surgery on testicular hypotrophy included 14 studies (1,475 adolescents) that used orchidometers or US before and after treatment to determine volume, and reported either 10 % or 20 % size discrepancy preoperatively. All but one were retrospective. Findings reported included:

- There was no difference in response between those with 10 or 20 % discrepancies.
- Together, the number of patients with persistent 10 or 20 % size difference significantly decreased with varicocelectomy, RR 4 (95 % CI 3–6).
- Catch-up growth was a mean of 76 % (53–94 %) the volume difference (Li et al. 2012).

A RCT identified boys aged 15–19 with grades 2 or 3 varicocele found during a school screening program and randomized 88 to open Paloma varicocelectomy vs. 36 to no therapy. Testicular measurements were obtained by US, with follow-up studies in both cohorts done at 12 months. There was no difference in mean percent volume discrepancy preoperatively (surgery: 19±17 %; observation 15±13 %), whereas at 12 months there was significant growth in surgical patients from a mean 12.6 % volume difference to only 3.0 % difference but no significant change in controls (9.5–8.7 %) (Paduch and Niedzielski 1997).

Pain Resolution

A retrospective review included 38 adolescents aged 14–16 with left grades 2 and 3 varicoceles and no testicular volume discrepancy who all had pain. All failed "conservative management for at least 2 months" (treatment not described) before varicocelectomy. Six months postoperatively, pain resolved in 26 (68 %). No mention was made regarding persistent varicoceles, if any (Zampieri and Cervellione 2008); Zampieri et al. 2008.

In another retrospective review of varicocelectomy with 230 males aged 8–40 years, 119 (52 %) had pain, of which postoperative follow-up was available in 82 (69 %) at 3 months. While awaiting surgery, all used scrotal support and nonsteroidal anti-inflammatory medication for mean 4 weeks (3–5), with pain resolution in 5/119. Of the 82 postoperative patients with follow-up, pain resolved in 72 (88 %), while others reported either decreased pain or persistent pain that was unchanged. Two with persistent pain were found by US to have persistent varicocele (Yaman et al. 2000).

A retrospective analysis involved 215 patients mean age 20±8.5 years undergoing varicocelectomy for grades 2 and 3 varicoceles, of which left scrotal pain was the primary indication in 59 (27 %). At median follow-up of 59 months (5–130), 2/59 (3 %) had persistent pain (May et al. 2006).

Cosmetic Improvement

One retrospective study reported varicocelectomy was done in a subset of 23 adolescents for complaints of a palpable scrotal mass. At median follow-up of 19 months for the entire study group, 20 (87 %) had resolution (Lee et al. 2011).

Management of Persistent Varicocele

Retrospective series report reoperative varicocelectomy can be performed by a variety of methods with low risk for testicular atrophy.

A retrospective review specifically concerned reoperative varicoceles, occurring in 19 patients, with known artery-sparing initially in 8. All had persistent grade 2 or 3 varicocele at a mean of 16 months after original surgery. Reoperative surgery was done inguinally following prior laparoscopic procedures ($n=13$), open Paloma ($n=2$), or microscopic inguinal ($n=1$), while the others had embolization ($n=2$) after prior inguinal surgery or a laparoscopic procedure after a prior inguinal approach ($n=1$). At mean follow-up of 23 months (6–53), one had persistent varicocele, one had testicular atrophy, and three developed a hydrocele. Eight of nine with volume discrepancy >10 % had improved growth to a testicular volume <10 % (Glassberg et al. 2011).

Another retrospective study concerned 106 patients referred for embolization from 1992 to 2010, 46 for primary therapy and 60, with mean age 21 years (12–43), as salvage procedures. Eighty-nine percent of salvage cases had a patent gonadal vein; 41 %, retroperitoneal collaterals; 28 %, inguinal collaterals; and 8.5 %, both retroperitoneal and inguinal collateral branches. Compared to primary embolizations, there were significantly more inguinal and combined inguinal/retroperitoneal collaterals in salvage cases (Rais-Bahrami et al. 2012).

Twenty-eight males aged 13–55 years with recurrent varicocele at a mean of 6.6 months (0–48) were all found to have venous drainage from the pampiniform plexus to the left renal vein treated with retrograde embolization. Initial varicocelectomy was laparoscopic in 11, open retroperitoneal in 7, inguinal in 7, and unknown in 3. Persistent/recurrent varicocele was grade 1 in 1, grade 2 in 3, and grade 3 in 24. In two cases, the procedure could be performed, and one had no follow-up. One had left scrotal pain due to phlebitis from the sclerosing agent. In the remaining 25, resolution was observed in 20 (80 %) at median follow-up 7 months (5 days-54 months) (Kim et al. 2012).

Another retrospective review included mention of 25 reoperative varicocelectomies in adults. Of these, 22 followed prior ligations and were recommended for retrograde embolization plus sclerotherapy, of which the procedure was technically possible in 18 and reported successful in 14. Three others had failure of initial embolization and underwent surgical ligation with results not stated (Feneley et al. 1997).

References

Abdel-Meguid TA, Al-Sayyad A, Tayib A, Farsi HM. Does varicocele repair improve male infertility? An evidence-based perspective from a randomized, controlled trial. Eur Urol. 2011;59(3):455–61.

Akbay E, Cayan S, Doruk E, Duce MN, Bozlu M. The prevalence of varicocele and varicocele-related testicular atrophy in Turkish children and adolescents. BJU Int. 2000;86(4):490–3.

Anderson JE, Farr SL, Jamieson DJ, Warner L, Macaluso M. Infertility services reported by men in the United States: national survey data. Fertil Steril. 2009;91(6):2466–70.

Andrade-Rocha FT. Significance of sperm characteristics in the evaluation of adolescents, adults and older men with varicocele. J Postgrad Med. 2007;53(1):8–13.

Arai T, Kitahara S, Horiuchi S, Sumi S, Yoshida K. Relationship of testicular volume to semen profiles and serum hormone concentrations in infertile Japanese males. Int J Fertil Womens Med. 1998; 43(1):40–7.

Baek M, Park SW, Moon KH, Chang YS, Jeong HJ, Lee SW, et al. Nationwide survey to evaluate the prevalence of varicoceles in South Korean middle school boys: a population based study. Int J Urol. 2011;18(1):55–60.

Beutner S, May M, Hoschke B, Helke C, Lein M, Roigas J, et al. Treatment of varicocele with reference to age: a retrospective comparison of three minimally invasive procedures. Surg Endosc. 2007;21(1):61–5.

Borruto FA, Impellizzeri P, Antonuccio P, Finocchiaro A, Scalfari G, Arena F, et al. Laparoscopic vs open varicocelectomy in children and adolescents: review of the recent literature and meta-analysis. J Pediatr Surg. 2010;45(12):2464–9.

Cayan S, Acar D, Ulger S, Akbay E. Adolescent varicocele repair: long-term results and comparison of surgical techniques according to optical magnification use in 100 cases at a single university hospital. J Urol. 2005;174(5):2003–6. discussion 6–7.

Diamond DA, Paltiel HJ, DiCanzio J, Zurakowski D, Bauer SB, Atala A, et al. Comparative assessment of pediatric testicular volume: orchidometer versus ultrasound. J Urol. 2000;164(3 Pt 2):1111–4.

Evers JH, Collins J, Clarke J. Surgery or embolisation for varicoceles in subfertile men. Cochrane Database Syst Rev (Online). 2009;(1):CD000479.

Feneley MR, Pal MK, Nockler IB, Hendry WF. Retrograde embolization and causes of failure in the primary treatment of varicocele. Br J Urol. 1997;80(4):642–6.

Ficarra V, Sarti A, Novara G, Dalpiaz O, Galfano A, Cavalleri S, et al. Modified antegrade scrotal sclerotherapy in adolescent patients with varicocele. J Pediatr Surg. 2004;39(7):1034–6.

Glassberg KI, Poon SA, Gjertson CK, DeCastro GJ, Misseri R. Laparoscopic lymphatic sparing varicocelectomy in adolescents. J Urol. 2008;180(1):326–30. discussion 30–1.

Glassberg KI, Badalato GM, Poon SA, Mercado MA, Raimondi PM, Gasalberti A. Evaluation and management of the persistent/recurrent varicocele. Urology. 2011;77(5):1194–8.

Granata C, Oddone M, Toma P, Mattioli G. Retrograde percutaneous sclerotherapy of left idiopathic varicocele in children: results and follow-up. Pediatr Surg Int. 2008;24(5):583–7.

Keene DJ, Sajad Y, Rakoczy G, Cervellione RM. Testicular volume and semen parameters in patients aged 12 to 17 years with idiopathic varicocele. J Pediatr Surg. 2012;47(2):383–5.

Kim J, Shin JH, Yoon HK, Ko GY, Gwon DI, Kim EY, et al. Persistent or recurrent varicocoele after failed varicocoelectomy: outcome in patients treated using percutaneous transcatheter embolization. Clin Radiol. 2012;67(4):359–65.

Korets R, Woldu SL, Nees SN, Spencer BA, Glassberg KI. Testicular symmetry and adolescent varicocele—does it need followup? J Urol. 2011;186 (4 Suppl): 1614–8.

Kumanov P, Robeva RN, Tomova A. Adolescent varicocele: who is at risk? Pediatrics. 2008;121(1):e53–7.

Lee HJ, Cheon SH, Ji YH, Moon KH, Kim KS, Park S. Clinical characteristics and surgical outcomes in adolescents and adults with varicocele. Korean J Urol. 2011;52(7):489–93.

Li F, Chiba K, Yamaguchi K, Okada K, Matsushita K, Ando M, et al. Effect of varicocelectomy on testicular volume in children and adolescents: a meta-analysis. Urology. 2012;79(6):1340–5.

Liang Z, Guo J, Zhang H, Yang C, Pu J, Mei H, et al. Lymphatic sparing versus lymphatic non-sparing laparoscopic varicocelectomy in children and adolescents: a systematic review and meta-analysis. Eur J Pediatr Surg. 2011;21(3):147–53.

May M, Johannsen M, Beutner S, Helke C, Braun KP, Lein M, et al. Laparoscopic surgery versus antegrade scrotal sclerotherapy: retrospective comparison of two different approaches for varicocele treatment. Eur Urol. 2006;49(2):384–7.

Mazzoni G, Fiocca G, Minucci S, Pieri S, Paolicelli D, Morucci M, et al. Varicocele: a multidisciplinary approach in children and adolescents. J Urol. 1999;162(5):1755–7. discussion 7–8.

Mori MM, Bertolla RP, Fraietta R, Ortiz V, Cedenho AP. Does varicocele grade determine extent of alteration to spermatogenesis in adolescents? Fertil Steril. 2008;90(5):1769–73.

Mottrie AM, Matani Y, Baert J, Voges GE, Hohenfellner R. Antegrade scrotal sclerotherapy for the treatment of varicocele in childhood and adolescence. Br J Urol. 1995;76(1):21–4.

Paduch DA, Niedzielski J. Semen analysis in young men with varicocele: preliminary study. J Urol. 1996;156(2 Pt 2):788–90.

Paduch DA, Niedzielski J. Repair versus observation in adolescent varicocele: a prospective study. J Urol. 1997;158(3 Pt 2):1128–32.

Paltiel HJ, Diamond DA, Di Canzio J, Zurakowski D, Borer JG, Atala A. Testicular volume: comparison of orchidometer and US measurements in dogs. Radiology. 2002;222(1):114–9.

Pasqualotto FF, Lucon AM, de Goes PM, Sobreiro BP, Hallak J, Pasqualotto EB, et al. Semen profile, testicular volume, and hormonal levels in infertile patients with varicoceles compared with fertile men with and without varicoceles. Fertil Steril. 2005;83(1):74–7.

Podkamenev VV, Stalmakhovich VN, Urkov PS, Solovjev AA, Iljin VP. Laparoscopic surgery for pediatric varicoceles: randomized controlled trial. J Pediatr Surg. 2002;37(5):727–9.

Poon SA, Gjertson CK, Mercado MA, Raimondi PM, Kozakowski KA, Glassberg KI. Testicular asymmetry and adolescent varicoceles managed expectantly. J Urol. 2010;183(2):731–4.

Preston MA, Carnat T, Flood T, Gaboury I, Leonard MP. Conservative management of adolescent varicoceles: a retrospective review. Urology. 2008;72(1):77–80.

Rais-Bahrami S, Montag S, George AK, Rastinehad AR, Palmer LS, Siegel DN. Angiographic findings of primary versus salvage varicoceles treated with selective gonadal vein embolization: an explanation for surgical treatment failure. J Endourol. 2012;26(5):556–60.

Sakamoto H, Saito K, Ogawa Y, Yoshida H. Testicular volume measurements using Prader orchidometer versus ultrasonography in patients with infertility. Urology. 2007a;69(1):158–62.

Sakamoto H, Saito K, Oohta M, Inoue K, Ogawa Y, Yoshida H. Testicular volume measurement: comparison of ultrasonography, orchidometry, and water displacement. Urology. 2007b;69(1):152–7.

Sakamoto H, Ogawa Y, Yoshida H. Relationship between testicular volume and varicocele in patients with infertility. Urology. 2008;71(1):104–9.

Schiff JD, Li PS, Goldstein M. Correlation of ultrasonographic and orchidometer measurements of testis volume in adults. BJU Int. 2004;93(7):1015–7.

Schwentner C, Radmayr C, Lunacek A, Gozzi C, Pinggera GM, Neururer R, et al. Laparoscopic varicocele ligation in children and adolescents using isosulphan blue: a prospective randomized trial. BJU Int. 2006;98(4):861–5.

Shiraishi K, Takihara H, Matsuyama H. Effects of grade 1 varicocele detected in the pediatric age-group on testicular development. J Pediatr Surg. 2009;44(10):1995–8.

Sigman M, Jarow JP. Ipsilateral testicular hypotrophy is associated with decreased sperm counts in infertile men with varicoceles. J Urol. 1997;158(2):605–7.

Spinelli C, Di Giacomo M, Lo Piccolo R, Martin A, Messineo A. The role of testicular volume in adolescents with varicocele: the better way and time of surgical treatment. J Urol. 2010;184(4 Suppl):1722–6.

Thomas JC, Elder JS. Testicular growth arrest and adolescent varicocele: does varicocele size make a difference? J Urol. 2002;168(4 Pt 2):1689–91.

WHO (World Health Organization). The influence of varicocele on parameters of fertility in a large group of men presenting to infertility clinics. Fertil Steril. 1992;57(6):1289–93.

Yaman O, Ozdiler E, Anafarta K, Gogus O. Effect of microsurgical subinguinal varicocele ligation to treat pain. Urology. 2000;55(1):107–8.

Zampieri N, Cervellione RM. Varicocele in adolescents: a 6-year longitudinal and followup observational study. J Urol. 2008;180(4 Suppl):1653–6. discussion 6.

Zampieri N, Zuin V, Corroppolo M, Chironi C, Cervellione RM, Camoglio FS. Varicocele and adolescents: semen quality after 2 different laparoscopic procedures. J Androl. 2007;28(5):727–33.

Zampieri N, Ottolenghi A, Camoglio FS. Painful varicocele in pediatric age: is there a correlation between pain, testicular damage and hormonal values to justify surgery? Pediatr Surg Int. 2008;24(11):1235–8.

Zaupa P, Mayr J, Hollwarth ME. Antegrade scrotal sclerotherapy for treating primary varicocele in children. BJU Int. 2006;97(4):809–12.

Zucchi A, Mearini L, Mearini E, Fioretti F, Bini V, Porena M. Varicocele and fertility: relationship between testicular volume and seminal parameters before and after treatment. J Androl. 2006;27(4):548–51.

Hypospadias

9

Warren T. Snodgrass and Nicol C. Bush

Primary goals in hypospadias repair:

1. **Restore normal penile function**
2. **Restore normal genital appearance**

Normal function includes forceful, straight urination without spraying or dribbling, straight erection, and normal ejaculation.

Normal genital appearance includes the following:

- **A vertical slit urethral meatus correctly positioned within the glans.**
- **Circumcision or foreskin reconstruction.**
- **A symmetric scrotum without transposition, midline cleft, or encroachment onto the penile shaft.**

A secondary aim is to complete repair in as few stages with as few complications as possible.

Summary of evidence for these goals:

- **Uroflowometry consistently demonstrates decreased Q_{max} in patients after repair compared to nomograms. No study reports uroflows comparing patients and controls.**
- **Adults repaired as children more often complain of obstructive voiding, spraying, and/or deviated stream than controls.**
- **Ventral penile curvature (VC) occurs in approximately 10 % of distal and over 50 % of proximal hypospadias. Short-term studies indicate that dorsal plication and ventral lengthening used according to extent of curvature reliably achieve straightening.**
- **Studies of dorsal plication done in adults with congenital curvature report persistence in <10 %.**
- **The few surveys of adults operated as children find similar prevalences of penile curvature in patients and controls.**
- **Ejaculation is more often reported by patients to have weak force with need to milk semen than controls.**
- **Objective assessment of postoperative penile appearance indicates that tubularized incised plate (TIP) operation creates a more normal meatus and glans than flap procedures (Mathieu and onlay preputial flap). One study reported that parents of hypospadias patients scored outcomes after distal and proximal TIP similarly to parents of normal boys after circumcision.**
- **Questionnaires of adults operated in childhood, sometimes by techniques no longer in use, find patients have less satisfaction with genital appearance than controls.**
- **Distal hypospadias repair has short-term complication rates <10 %.**
- **A reduction in proximal TIP complications from 53 to 13 % was reported in one study after a series of technical modifications.**
- **Onlay and tubularized preputial flap proximal hypospadias repairs have complications of approximately 15–45 %.**

W.T. Snodgrass, M.D. (✉) • N.C. Bush, M.D., M.S.C.S.
Department of Pediatric Urology, University of Texas Southwestern Medical Center and Children's Medical Center Dallas, 1935 Medical District Drive, MS F4.04, Dallas, TX 75235, USA
e-mail: warren.snodgrass@childrens.com

W.T. Snodgrass (ed.), *Pediatric Urology: Evidence for Optimal Patient Management*,
DOI 10.1007/978-1-4614-6910-0_9, © Springer Science+Business Media New York 2013

- **There are few reported data for complications after various staged repairs.**
- **Multiple logistic regression analyses find proximal meatal location and reoperation to be independent risk factors for complications, whereas suture materials and methods (interrupted vs. continuous) and stent or not (distal repair) did not impact outcomes.**
- **Age at surgery >4 years was an independent risk factor in one study, but age was not a factor in two other analyses.**
- **Most urethroplasty complications are diagnosed within 1 year of repair. Two studies of patients dismissed from childhood follow-up reported that 8 and 17 % had a complication when evaluated again as teens or adults.**

Preoperative Assessment and Management

Prevalence and Familial Risk

Hypospadias occurs in ≤0.5 % of males.

Relative risk for hypospadias recurrence in first-degree relatives is approximately 13×, found in from 9 to 17 % of brothers and 1 to 3 % of fathers in case–control studies.

Risk ratios for relatives of a proband with hypospadias were determined from analysis of all boys born in Denmark between 1973 and 2005, of which 5,380 (0.45 %) were diagnosed with the condition. Of these patients, 228 (4.2 %) had another family member with a history of hypospadias. The relative recurrence risk for first-degree relatives was the same: for a brother to have hypospadias it was 13.4 (95 % CI 11.0–16.4), and for offspring of an affected male 10.4 (95 % CI 7.54–14.4), $p=0.16$. Risk in same-sex twins was 50.8 (95 % CI 34.2–75.5) (Schnack et al. 2008).

A case–control study of all males born in Alsace from 1979 to1987 found 176 hypospadias cases in 60,847 births, a prevalence of 2.9/1000. Hypospadias was described as glanular/coronal ($n=121$, 69 %), penile ($n=44$, 25 %) or perineal ($n=11$, 6 %). Of the 176 cases, 2 (1 %) had fathers with hypospadias, as did 8/47 (17 %) brothers (Stoll et al. 1990).

Another case–control study was performed in northern Italy on boys born from 1978 to 1983. There were 168 identified cases with hypospadias in 41,078 male births, a prevalence of 4.1/1000. Of these, 3/33 (9 %) brothers also had hypospadias, as did 5/166 (3 %) fathers (Calzolari et al. 1986).

Isolated vs. Syndromic Hypospadias

Case–control studies report additional nongenital anomalies in from 9 to 15 % of boys with hypospadias.

In the case–control study by Stoll et al. (1990) described above, 27/176 (15 %) newborns with hypospadias (4 distal, 17 penile, 6 perineal) had two or more nongenital malformations. Ten of 27 had other urinary tract anomalies, including renal agenesis, vesicoureteral reflux (VUR), and horseshoe kidney. Cardiac and intestinal malformations were the next most frequent.

The case–control study by Calzolari et al. (1986) reported 15/168 (9 %) cases of newborn hypospadias were associated with additional nongenital anomalies.

Karyotyping

No published series performed karyotyping in consecutive boys with hypospadias; consequently, selection bias likely overestimates prevalence of abnormalities.

Sex chromosome abnormalities are reported in <10 % of patients with isolated hypospadias.

Several case series report patients with hypospadias and undescended testicle (UDT) have a 4–33 % likelihood for sex chromosome abnormalities.

Karyotyping was performed in 984 patients 0–35 years of age that included 68 with hypospadias and 33 with both hypospadias plus UDT. Sex chromosome abnormalities were found in 2/67 (3 %) and 5/33 (15 %). Of the seven patients, four had dysmorphic features. Selection of patients for study inclusion was not described (Moreno-Garcia et al. 2002).

Twenty-six males with hypospadias that was glanular ($n=5$), penile ($n=14$), penoscrotal ($n=6$), or scrotal ($n=1$), and one with chordee without hypospadias had chromosome analysis. Of these, hypospadias was isolated in 14, associated with other congenital anomalies (not described) in 4, and associated with UDT in 9, of which 5 had additional anomalies. Sex chromosome abnormalities were found in 1/14 (7 %) isolated hypospadias patients, 0/4 hypospadias patients with other anomalies, and 2/9 (22 %) patients with hypospadias plus UDT (1/4 without and 1/5 with other anomalies). Selection for study inclusion was not stated; cases of "male pseudohermaphroditism and gonadal intersex disorders" were not included (Yamaguchi et al. 1991).

Retrospective chart review was done in databases for hypospadias ($n=1,057$) and UDT ($n=2,105$) registered between 1982 and 1996 to identify 79 with both conditions. Karyotyping was done in 54 (68 %) (reasons for selective testing not stated), of which 23 (43 %) were diagnosed with sexual development disorders, including mixed gonadal dysgenesis ($n=11$), ovatesticular DSD ($n=5$), 5-alpha reductase deficiency ($n=2$), Klinefelters ($n=2$), and partial androgen resistance ($n=3$). Assuming normal sex chromosomes in the two with 5-alpha reductase deficiency and three with partial androgen resistance (and assuming that all with ovotesticular DSD (disorder of sex development) had abnormal sex chromosomes), karyotyping revealed abnormal sex chromosomes in 18 (33 %) (Kaefer et al. 1991).

Retrospective chart review of patients seen between 1986 and 1999 was done, identifying 113 with hypospadias plus UDT. Of these, only 48 (42 %) had karyotyping (selection not described), with 8 (17 %) demonstrating a chromosome abnormality that was autosomal in 6 and involved sex chromosomes in 2 (mixed gonadal dysgenesis in 1 and ovatesticular DSD in 1) (McAleer and Kaplan 2001).

Another retrospective chart review was done for patients between 1994 and 2006, finding 44 with hypospadias plus UDT. Karyotyping had been done in 25 (57 %) (selection basis not discussed), of which 6 (24 %) had autosomal ($n=3$) or sex chromosome ($n=3$) abnormalities. The latter all had mixed gonadal dysgenesis (Cox et al. 2008).

Imaging

Renal abnormalities are reported in approximately 20 % of hypospadias patients. Most are ureteral duplications, malrotations, or minor hydronephrosis not requiring interventions.

Voiding cystourethrogram (VCUG) in two studies reported VUR in approximately 10 % of cases with cystography.

A prospective study between 1972 and 1983 obtained intravenous pyelogram (IVP) and VCUG in 153 boys <2 years of age with hypospadias (93 [61 %] glanular/coronal, 12 [8 %] penile shaft, 48 [31 %] penoscrotal/perineal). Of these, 36/153 (24 %) patients had abnormal imaging: VUR in 18 patients, horseshoe kidney, solitary kidney, hydronephrosis, ureterovesical junction obstruction (UVJO), ureteral duplications in the others. Of these, 18/153 (12 %) were judged to require surgery (Moore 1990).

Retrospective chart review was done to identify patients with hypospadias, finding 400 cases of which 163 (41 %) had imaging. Selection criteria for upper tract imaging were not described, but case distribution (26 % glanular, 22 % penile, 47 % penoscrotal) suggests it was weighted towards more severe forms. Upper tract imaging was done by IVP ($n=65$) or US ($n=98$), with 31 (19 %) abnormal, mostly malrotations or positional anomalies with "mild" hydronephrosis/hydroureter in 6 (4 %). Cystography was obtained in 68 patients, finding VUR in 6 and a bladder diverticulum in 2. No mention was made of prostatic utricle (Friedman et al. 2008).

Retrospective review of IVP was done in 87/121 (72 %) patients undergoing hypospadias repair from 1969 to 1974. Sixteen of 87 (18 %) were abnormal, but of these only 1 with UPJO had upper tract surgery. These 16 abnormalities (ureteral duplications, malrotation, horseshoe kidney, ureteral "ectasia," UPJO) occurred in 21 % with glanular/coronal, 12 % with penile shaft, and 23 % with penoscrotal/perineal hypospadias (Lutzker et al. 1977).

Adjuvant Hormonal Therapy

One cross-sectional study reported glans width in normal neonates at median age 1 month

was a mean of 14 mm (11–19), while mean glans width in patients at median age 8 months with proximal hypospadias was significantly smaller, 13 mm (9–16).

Several prospective studies demonstrate androgens increase penile length and glans circumference. Two report that both IM and topical androgens delivering 2 mg/kg achieve similar effects.

Objective endpoints for therapy have not been described, so published regimens are empiric.

One study treated consecutive boys with proximal hypospadias and glans width ≤14 mm with an escalating dose of IM testosterone to achieve width ≥16 mm, reporting one injection of 2 mg/kg was sufficient in approximately 50 %, while the others had additional monthly injections increasing from 4 to 16 mg/kg.

One RCT reported decreased urethroplasty complications in patients receiving preoperative topical DHT vs. no therapy.

One prospective observational study found adjuvant testosterone therapy not only failed to decrease urethroplasty complications, but was a risk factor predicting complications.

There are few data concerning advanced bone age following androgen stimulation, but no increased bone age has been reported.

One prospective study measured glans width in 201 consecutive neonates undergoing circumcision, used to compare with older boys undergoing distal ($n=165$) and proximal ($n=26$) hypospadias repair. Median ages were 1.3 months (0.1–3.2), 8 months (3–117), and 8.5 months (2.5–83), respectively, and median glans width for each group was 14 mm (11–19), 15 mm (10–21), and 13 mm (9–16), which were significantly different. Although there was overlap in glans width between all groups, the cohort of boys with proximal hypospadias had a significantly smaller glans than did normal newborns (Dajusta et al. 2011).

Response to Androgens

A prospective study randomized 25 patients with microphallic (penile length <2 SD) hypospadias to receive a mixture of testosterone propionate and enanthate, providing a dose of 2 mg/kg/week administered twice daily topically for 3 weeks or intramuscularly weekly 3×. Meatal location was distal ($n=8$), midshaft ($n=3$), and proximal ($n=14$). Mean pre-therapy/post-therapy length was 2/3 cm for topical vs. 1.85/3 cm for intramuscular treatment, reported as nonsignificant differences. Nonresponders were not clearly described, except to state that one patient with topical application had no growth. Elevated serum levels >10 ng/mL were only noted after topical therapy, occurring in 2/13 patients, possibly from excessive application (Chalapathi et al. 2003).

Another prospective trial randomized 21 boys with proximal hypospadias and "a significantly small penis" to either testosterone cream 2 mg/kg/week for 3 weeks or 2 mg/kg testosterone enanthate injections monthly for 3 months. Mean pre-therapy/post-therapy length (cm) was 2.1/2.4 vs. 2/2.4 cm for those receiving topical vs. IM testosterone. Similar pre- and post-therapy glans circumference measurements (cm) were 2.7/3.8 vs. 2.8/3.8, which would correspond to mean glans diameter changes of approximately 9–12 mm. The authors stated that there were no differences in the two groups and that the increased penile length and glans circumferences observed were all statistically significant. Two patients in each group did not respond (Nerli et al. 2009).

A study prospectively selected 40 patients, mean age 27 months (13–74), from a total of 170 with primary hypospadias (selection methods not described; hypospadias severity not stated) to receive testosterone 2 mg/kg IM 5 and 2 weeks preoperatively. Mean pre-stimulation penile length was 3.5 ± 1.1 cm, which significantly increased to 5.9 ± 1.1 cm before partially regressing 12 months later to 4.9 ± 1.1 cm (Davits et al. 1993).

Thirty-six boys with hypospadias, 4 coronal, 7 distal shaft, 16 midshaft, 3 penoscrotal, and 6 with failed repair, received 2 mg/kg testosterone enanthate IM 5 and 2 weeks preoperatively. Mean increased penile length was 4.7–7.4 cm, returning to 4.9 "postoperatively" (time not stated); mean increased glans circumference was 3.8–5.5 cm, then 4.0 cm postoperatively (12–17 mm, then 13 mm) (Gearhart and Jeffs 1987).

An observational study involved 25 patients 9–12 months of age, 8 with penile, 14 with penoscrotal, and 2 with perineal hypospadias who were considered to have a penis "significantly smaller than usual" and so were scheduled to receive testosterone enanthate 25 mg IM monthly for 3 months. Twenty-three out of 25 responded, with mean increase in glans circumference (cm) from 2.70 ± 0.01 to 3.74 ± 0.02 (9–12 mm) and penile length (cm) from 1.98 ± 0.02 to 2.38 ± 0.02, both $p < 0.001$. Of the 23 responders, 4 were considered to have sufficient increases after one injection and another 6 after two injections (Luo et al. 2003).

Another study recommended preoperative testosterone for glans width (at the widest point) ≤14 mm, and used width ≥16 mm as the endpoint for treatment. Consecutive patients were given an escalating dose beginning at 2 mg/kg with remeasurement 1 month later. There were 25 consecutive patients with proximal hypospadias; 13 (52 %) needed only one injection of 2 mg/kg to achieve target growth, while the others needed 4 mg/kg ($n = 6$), 8 mg/kg ($n = 5$), and 16 mg/kg ($n = 1$) (Granberg et al. 2012).

Impact on Hypospadias Outcomes

A RCT allocated 75 consecutive boys mean age 33 months (10–159) to preoperative topical DHT (2.5 % transdermal gel to glans and shaft daily for 3 months, ending 5 weeks preoperatively) vs. no androgens. Treated vs. control patients had coronal (70 % vs. 84 %), penile (24 % vs. 16 %), and penoscrotal (5 % vs. 0 %) hypospadias. All had TIP repair, with fewer urethroplasty complications in those with preoperative stimulation (1/37 vs. 9/38, $p = 0.01$) (Kaya et al. 2008).

A prospective observational trial measured glans width preoperatively at the widest point and then gave IM testosterone cyprionate for diameter ≤14 mm with proximal and ≤12 mm with distal hypospadias. Injections began with 2 mg/kg with remeasurement in 1 month and dose escalation to 4, 8 mg/kg, and so on, until a predetermined target width of ≥15 mm was achieved. There were 279 patients with distal ($n = 231$), midshaft ($n = 10$), and proximal ($n = 29$) hypospadias, of which 41 (15 %) received adjuvant therapy. Mean glans diameter in those injected with testosterone was 12 mm, increasing to 16.5 mm, vs. 15.4 mm in those not treated. Although glans size increased, urethroplasty complications remained significantly greater in those with adjuvant therapy, 34 % vs. 11 %, $p < 0.001$. Multiple logistic regression analysis showed that adjuvant therapy was an independent risk factor for complications when controlling for meatal location, age, and primary repair vs. reoperation (Bush et al. 2012).

Side Effects

Appearance of pubic hair was reported in 2/25 (Chalapathi et al. 2003), 5/21 (Nerli et al. 2009), 2/40 (Davits et al. 1993), and 0/25 (Luo et al. 2003).

Pre-and 12-month post-stimulation bone age was determined in all 40 patients in one study (Davits et al. 1993), and only 12 month post-stimulation in 20/36 patients in another (Gearhart and Jeffs 1987), with neither reporting bone age advancement.

Timing of Surgery

The commonly quoted ideal age of 6–18 months was based on expert opinion.

Several retrospective studies using logistic regression suggest that increasing patient age >6 months, >1.5 years, or >4 years predicts increased risk for urethroplasty complications after TIP repair.

One prospective study of consecutive prepubertal patients undergoing TIP using multiple logistic regression reported that age was not an independent risk factor for urethroplasty complications.

Surgery at ≥3 months of age in full-term infants was not associated with anesthetic complications in one study.

Age guidelines for hypospadias repair were derived from expert opinion. The 1996 committee for the American Academy of Pediatrics Section on Urology reviewed psychological factors, anesthetic considerations, and technical aspects of repair before recommending surgery be performed between 6 and 12 months, assuming the surgeon, anesthesiologist, and facility were experienced in care of infants (AAP Section on Urology, Pediatrics 1996).

The 2012 EAU guidelines similarly state repair is usually between 6 and 18 months of age, based on evidence level 4 (case series), and noted one report of surgery between 4 and 6 months.

To test the hypothesis that the preferred age for repair is <18 months for psychological adjustment and health-related quality of life, patients 6–17 years of age were enrolled and divided into those having final surgery at age <18 vs. >18 months. Of 102 eligible patients operated over a 14-year period, 77 consented to psychological assessment using questionnaires and interviews. No differences were found between the two cohorts regarding health-related quality of life, psychological adjustment, gender-role behavior, or penile self-perception (Weber et al. 2009).

Multivariable analysis of prospective data for 669 consecutive boys aged 3–144 months undergoing TIP repair by a single surgeon reported that age <6 months, >1 year, >5 years, log age, or age quartiles did not predict risk for urethroplasty complications. Furthermore, anesthetic risks were not increased in infants aged 3–5 months vs. older patients (Bush et al. 2012).

A retrospective review of 316 distal hypospadias repairs by a single surgeon between 1999 and 2005 included 194 (60 %) TIP, 69 (21 %) meatal advancement and glanuloplasty (MAGPI), and 53 (9 %) glans approximation procedure (GAP). Of these, 92 (29 %) were <6 months of age at surgery, and urethroplasty complications were less than in older patients (2/92 [2 %] vs. 23/224 [10 %], $p=0.006$). Considering only TIP repairs, complications in those <6 months (2/55 [4 %]) were significantly less than those >6 months of age (19/139 [14 %], $p=0.027$). Age was not related to outcomes after MAGPI or GAP repairs (Perlmutter et al. 2006).

Patients undergoing TIP between 2005 and 2007 were analyzed, a younger cohort mean age 1.6 years (95 % CI 1.5–1.7) vs. older patients at mean age 5 years (95 % CI 4.8–5.2). These represented the first patients to undergo TIP by the two surgeons involved. Complications included fistula and/or "stenosis" (not defined) and/or foreskin reconstruction problems (dehiscence, phimosis). Total complications were 4/57 (7 %) in those 1.5 years old vs. 21/65 (32 %) in older boys, $p=0.0006$. Year of surgery and surgeon did not predict outcomes (Korvald and Stubberud 2008).

Multivariable analysis was done on data from retrospective chart review of 391 patients with median age 2 years undergoing TIP over a 10-year period ending 2007. Age was analyzed as a continuous variable and reported for those less than vs. greater than 4 years at repair. There was a 3.25 relative risk (95 % CI 1.44–7.35) for complications in older boys (Eassa et al. 2011).

Intraoperative Assessment and Management

Sutures

Few studies compare suture material used in hypospadias surgery. One RCT used polyglytone vs. polydioxanone to analyze relatively faster vs. slower suture absorption, finding no difference in fistulas.

Another RCT compared continuous vs. interrupted sutures for distal to midshaft TIP and reported no difference in overall complications, but did not specifically report differences, if any, in fistula rates.

A RCT allocated 100 patients to distal TIP repair using either polyglytone (rapid absorption) or polydioxanone (slow absorption) for urethroplasty done in two layers, with running subepithelial stitches. All operations were done by one surgeon. Follow-up assessment was blinded. There was no difference in fistula rates between the two cohorts to 2 years postoperatively: 4/50 (8 %) polyglytone vs. 6/50 (12 %) polydioxanone (Guarino et al. 2009).

A RCT studied 80 boys, mean age 4.5 years (3–7), with primary distal ($n=64$) and midshaft ($n=16$) hypospadias to TIP repair using subepithelial 6–0 or 7–0 polyglactin, randomized to continuous vs. interrupted sutures, finding no difference in overall complications (Sarhan et al. 2009). All urethroplasty complications were considered, with a total of 8 fistulas, 2 glans dehiscences, and 3 meatal stenoses.

Perioperative Antibiotics

Our review found no trials comparing preoperative antibiotics to no antibiotics before hypospadias surgery.

One RCT reported that febrile UTI was less in patients receiving postoperative oral antibiotics vs. no antibiotic.

One RCT comprising 101 patients undergoing TIP compared intraoperative intravenous cefonicid to intraoperative cefonicid plus postoperative oral cephalexin (TID) for 8 days (duration of catheterization). There were no differences in the two groups regarding surgical complications, but both asymptomatic bacilluria (11/52 [21 %] vs. 25/49 [51 %], $p<0.05$) and febrile UTI (3/52 [6 %] vs. 12/49 [23 %], $p<0.05$) were more common without postoperative oral antibiotics. Time of febrile UTI postoperatively was not stated (Meir and Livne 2004).

Urethral Plate

One study asked pediatric urologists to judge urethral plate (UP) suitability for incision and tubularization from photographs, reporting poor agreement.

Two studies report that UP characteristics impact TIP outcomes. A "shallow" UP was associated with increased urethroplasty complications in one study but not the other. Both stated that a pre-incision plate width <8 mm increased complications.

One article analyzed TIP used in 426 consecutive patients with distal hypospadias and found no difference in outcomes based on description of the UP groove as "flat," "cleft," or "deep."

A study asked 21 pediatric urologists to rate urethral plate quality based on photographs using a Likert scale from "very unfavorable" to "very favorable" for incision and tubularization, reporting poor to slight agreement regardless of meatal position (distal vs. midshaft vs. proximal) or years of surgical experience, Kappa = 0.06 (El-Hout et al. 2010).

Analysis of outcomes in 426 consecutive boys, mean age 17 months (3–140), with distal hypospadias using prospectively collected data in a database reported urethroplasty complications in 19 (4 %), comprising 9 fistulas, 9 glans dehiscences, and 1 meatal stenosis during follow-up a mean of 8 months. All had TIP repair regardless of UP appearance. Excluding 30 MIP variants, the UP was described in 337 as "flat" ($n=137$, 41 %), "cleft" ($n=140$, 42 %), or "deep"($n=60$, 18 %), with no difference in outcomes. Calibration was done in 263 (62 %) postoperatively, with all ≥8 Fr (Snodgrass et al. 2010).

Retrospective review was done in 48 patients, median age 14 months (6–45), after distal TIP repair, with median follow-up 28 months (5–33). The UP was described as "shallow" ($n=15$, 31 %), "moderate" ($n=20$, 42 %) and "deep" ($n=13$, 27 %), of which six (12.5 %) had fistulas with no difference between groups. The UP was also analyzed by pre-incision width at its widest point <8 mm ($n=11$) or >8 mm. All fistulas and meatal stenoses ($n=2$) occurred in those <8 mm. The final neourethra calibrated intra-operatively <6 Fr in 9/48 (19 %) (Holland and Smith 2000).

A RCT randomized 80 boys, mean age 4.5 years (3–7), with primary hypospadias (64 distal, 16 midshaft) into two equal groups based on continuous vs. interrupted urethroplasty suture method. Additionally, the UP was described as "shallow" ($n=20$, 25 %), "intermediate" ($n=34$, 42.5 %), and "deep" ($n=26$, 32.5 %), and was measured under stretch at its widest point before incision and categorized as <8 mm ($n=39$) or >8 mm ($n=41$). There was no difference in outcomes for the primary endpoint (suture method), or based on UP description (shallow, intermediate, or deep). UP width <8 mm before incision had 9/39 (23 %) complications vs. >8 mm with 2/41 (5 %), $p=0.048$. However, plate width after incision <12 mm vs. >12 mm did not correlate with complications (7/47 [15 %] vs. 4/33 [12 %], $p=0.49$) (Sarhan et al. 2009). Severity of hypospadias was not reported to be evenly distributed between the groups with <8 mm vs. >8 mm UP widths, adding a potential confounder to the result, since the same author earlier reported meatal location a significant variable in TIP outcomes (Sarhan et al. 2009).

Ventral Curvature

Distal Hypospadias

Approximately 10 % of distal hypospadias patients have ventral curvature (VC) <30°, with none >30° after degloving.

A series of 440 consecutive distal hypospadias repairs that included artificial erection reported that 11 % had VC after degloving and ventral dartos dissection that always was <30°. This extent of curvature was corrected with a single dorsal midline plication of the tunica albuginea using 6–0 polypropylene (Snodgrass et al. 2009).

Proximal Hypospadias

Prevalence

One study reported VC in consecutive proximal hypospadias cases, finding 50 % had either no or <30° curvature after degloving and ventral dartos dissection, while the other 50 % had >30° curvature.

In 70 consecutive boys with proximal shaft to perineal hypospadias, 13 (19 %) had no VC after degloving the penis and dissecting ventral dartos. Another 22 (31 %) had curvature <30° corrected by a single dorsal plication. The remaining 35 (50 %) had VC>30° (Snodgrass and Prieto 2009).

Dorsal Plication

Two retrospective reviews of dorsal plication in children, one of which reported use for VC>30°, found recurrent VC in 7 %.

Reports of adult patients undergoing plication for penile curvature indicate persistent/recurrent curvature in <10 %.

One study reported (non-validated) questionnaire responses by adults after plication for VC a mean of 55°, with 74 % noting the penis was shorter but 77 % stating they were "modestly to very satisfied" with surgery. Another study of adults including questionnaires stated 95 % reported "good or excellent" results.

Retrospective review was done in 43 patients median age 25 months (6–163) for VC<30° (*n*=20) or >30° (*n*=23), associated with hypospadias in 37 and congenital curvature in 6. Plication was done in the dorsal midline using one or two (*n*=2) 4–0 or 5–0 polypropylene sutures. At median follow-up of 16 months (3–34), 3/43 (7 %) had recurrent VC>30°, including 2 with initial VC>30° (Bar-Yosef et al. 2004).

Another retrospective review included 70 hypospadias patients and 13 with isolated VC median age 2 years who had dorsal plication using three 5–0 polypropylene sutures placed at 1, 12, and 11 o'clock. Extent of VC was not stated. During mean follow-up 6 years (6 months–10 years), repeat erection testing was done in 28 (34 %%) during reoperations with 6 (7 % of the entire cohort) having repeated plication. Parents reported that the other children all had straight erection (Chertin et al. 2004).

Retrospective review was done in adult men, mean age 43 years (16–77), with VC>30°, including 25 with congenital curvature and 5 with curvature after prior hypospadias repair. Plication was done with 3–0 polypropylene sutures into the tunica albuginea without corporal incision. At mean follow-up of 18 months, all these patients reported ability to have sexual intercourse and satisfaction with penile appearance (Thiounn et al. 1998).

Nineteen patients, mean age 19 years, with congenital curvature >30° underwent correction using one to three pairs of 2–0 polypropylene for plication, and then answered a (non-validated) questionnaire a mean of 22 months later. Eighteen of 19 reported "good or excellent" results and 1 (5 %) had recurrent curvature (extent not stated) (Friedrich et al. 2000).

Fifty of 59 patients mean age 40 years (18–71) at time of surgery responded to a (non-validated) questionnaire regarding outcomes of plication for curvature a mean of 55° (30–90°), including 22 with congenital curvature. Straightening was done using six 3–0 polypropylene or Goretex sutures without tunica incision. At a mean of

30 months after surgery, 2/22 (9 %) reported no improvement in VC. Of the 50 respondents, 74 % noted the penis was shorter. Of the 22 with congenital curvature, 17 (77 %) were "moderately to very satisfied" with their outcome and 5 were dissatisfied (van der Horst et al. 2003).

Ventral Lengthening vs. Dorsal Plication

One retrospective study found reoperation for recurrent VC was the same after dorsal plication vs. ventral lengthening in proximal hypospadias patients.

A retrospective analysis identified 100 consecutive patients with proximal hypospadias operated between 1994 and 2004. Decision-making for VC correction was not standardized, but done according to surgeon preference (number of surgeons not stated). Of these 100 patients, 32 had ventral lengthening by UP transection and corporotomy with graft or flap, and 68 had dorsal plication using one or two (numbers not reported) 4–0 or 5–0 polypropylene sutures with UP transection also done in 16 (23 %). At mean follow-up of 2 years, recurrent curvature was more likely after dorsal plications vs. ventral corporal lengthening (19/68 vs. 3/32, $p=0.03$). Among patients with dorsal plication, recurrent VC was more likely in those with UP preservation vs. UP transection (19/52 vs. 0/16, $p=0.002$). Of the 22 patients described with recurrent VC, the extent of curvature was considered sufficient to warrant reoperation in 13, and if only these patients are analyzed, there was no difference in corporal lengthening vs. dorsal plication (1/32 vs. 11/68, $p=0.09$) (Braga et al. 2008).

Dermal Graft

Three retrospective studies reported ventral corporotomy with dermal grafting corrected VC with no or insignificant persistent bending.

One adult with prior corporotomy and grafting reported poor erections requiring medical therapy.

A retrospective review was reported for 16 patients, mean age 7 years (1–19), with corporotomy and dermal grafting who had follow-up a mean of 10 years (6–15). At last review, all were postpubertal, with 13 reporting straight erection, 1 having dorsal curvature from overcorrection, and 2 having persistent VC described as "mild" and not requiring further surgery. Three had known sexual activity, with one having poor-quality erection requiring intracorporeal vasoactive drug injection (Badawy and Morsi 2008).

A two-institution retrospective review identified 41 patients with VC > 15° after degloving, dartos dissection, and UP transection who underwent ventral corporotomy and dermal grafting at median age 13 months (5–70). None had recurrent VC on artificial erection during a second-stage procedure or reported during follow-up a mean of 27 months (Pope et al. 1996).

Retrospective chart review found 23 patients with ventral corporotomy and dermal grafting in 6 primary repairs and 17 reoperations after degloving, dorsal plication, and UP transection. At mean follow-up of 2 years, no patient had recurrent VC (Caesar and Caldamone 2000).

SIS Graft

One- and four-ply SIS have been reported to be effective for grafting the ventral corporotomy with <10 % recurrent VC. One review stated that several patients developed palpable fibrosis after four-ply SIS grafting.

A retrospective review included 28 patients with ventral corporotomy and SIS grafting for VC > 30° after degloving, dartos dissection, and UP transection. Grafts were four-ply in 21 and one-ply in 7. At follow-up a mean of 38 months (6–61) in 26 patients, there was no recurrent VC (Elmore et al. 2007).

Another retrospective review involved nine patients with proximal hypospadias and VC > 30° after degloving and UP transection. Ventral corporotomy and single-ply SIS grafting was done, and at follow-up at 16–21 months, no recurrent VC occurred (Weiser et al. 2003).

Retrospective review of 12 patients with proximal hypospadias who underwent ventral corporotomy and four-ply SIS grafting stated that two (17 %) had either a palpable fibrotic mass over the graft site deemed necessary to excise, or recurrent VC. Another two also had palpable fibrosis that was not treated (Soergel et al. 2003).

Tunica Vaginalis Graft

Ventral corporotomy grafting using tunica vaginalis has <10 % VC recurrence.

A retrospective review stated that 11 patients, mean age 3 years (16–62 months), with proximal hypospadias had ventral corporotomy with tunica vaginalis grafting. At mean follow-up of 14 months (maximum 37), one (9 %) had persistent VC "of some degree" (Perlmutter et al. 1985).

Retrospective review was done in 25 patients, median age 8 months (5 months–16 years), with scrotal to perineal hypospadias who had VC after degloving, dartos dissection, and UP transection and underwent corporotomy with tunica vaginalis grafting. At follow-up of 1–5 years, one (4 %), the 16-year-old, had recurrent VC requiring surgery (Ritchey and Ribbeck 2003).

Another retrospective study included 18 patients with proximal hypospadias: 13 had UP elevation with ventral corporal incision and tunica vaginalis grafting, 5 had only UP transection. At mean follow-up of 27 months (14–41), two (11 %) had recurrent VC < 20°, one with UP elevation and one with UP transection (Kajbafzadeh et al. 2007).

Tunica Vaginalis Flap

Ventral corporotomy coverage was also reported using tunica vaginalis flaps, rather than the various grafts mentioned above. In one analysis, recurrent VC developed in <10 %.

A retrospective review reported ventral corporotomy with tunica vaginalis flap in 23 patients with proximal hypospadias and VC > 45°. At median follow-up of 5 years, recurrent VC > 30° occurred in 1 (4 %) (Braga et al. 2007a).

UP ± Urethral Elevation

Dissection of the UP from the corpora cavernosa potentially reduces the extent of VC, and can be continued proximally along the formed urethra to near the membranous segment to gain additional straightening.

Twenty-five consecutive boys with proximal hypospadias had VC > 30° after degloving and dartos dissection. UP elevation reduced VC to <30° in four boys such that straightening was completed by dorsal plication. UP elevation and continued dissection to mobilize the urethra proximally to near the membranous segment similarly reduced curvature in another 4, leaving 17 with persistent VC > 30°. Three ventral corporotomies were next done without grafting, which achieved straightening while maintaining the UP in eight. The other nine still had VC requiring UP transection. During follow-up a mean of 12 months (2–38), there was no recurrent VC (Snodgrass and Bush 2011).

A retrospective study identified 34 patients with proximal hypospadias (18 proximal shaft, 10 penoscrotal, 6 scrotal), finding VC after degloving was <30° in 6, 30°–60° in 12, and >60° in 16. The next step was dissection of the UP and proximal urethra from the corpora cavernosa, which was reported to achieve straightening in 30 (88 %). Another two also had dorsal plication, while two others had UP transection (Bhat 2007).

Single vs. Multiple Ventral Corporotomies

One study reported no recurrent VC with either single ventral corporotomy with dermal grafting or three ventral corporotomies without grafting.

One study reported prospectively collected data analyzing straightening maneuvers in 70 consecutive patients with primary proximal hypospadias. Of these, 18 had persistent VC > 30° after degloving, dartos dissection, and either UP transection or elevation, with 7 undergoing single corporotomy and dermal grafting vs. 11 straightened by three corporotomies without grafting. No recurrent curvature was apparent with follow-up of 27 months vs. 19 months, respectively (Snodgrass & Prieto 2009).

Urethroplasty

Distal Hypospadias

A prospective case series by one surgeon using only TIP to repair distal hypospadias in 426 consecutive patients reported complications in 4 %, fistulas and glans dehiscences.

A systematic literature review reported a total of 1,872 TIP repairs, with fistulas in 4 %, meatal stenosis in 3 %, and no urethral strictures. Another review found complications ranged from 0 to 24 %, with most articles reporting <10 %.

Two RCTs compared TIP to Mathieu, reporting no difference in urethroplasty complications but improved meatal appearance with TIP.

One systematic literature review reported fistulas more common after Mathieu and meatal stenosis more likely after TIP.

TIP

Five-hundred fifty-one consecutive patients, mean age 17 months (3–140), with distal hypospadias all underwent TIP repair by a single surgeon. Meatal location was glanular/coronal/subcoronal in 445 and distal shaft in 106; 83 (15 %) were MIP variants. Follow-up in 426 was a mean of 8 months, and included calibration, uroflowometry, and/or urethroscopy in 279 (65 %). Complications occurred in 19 (4 %), comprising 9 fistulas, 9 glans dehiscences, and 1 late presentation of meatal balanitis xerotica obliterans (BXO). Otherwise, there were no strictures or meatal stenoses (Snodgrass et al. 2010).

A systematic review of outcomes for distal TIP repair included 15 articles published before December 2009, totaling 1,872 patients. Rates of three complications were reported: fistulas (72, 4 %), meatal stenosis (57, 3 %), and urethral stricture (0) (Wilkinson et al. 2012).

Review of 35 English publications between 1994 and 2009 concerning distal TIP found overall complications ranged from 0 to 24 %, with 25 series reporting ≤10 %. Nearly all of these were fistulas or meatal stenoses (Snodgrass 2011).

A retrospective review included 324 distal TIP repairs done by seven surgeons from 1997 to 2002, during which time another 54 had MAGPI. At follow-up ranging from 6 months to 5 years, complications developed in 75 (23 %), comprising 28 (9 %) with fistulas, 21 (7 %) with meatal stenosis, 11 (3 %) with both fistulas and meatal stenosis, 12 (4 %) with dehiscences, and 3 with strictures (1 %) (Elicevik et al. 2004).

TIP vs. Mathieu

A RCT allocated 30 patients, mean age 24 months, to TIP or Mathieu performed by one surgeon. Mean follow-up was 15 months, with urethroplasty complications in 1 (3 %) TIP and 3 (10 %) Mathieu, $p=0.6$. The meatus was described as slit in all TIP and round in "most" Mathieu (means to determine appearance was not stated) (Oswald et al. 2000).

Another prospective RCT resulted in 30 Mathieu and 37 TIP repairs in children at mean age 23 months, with follow-up scheduled to 6 months (mean not stated). Only fistulas and meatal stenoses were reported, with 3/30 (10 %) Mathieu and 8/37 (22 %) TIP having complications, $p=0.3$. Meatal appearance was determined by a urologist blinded to the repair type, who rated all Mathieu rounded and all TIP slit (Elganainy et al. 2010).

A systematic review of published articles from 1990 to 2009 reviewed a total of 23 papers, with 1,872 distal TIP and 1,496 Mathieu repairs. Fistulas occurred in 4 % of TIP and 5 % of Mathieu, $p=0.028$; meatal stenosis was reported in 3 % of TIP and 0.7 % of Mathieu, $p<0.001$(Wilkinson et al. 2012).

Proximal Hypospadias

Urethroplasty options for proximal hypospadias repair depend in part on whether or not the UP is transected during penile straightening, discussed above.

When the UP is preserved, both TIP and onlay preputial flap are options.

When the UP is transected, urethroplasty options include one-stage tubularized preputial flaps or grafts, or two-stage preputial flaps or grafts.

TIP

One surgeon reported technical modifications (chromic to polyglactin/polydiaxone sutures, one-layer running epithelial to two-layer interrupted and running subepithelial tubularization, and dartos barrier flap to tunica vaginalis flap) that reduced proximal TIP complications from 53 to 13 % in consecutive patients.

One retrospective study similarly found 12 % complications with proximal TIP, while another compared proximal TIP to onlay preputial flap and found no difference in urethroplasty complications (60 % vs. 45 %).

Prospectively recorded data was used to evaluate 49 consecutive boys with TIP repair for proximal hypospadias by a single surgeon. Fifty-three percent of complications occurred in the first 15, 25 % in the next 20, and 13 % in the final 24 patients ($p=0.02$), including fistulas ($n=7$, 44 %), glans dehiscence ($n=5$, 31 %), and meatal stenosis or urethral stricture (1 each, 12.5 %). Technical modifications made to reduce fistulas included:

- Change in urethroplasty sutures from chromic to polyglactin/polydiaxone.
- Change in urethroplasty suturing method from one layer running epithelial to two-layer subepithelial tubularization, the first interrupted polyglactin and the second running polydiaxone.
- Addition of spongioplasty.
- Substitution of tunica vaginalis for dartos as a barrier flap over the neourethra.

No fistulas occurred in the last 24 patients (Snodgrass and Bush 2011).

A review was done in 49 patients, mean age 23 months (16–72), undergoing proximal TIP repair (dates of study period, number of surgeons, number of alternative repairs not stated). Urethroplasty was done using 6–0 polyglactin subepithelial continuous suture in one layer covered by a dorsal dartos flap. During follow-up a mean of 3 years (14 months–6 years), urethroplasty complications developed in six (12 %), including four fistulas, one meatal stenosis, and one glans dehiscence (Ghanem and Nijman 2011).

A retrospective review compared 35 proximal TIP to 40 onlay preputial flap repairs done from 1998 to 2006 in children a mean age of 17 months (9–91). The number of surgeons involved was not stated. At mean follow-up of approximately 3 years, there was no significant difference in urethroplasty complications, 21/35 (60 %) TIP and 18/40 (45 %) onlay (Braga et al. 2007b).

Onlay Preputial Flap

Several retrospective studies report urethroplasty complications in 17–45 % after proximal onlay preputial flap repair (Table 9.1).

A retrospective review concerned patients with "proximal division of the corpus spongiosum after degloving and marked hypoplasia of ventral tissues" operated by one surgeon from 1997 to 2007. There were 126 primary onlay repairs done at mean age 23 months (8–96), with follow-up a mean of 22 months (1–97). Of these, only 13 (10 %) had VC corrected by dorsal plication. Urethroplasty complications developed in 34 (27 %), including 18 fistulas, 13 dehiscences, 2 strictures, and 1 diverticulum (de Mattos e Silva et al. 2009).

The retrospective review by Braga et al. (2007b) described above included 40 onlay repairs for children mean age 17 months with proximal hypospadias. Of these, 18 (45 %) had VC > 30° corrected by dorsal plication. With follow-up a mean of 39 months, complications occurred in 18 (45 %), including 8 fistulas, 2 dehiscences, 2 strictures, 1 meatal stenosis, and 5 recurrent VC, of which 2 had subsequent dorsal plication.

A retrospective chart review considered patients operated for proximal hypospadias from 1981 to 1997, identifying 142 with follow-up of which 20 had an onlay flap repair. Median age for the entire series was 11 months, and follow-up was a median of 9 months (1–79). Urethroplasty complications after onlay flap occurred in six (30 %), including three fistulas, one stricture, one meatal stenosis, and one diverticulum (Powell et al. 2000).

Table 9.1 One-stage proximal hypospadias repair using preputial flaps

	No. patients	Mean f/u (mos)	Complications/Rate (%)	F	MS	Stx	GD	D	VC
Onlay preputial flap									
Powell et al.	20	9 (median)	6/30	3	1	1	–	1	–
Braga et al.	40	39	18/45	8	1	2	2	–	5
de Mattos e Silva et al.	126	22	34/27	18	–	2	13	1	–
Hayashi et al.	52	NS	9/17	3	–	–	9	–	–
Tubularized preputial flap									
Powell et al.	27	9 (median)	9/33	7	1	1		0	
Shukla et al.	12	24.5	2/17	1	1			1	
Chuang et al.	86	6	22/39	16[a]	–	–	–	–	–
Aoki et al.	22	24	3/14	1	2	–	–	–	–

F fistula, *MS* meatal stenosis, *Stx* stenosis, *GD* glans dehiscence, *D* diverticulum, *VC* ventral curvature
[a]Other complications not described

Retrospective analysis was done in 52 patients after onlay preputial flap repair for proximal hypospadias at median age of approximately 2 years (10–132 months). Duration of follow-up was not stated. Urethroplasty complications occurred in a total of 9 (17 %) boys, including 9 glans dehiscences and 3 fistulas (Hayashi et al. 2007).

Tubularized Preputial Flap

Four retrospective studies report urethroplasty complications in from 14 to 39 % after tubularized preputial flap repairs for proximal hypospadias (see Table 9.1).

One study reported that two-layer tubularization of the flap had significantly fewer complications that did one-layer repair.

The two studies reporting the lowest complication rates both anchored one edge of the flap to the corpora cavernosa and then stretched and fashioned it into a tube.

A retrospective review analyzed 56 patients with proximal hypospadias undergoing tubularized preputial flap repair from1986 to 1993 within a cohort of 103 total patients mean age 4 years (5 months–14 years) who underwent that repair, the others having distal hypospadias. Follow-up was at least 6 months. Of the 56 cases, the flap was tubularized in one layer in 29 and in two layers in 27, the authors stating most the one-layer closures were done earlier in the series and then gradually phased out in favor of a two-layer technique. Complications occurred in 17 (59 %) and 5 (19 %), for a total rate of 22 (39 %). These included mostly fistulas, as well as urethral stricture, meatal stenosis, glans dehiscence, and urethra diverticulum, but those specifically occurring after proximal hypospadias repair were not stated (Chuang and Shieh 1995).

The retrospective chart review by Powell et al. (2000) described above with 142 patients operated for proximal hypospadias from 1981 to 1997 reported outcomes for 27 tubularized preputial flaps. Median age for the entire series was 11 months, and follow-up was a median of 9 months (1–79). Urethroplasty complications developed in nine (33 %)—seven fistulas, one stricture, one meatal stenosis, and 0 diverticulum.

Another retrospective study of patients operated with proximal hypospadias between 1997 and 2001 by one surgeon found 12 corrected using a tubularized preputial flap vs. 10 undergoing two-stage repairs. All had UP transection while straightening VC. Rather than tubularizing the preputial flap over a catheter, the flap was anchored length-wise to the corpora cavernosa and then tailored into a tube. During follow-up at a mean of 24 months (20–33), two (17 %) with tubularized preputial flap had complications—one fistula and one meatal stenosis (Shukla et al. 2004).

Twenty-two boys, mean age 17 months (10–156), with proximal hypospadias had tubularized preputial flap repair in 2005 and 2006. The flap was first sutured to the corpora and then folded into a tube. At follow-up a mean of 24 months

Table 9.2 Proximal Byar's flap outcomes

	No. patients	Mean f/u (mos)	Complications/rate (%)	F	MS	Stx	GD	D	VC
Gershbaum et al.[a]	11	60–180	2/18	1	–	–	–	1	–
Cheng et al.[b]	14	6–36	2/14	1	–	–	–	2	–
Shukla et al.	10	43.5	7/70	7	3	–	–	1	–

F fistula, *MS* meatal stenosis, *Stx* stenosis, *GD* glans dehiscence, *D* diverticulum, *VC* ventral curvature
[a]Surgical technique not stated
[b]Combined with distal TIP

(18–30), complications developed in three (14 %)—two meatal stenoses and one fistula (Aoki et al. 2008).

Two-Stage Preputial Flaps (Byar's Flaps)

Our review found only three reports with information regarding outcomes after two-stage preputial flap repairs, comprising 35 patients. Complications ranged from 14 to 70 % (Table 9.2).

The study by Shukla et al. (2004) described above included ten patients who underwent two-stage preputial flap repair. During follow-up a mean of 43 months (33–60), seven (70 %) had urethroplasty complications that included fistulas in all seven, meatal stenosis in three, and a urethral diverticulum in one.

A retrospective study of patients operated between 1980 and 1995 reported 1,934 hypospadias repairs, of which 51 (3 %) had scrotal/perineal defects. Of these, 11 had two- stage preputial flap repair. Follow-up was only described as from 5 to 15 years. None had recurrent VC. Urethroplasty complications occurred in two (18 %), a fistula and a diverticulum, but only seven were described as voiding with a "normal stream"; four had "difficulty with terminal voiding and spraying" (Gershbaum et al. 2002).

Four surgeons reported results of two-stage preputial flaps interposed between the glanular UP and a more proximal urethral meatus in 14 patients. At follow-up of between 6 months and 3 years, complications developed in two (14 %)—two diverticula and a fistula (Cheng et al. 2003).

One- and Two-Stage Preputial Grafts

One study reported one-stage tubularized preputial grafts had 34 % complications, including 13 % strictures.

Two retrospective studies reported complications after two-stage preputial graft repairs in 6 and 26 %.

The retrospective study by Powell et al. (2000) discussed above included 61 one-stage tubularized preputial skin grafts. At median follow-up of 9 months for the entire study group, there were 21 (34 %) complications after these grafts, including 11 fistulas, 8 strictures, 1 meatal stenosis, and 1 diverticulum. However, glans dehiscence was also stated to occur in three patients not listed among these complications.

Two-stage preputial grafts were the subject of a retrospective review including 32 patients, of which 8 (25 %) had midshaft hypospadias and the remainder, proximal hypospadias. Initial surgery was performed at median age 21 months (15–26), and follow-up after the second stage was a median of 35 months (20–55) in 31 cases. The authors reported that one developed a fistula and one had "mild residual" VC for a complication rate of 2/31 (6 %), although the authors did not specifically state there were no other problems such as glans dehiscence or diverticula (Springer and Subramaniam 2012).

Another retrospective study reported two-stage preputial grafts in 43 patients with proximal penile to perineal hypospadias and "significant chordee" at median age 1 year (7 months–17 years). Of these, six were reoperations, and there was follow-up of 1 month to 4 years (mean not stated) in 34 (number with primary vs. reoperative repairs not stated). Penile straightening was not described, and 6/37 (16 %) primary repairs had additional subsequent correction with dorsal plication. Complications after the second stage occurred in nine cases (26 %), including four glans dehiscences, two fistulas, one diverticulum, one "long urethral stenosis with BXO" and one "meatal retraction" (Ferro et al. 2002).

Postoperative Management and Assessment

Urinary Diversion

One RCT reported no differences in urethroplasty outcomes following distal TIP repair with vs. without urinary diversion in toilet-trained boys. However, there were significantly more complications, including dysuria, urinary retention, and urinary extravasation without stents, with 40 % of those not stented having a catheter subsequently placed.

TIP urethroplasty without stent was reported in 32 consecutive non–toilet-trained boys with distal, midshaft, and proximal hypospadias, with one developing extravasation with subsequent catheter placement.

There are no data indicating optimal size or duration of use of stents. No report compares urinary diversion by suprapubic vs. urethral catheters in otherwise similar patients.

One RCT comprised 64 toilet-trained boys (median age 6 years, range 2–17) undergoing distal TIP repair by a single surgeon, randomized at the end of the procedure to postoperative bladder catheterization vs. no urinary diversion. There were no differences in urethroplasty complications (3/35 vs. 6/29, $p=0.3$); however, dysuria (14 % vs. 45 %, $p<0.01$), urinary retention (0 % vs. 24 %, $p<0.05$), and urinary extravasation (0 % vs. 17 %, $p<0.05$) occurred significantly more often in the unstented group. Of 29 unstented patients, 12 (41 %) had a catheter placed for urinary retention or extravasation ≤3 days postoperatively (El-Sherbiny 2003).

A prospective study involved 32 consecutive non–toilet-trained boys (mean age 18±6 months) undergoing TIP by one surgeon for distal-midshaft ($n=26$) and proximal shaft ($n=6$) hypospadias with no urinary diversion. Urinary extravasation developed in one patient (distal vs. proximal defect not stated) the second postoperative day, resulting in catheter placement. There was 1 (3 %) urethroplasty complication, meatal stenosis, during mean follow-up of 9±6 months (Almodhen et al. 2008).

Bandages

Two RCTs reported no differences in urethroplasty complications related to use or nonuse of postoperative bandages.

One hundred consecutive patients undergoing distal to proximal primary and reoperative hypospadias repair were eligible for randomization in a study comparing a transparent waterproof adhesive bandage around the penis for 2 days or no bandage (randomization pre- or intra-operatively was not stated). Two were excluded for bleeding at the end of the procedure. Parents of those with a bandage were told to remove it on the second day "or sooner if it was soiled." Mean follow-up was 1 year, with urethroplasty complications occurring in 4/49 with vs. 3/49 without a bandage. Telephone calls from patients were significantly greater in those without bandages (0.3 vs. 0.8 calls/patient, $p=0.02$), but the authors did not state if these calls related specifically to bandages or wound appearance vs. other questions (Van Savage et al. 2000).

One-hundred twenty boys mean age 2 years with distal and proximal ($n=60$) hypospadias underwent repair by four surgeons and were randomized at the end of the procedure to a transparent biomembrane adhesive film, compression wrap, or no bandage (polymixin B and bacitracin zinc in a white petrolatum applied with diaper change or TID for 7 days). Three were withdrawn due to bleeding that resulted in a compressive wrap. Bandages were removed at ≥3 days when bathing resumed and they soaked off, with subsequent white petrolatum applied until 7 days. Urethroplasty complications developed in 16 (14 %) with no differences among the three groups (McLorie et al. 2001).

Preventing Erections

One RCT found oral ketoconazole was no more effective than placebo in preventing

postoperative erections, but did cause increased nausea and transient liver dysfunction in one patient. No medication therapy has been reported effective to temporarily reduce or prevent postoperative erections.

One placebo-controlled double-blinded RCT enrolled 40 men at mean age 28 years undergoing penile surgeries, such as circumcisions and urethroplasties, to either perioperative oral ketoconazole 400 mg TID or placebo for 1 week. There was no reduction in either erections or painful erections (both occurring in >80 %) using ketoconazole, but three (16 %) treated patients withdrew due to nausea and another developed transient liver dysfunction (DeCastro et al. 2008).

Duration of Follow-up

The minimum duration of follow-up needed to encounter the majority of complications has not been established for hypospadias repair. Two studies report that >70 % are diagnosed within 1 year of repair.

No case series include continuous follow-up into adulthood of patients after childhood hypospadias repair.

One review concerning glans dehiscence reported diagnosis in 32 patients a mean of 3.9 months after surgery, with 88 % found at the first postoperative visit (Snodgrass et al. 2011).

Another analysis considered time to diagnosis of urethroplasty complications after TIP repair using prospectively maintained databases. There were 752 primary and 139 reoperations with complications in 78 and 37, respectively. These were diagnosed at the first postoperative visit in 73 (64 %) and/or within the first year in 89 (78 %), with median time 3 months. After 12 months, 35 patients would need indefinite follow-up to detect an additional urethroplasty complication (Villanueva et al. 2012).

A retrospective review of 26 patients with fistulas reported that approximately 60 % were diagnosed within 1 month after surgery, and 70 % within 1 year. However, time for follow-up to detect over 90 % of fistulas was 93 months after primary hypospadias repair, since patients sometimes present years after surgery with apparently new onset of a fistula (Wood et al. 2008). The total number of patients undergoing hypospadias repair that would need postoperative follow-up to as long as 8 years to detect these occasionally late-appearing fistulas was not calculated.

Calibration

Sounding the neomeatus and urethra provides objective evidence for the lack of anatomic obstruction.

The minimum caliber of the urethra in normal boys varies in published reports. One study found that 14 % of boys < 3 years of age were <8 Fr, while two others performing calibrations under general anesthesia stated minimum size encountered was 10 Fr.

Meatal size was determined in 100 consecutive full-term newborns using bougie a boules or olive-tipped catheters on the second day of life. The mean and median was 8 Fr. The meatus was less than 8 Fr in 51, the smallest reported as 4 Fr in 9 patients. The largest caliber was 12 Fr in a single newborn (Allen et al. 1972).

Another study similarly used bougie a boules to determine meatal size in 200 boys referred to urology "with no voiding complaints." Of 160 <1 year of age, 22 (14 %) were <8 Fr, while the remainder were 10 Fr. Results were the same for boys 1–3 years of age. From ages 4–10 years, the meatus was "tight 8 Fr" in <10 % and 12 Fr in the remainder (Litvak et al. 1976).

Calibration using sounds under general anesthesia was done in 88 uncircumcised boys aged 0–14 years with non-urethral conditions. The cohort included 10 patients <1 year, and 66 <4 years of age. None had urethral caliber <10 Fr (Yang et al. 2001).

Sixty uncircumcised boys aged 5 months–16 years undergoing hernia repairs or appendectomies were calibrated with Hegar dilators under general anesthesia. Considering those 5 months–12 years, mean width was 4 mm (3.5–4.5), which corresponds to approximately 10–12 Fr. The number of boys calibrated in various age groups was not stated (Orkiszewski and Madej 2010).

Uroflowometry

Most reported data compare patients to various nomograms rather than to controls.

Two studies reported uroflow in infants using ultrasound probes, one finding mean preoperative and postoperative Q_{max} no different than controls and the other reporting preoperative infants with distal hypospadias had median Q_{max} less than controls.

Flow rates after hypospadias repair frequently cluster below the fiftieth percentile for age compared to nomogram, regardless of urethroplasty technique, indicating that the neourethra is not a normal urethra. Significance of diminished flow velocity in asymptomatic boys without anatomic obstruction is uncertain.

Preoperative

A study compared preoperative uroflow data in 42 patients with distal hypospadias at mean age 16±6 months to 51 controls with mean age 11±11 months, obtained using an ultrasound flow probe affixed around the penile base. There was no significant difference in mean Q_{max} in patients vs. controls (7.5±2.5 cc/s vs. 6.8±4.1 cc/s). Plateau curves occurred in 6 % of patients and 3 % of controls. Postoperative studies after 53 distal TIP and 10 proximal TIP repairs were not significantly different than controls (7.3±5.5 cc/s, 8.2±4.6 cc/s vs. 10.9±10.9 cc/s) (Wolffenbuttel et al. 2006).

Another study compared uroflow data in 21 unoperated infants with distal hypospadias at mean age 14 months (13–22) to 19 normal infants at mean age 12 months (9–20) using an ultrasound flow probe fixed around the base of the penis. Median Q_{max} was significantly less in patients vs. controls (2.4 [0.9–10] vs. 4.4 [0.6–10], $p<0.01$). Bell-shaped curves were noted in 43 % of patients and 63 % of controls, while plateau curves were found in 38 % of patients but in no controls. The hypospadias meatus calibrated to a median 10 Fr (6–12) and did not correlate with Q_{max} (Olsen et al. 2011).

Postoperative TIP

Q_{max} <2 SD from normal has been reported in 0–22 % of toilet-trained patients having uroflowometry after TIP.

One study that reported that 49 % were <2 SD stated that all had Q_{max} > 5 cc/s, and that had an alternative nomogram been used (Toguri rather than Miskolc), the percentage <2 SD would change to 11 %.

Seventeen (34 %) of the first 50 patients who had TIP repair and were toilet-trained during follow-up had uroflowometry at a mean of 45 months (6 months–7 years) postoperatively. Fourteen had distal and three had proximal repairs, and all Q_{max} were within 2 SD of normal for "standard curves" (nomogram used was not stated). All Q_{max} exceeded 5 cc/s. Curve patterns were not reported (Snodgrass 1999).

A retrospective study identified 48 patients who were toilet-trained and had uroflowometry >6 months postoperatively after distal hypospadias repair, from a cohort of 412 boys undergoing TIP from 1996 to 2000. Q_{max} were above 2 SD from normal in 33 (78 %) using an institutional nomogram. The curve was described as "flat" in 31 with normal peak flows, to distinguish it from either bell-shaped or plateau patterns (Hammouda et al. 2003).

Another retrospective study reported uroflow data from 28 of a total of 70 patients who underwent TIP for distal to midshaft hypospadias, excluding those not toilet trained or having fistula, meatal stenosis, or urethral stricture. Follow-up was a mean of 18 months (10–40), and Q_{max} was compared to Toguri nomograms. Values <2 SD were found in two (7 %). Normal was defined as greater than the twenty-fifth percentile and occurred in 22 (78.5 %). A bell-shaped curve was reported in 23 (82 %) (Kaya et al. 2007).

Forty-eight patients with foreskin-preserving TIP repair, 38 distal and 10 proximal, who were toilet trained 1 year after surgery, had uroflowometry. Two to three determinations were made, the highest Q_{max} reported, and values then compared to Miskolc nomograms. A urotherapist additionally questioned the patients for obstructive voiding complaints. Eleven (23 %) had obstructive symptoms and were all diagnosed with meatal stenosis. For the remaining 37, mean Q_{max} was 14 cc/s (6–28). Eighteen (49 %) had Q_{max} below 2 SD, yet ≥5 cc/s. Calibration was done in 6 of these 18 without evidence for anatomic obstruction. Curves were described in

26/37 (70 %), bell-shaped in 14 (54 %) and plateau in 12. Repeated uroflows were obtained 6 years later, with a significantly greater mean Q_{max} 19 cc/s (17–36), and 12 (32 %) with flows less than the fifth percentile. Curves were stated for 24; bell-shaped in 11 (44 %) and plateau in the remainder. Considering all with flows less than the fifth percentile, all improved, with 28 % moving above the fifth percentile. Two others with initial flow rates greater than the fifth percentile were later less than the fifth percentile, but were asymptomatic and not further evaluated. Boys having proximal repairs were more likely than those with distal repairs to have Q_{max} less than the fifth percentile. The authors noted that the number of patients less than the fifth percentile 1 year after surgery would have been less (4 vs. 18) had they used Toguri rather than Miskolc nomograms (Andersson et al. 2011).

A retrospective study reported uroflowometry after proximal TIP, in a series with urethroplasty complications in 21/35 (60 %). "All toilet-trained" patients had two uroflows, with the second used for analysis, but the number of patients this comprised was not stated. Mean Q_{max} was 8 cc/s (4–17), with 16/24 (67 %) having a plateau curve pattern (Braga et al. 2007b).

Postoperative Preputial Flaps

One study reported no difference in results on uroflowometry between onlay and tubularized preputial flaps, with 27 % having Q_{max}<2 SD. Most of the others had Q_{max} in the lower fiftieth percentile.

Retrospective review reported uroflow data in patients undergoing tubularized or onlay preputial flap repairs between 1986 and 1992, finding no significant differences between results obtained with these two methods. Of 51 boys without complications, 37 (73 %) had normal Q_{max} (>2 SD), while 14 (27 %) had Q_{max}<2 SD using an institutional nomogram. The authors reported that most normal Q_{max} were in the lower fiftieth percentile. Curves were not described (Jayanthi et al. 1995).

The retrospective study by Braga et al. (2007b) mentioned above included uroflow data on patients after proximal onlay repair, of which 18/40 (45 %) had urethroplasty complications. An unspecified number had uroflowometry, reporting mean Q_{max} 8 cc/s (4–17); 17/21(33 %) with curve description had a plateau pattern.

Another study evaluated patients who underwent tubularized and onlay preputial flap repair by one surgeon for proximal hypospadias between 1981 and 1992. Of 125 patients, medical information could only be retrieved for 73, of which 49 could be contacted for follow-up ≥10 years postoperatively, and 30 agreed to examination. These patients had been operated at mean age 17 months (8–74), and late follow-up was a mean of 14 years later (12–21). Uroflowometry was obtained in 25 of the 30, with mean Q_{max} of 11 tubularized flaps, 17 cc/s (15–21), and of 14 onlay flaps, 18 cc/s (7–36), $p=0.7$. Post-void residual by bladder scan ultrasound was a mean of 5 cc (0–21) for tubularized and 17.5 cm^3 (0–221) after onlay, $p=0.5$ (Patel et al. 2004).

Cosmesis

One study using (non-validated) questionnaires reported parents scored cosmetic outcomes after distal and proximal TIP repair similar to parents of normal boys undergoing circumcision.

No similar data comparing cosmetic hypospadias outcomes to normal controls have been published for flap-based repairs.

Blinded photographic assessment in two studies rated appearance after TIP superior than after Mathieu or preputial onlay flaps.

One study used photographs to judge postoperative appearance of the meatus after standard proximal onlay preputial flap vs. a modified version with ventral meatal slit to improve the appearance of the neomeatus. While the modification increased likelihood for a slit-meatal appearance (27 % vs. 55 %), the most reliable factor for optimal appearance of the neomeatus was an already deeply grooved UP.

A study administered Likert-scale questionnaires to parents of boys after 50 distal and 15 midshaft-to-proximal TIP, and 22 circumcisions (controls) in consecutive patients returning for 6-week follow-up. There were no significant differences in scores rating overall appearance or specific appearance of the meatus and penile skin by parents of patients vs. controls (Snodgrass et al. 2008).

Another study used postoperative standardized photographs obtained a median of 21 months (1–120) after surgery to compare 16 TIP (10 distal and 6 proximal) done by one pediatric urologist to 10 Mathieu (distal) and 6 onlay (proximal) repairs done by a second pediatric urologist. A blinded panel of three men and two women, comprising another four surgeons and a nurse, scored the photographs assigning 1–4 points each for the appearance of the meatus, glans, shaft, and overall appearance. All mean scores were significantly higher for TIP (Ververidis et al. 2005).

A study was done to determine if objective scoring by photographs or subjective assessments was superior. Twenty-seven patients with distal hypospadias repaired by one surgeon using TIP in 12 and Mathieu in 15 were assessed 6 months' postoperatively. Objective scoring considered five items assigned 0–2 points each: prepuce (reconstructed in approximately 50 % of both repairs), glans shape, meatal shape, meatal position, and shaft appearance. These photos were reviewed by a surgeon blinded to the surgical technique. Then the same photos were rereviewed by the same blinded surgeon, and the operating surgeon was asked to give only an overall subjective score of 0–10. A parent also subjectively scored an overall impression. The objective mean score was 7.4 ± 1.5, median 7 (5–10). Subjective scores by each observer were similar. Median scores were significantly better for TIP vs. Mathieu (8 [5–10] vs. 7.25 [5–10], $p = 0.02$) (Scarpa et al. 2009).

Retrospective analysis was done for two groups of patients at median age approximately 2 years (10–132 months) with proximal hypospadias undergoing the standard onlay procedure ($n = 30$) vs. a ventral slit modification ($n = 22$) designed to create a more slit-like neomeatus. Outpatient photographs were used to judge the meatus, which was considered slit-like in 8/30 (27 %) standard onlays vs. 12/22 (55 %) modified onlays, $p = 0.04$ (Hayashi et al. 2007). However, only those patients with a deeply grooved UP reliably had a slit-like neomeatus, while there was no significant difference in outcomes in the standard vs. modified technique for those with a flat or intermediately clefted UP.

Complications

General Risk Factors

Logistic regression analysis of prospectively collected data in over 600 consecutive patients undergoing TIP by one surgeon found increased urethroplasty complications predicted by meatal location (increasing with more proximal cases), and reoperation (vs. primary repair).

Similar analyses using retrospective data after TIP also reported proximal repair increased risk for complications.

Sutures (chromic, polyglactin, polydiaxone), suturing methods (interrupted vs. continuous), suture size (6–0,7–0), stents or not, and surgeon were not found to be independent risk factors. The presence or absence of a barrier layer was significant in one report, while another found spongioplasty an independent factor, but not when compared to a dartos flap.

One report demonstrated a learning curve (first 100 cases), while another did not (first 50 cases). One found age >4 years a risk factor, while two others did not find age at surgery a significant independent factor.

Multiple logistic regression was used to determine odds for TIP urethroplasty complications based upon potential risk factors, including age at surgery, meatal location, and primary vs. reoperative repair, in consecutive patients operated by a single surgeon. All data were prospectively collected in databases. From a total of 967 hypospadias repairs done from 1999 to 2011, 156 TIP had no follow-up, 124 boys underwent inlay or staged graft operations, and 18 were postpubertal, leaving the study cohort of 669 boys aged 3–144 months with meatal location distal in 540 (81 %), midshaft in 50 (7.5 %), and proximal in 79 (12 %). Reoperations comprised 73 (11 %) cases. Urethroplasty complications (fistula, glans dehiscence, meatal stenosis, urethral stricture) occurred in 77 (11.5 %). Meatal location (distal vs. midshaft vs. proximal) correlated with complication risk (OR 1.79 [95 % CI 1.34–2.40]), as did reoperative TIP (OR 3.07 [95 % CI 1.54–6.13]). Age, log age, age quartiles, age <6 months, age >1 year, and age >5 years did not contribute to risk for urethroplasty complications, nor was there a learning curve (first 50 cases) or difference in urethroplasty using chromic vs. polyglactin sutures (Bush et al. 2012).

A retrospective analysis was done to determine risk factors for urethroplasty complications after TIP in operations performed from 1997 to 2007 by five surgeons. During this time, a total of 777 children had repairs, of which 391 were TIP at median age 2 years (6 months–16 years). 347 (89 %) were primary repairs, while another 44 (11 %) were reoperations, and meatal location was distal-midshaft in 334 (85 %) and proximal in 57 (15 %). Urethroplasty complications occurred in 48/391 (12 %). Logistic regression identified proximal hypospadias (RR 2.81 [95 % CI 1.42–5.52]), age >4 years (RR 3.25 [95 % CI 1.44–7.35]) and no neourethra barrier layer (RR 6.23 [95 % CI 1.87–20.77]) as risk factors for urethroplasty complications. Surgeon, polyglactin vs. polydiaxone, continuous vs. interrupted suturing, 6–0 or 7–0 suture, and stent were not found to be independent risk factors (Eassa et al. 2011).

Another retrospective analysis also performed multivariable logistic analysis to determine risk factors for complications after TIP. There were 500 patients with mean age 6 years (1–18), of which 439 (88 %) had primary repair and 61 (12 %) a reoperation after one failed repair. The meatus was distal in 371 (74 %), midshaft in 78 (16 %), and proximal in 51 (10 %). Operations were done by five surgeons (with results for each reported). Variables evaluated included patient age, meatal location, primary vs. reoperation, continuous vs. interrupted urethroplasty suture methods, use of a stent or not, spongioplasty or not, dartos barrier flap or not, surgeon, and learning curve. Multivariable analysis found only proximal meatal location, no spongioplasty, and learning curve (first 100 cases) as independent risk factors for complications. However, the authors stated that spongioplasty vs. a dartos flap was not significantly different (Sarhan et al. 2009).

Fistulas

Prevention

One RCT indicated that one-layer subepithelial distal-midshaft TIP urethroplasty had the same outcomes whether suturing was interrupted or continuous.

One RCT found that a ventral dartos flap significantly reduced fistulas vs. no dartos flap in distal TIP.

Technical modifications, including suture change (chromic to polyglactin and polydiaxanone), change in suturing method (one-layer running epithelial to two-layer subepithelial, the first interrupted and second running), spongioplasty, and change in barrier flaps (tunica vaginalis rather than dartos) resulted in a significant reduction in fistulas after proximal TIP in consecutive patient cohorts.

Retrospective analyses report that one-layer subepithelial suturing had fewer fistulas than one-layer epithelial closures in Mathieu flap repairs, and two-layer epithelial suturing resulted in fewer fistulas than one-layer tubularized preputial flap in proximal repairs.

One RCT reported fibrin glue plus dartos flap reduced fistulas and decreased size of fistulas more than dartos flap alone in tubularized preputial flap repair.

One RCT equally allocated a total of 80 boys at mean age 4.5 years (3–7) with primary distal shaft ($n=64$) or midshaft ($n=16$) hypospadias to TIP urethroplasty using interrupted vs. running subepithelial 6–0 or 7–0 polyglactin sutures (number of layers not stated). There were no differences in fistulas, meatal stenosis, or wound dehiscence between patient groups (Sarhan et al. 2009).

Another RCT allocated 130 patients with primary distal hypospadias to TIP with vs. without a ventral dartos flap barrier layer over the neourethra. Operations were done by three surgeons; urethroplasty was the same in all patients using 6–0 continuous polyglyconate (epithelial vs subepithelial and number of layers was not stated), and postoperative care was also uniform. Median follow-up was 24 months (6–60), with fistulas noted in 15/65 (23 %) without a dartos flap vs. 5/65 (8 %), $p=0.03$. Meatal stenosis and glans dehiscence occurred equally in both cohorts for overall rates of 4 % and 5 %, respectively (Savanelli et al. 2007).

Statistically significant reduction in fistula occurrence after proximal TIP was reported from 33 to10 to 0 % in 15, 20, and 24 consecutive patients in sequential series operated by a single surgeon after making several technical changes:

- Urethroplasty sutures from chromic to polyglactin and polydioxanone.
- Suturing methods from one-layer running epithelial to two-layer subepithelial interrupted (polyglactin) and then running (polydiaxone).
- Addition of corpus spongiosum coverage over the neourethra.
- Replacement of dartos barrier flaps with tunica vaginalis flaps (Snodgrass and Bush 2011).

A retrospective review of primary Mathieu distal hypospadias repairs done from 1993 to 1995 found that 36 initial patients had one-layer urethroplasty using 6–0 polyglactin running epithelial sutures, while 61 subsequent patients had one-layer urethroplasty using 7–0 polydioxanone running subepithelial sutures. All other aspects of surgery and postoperative care were said to be similar. During follow-up, described as between 6 and 12 months, 6/36 (17 %) initial vs. 3/60 (5 %) later patients had fistulas, $p<0.01$, with no other complications noted in either group (Ulman et al. 1997).

Another retrospective review analyzed preputial flaps tubularized in one vs. two layers using running epithelial 6–0 or 7–0 polyglactin. Single-layer closures were more common initially and gradually replaced with two-layer repairs done from 1986 to 1993. Otherwise, surgical technique and postoperative care were described as similar. All patients were followed at least 6 months, but actual duration and timing of fistula diagnosis were not stated. There was no difference in fistula rates in patients with distal hypospadias regardless of methods, but there was a significant reduction of fistulas in proximal repairs with two-layer urethroplasty (12/29 [41 %] one-layer vs. 4/27 [15 %] two-layer, $p=0.04$) (Chuang and Shieh 1995).

Reduction of fistula rate by using fibrin glue was reported in a prospective randomized trial of 120 boys with proximal hypospadias undergoing tubularized preputial flaps by a single surgeon. Timing of randomization to receive fibrin glue vs. none was not stated. Those treated had the glue coated directly onto the neourethra suture line, and then also over the dartos flap covering the neourethra. Fistulas were found in 6/60 (10 %) with fibrin glue vs. 19/60 (32 %) without glue, $p=0.027$, and were more likely to be <2 mm with glue than without, 6/6 vs. 7/19, $p=0.015$ (Gopal et al. 2008).

Treatment

Three retrospective case series found recurrent fistulas in from 4 to 29 % despite barrier layer coverage over the repair and either universal or selective postoperative stenting.

There was no difference in recurrence for fistulas repaired after primary vs. reoperative hypospadias repair, or with first vs. subsequent fistula closures.

One study found recurrence greater in fistulas >2 mm.

One case series reported that one to seven topical applications of n-butylcyanoacrylate at diagnosis of fistula (as early as 3 days after catheter removal) successfully closed approximately 50 %.

One retrospective series reported outcomes for 113 fistula closures. Interval between hypospadias and fistula repair was not stated. At surgery, eight had distal obstruction, resulting in a simultaneous three meatal dilations, two meatotomies, two direct visual internal urethrotomies (DVIU), and one reoperative urethroplasty. All had subepithelial urethral closure and coverage with barrier tissues, and all were stented 1 week. Follow-up after the last surgery was a median 7.5 years (2–17). Thirty-three out of 113 (29 %) fistulas recurred after initial closure, 10/33 (30 %) after a second closure, and 5/10 (50 %) after a third closure, $p=0.4$. Fistulas ≤2 mm were less likely than those >2 mm to recur (22/92 vs. 11/21, $p=0.02$ (Shankar et al. 2002).

Another retrospective review reported outcomes for closure of 99 fistulas, all >6 months after hypospadias repair. Boys were divided into those with simple closure (epithelial or subepithelial not stated) including coverage with either a dartos flap or skin/dartos flap

($n=69$) or complex repairs that included reoperative urethroplasty or meatotomy ($n=25$). Stents were used "routinely" in complex but not in simple cases. Duration of follow-up after fistula closure was not stated. Recurrent fistula developed in 6/94 (4 %), including 3/69 simple and 3/25 complex closures, $p=0.3$ (Santangelo et al. 2003).

A third retrospective study identified 123 patients with fistulas, 100 after initial hypospadias repair and 23 failed fistula closures. Repair was a median 13 months postoperatively (4 months–12 years), and involved fistula closure (epithelial vs. subepithelial not stated) and coverage with dartos. Duration of follow-up after fistula closure was not stated. Successful closure occurred in 36/54 (68 %) with postoperative catheter (used for "larger" fistulas and "more complex" repairs) vs. 35/46 (76 %) without catheters, $p=0.3$. Successful repair was done at 4–6 months in 11/16 (73 %) vs. 55/90 (61 %) at >6 months, $p=0.4$ (total repair number of 106 rather than 123 was not explained). Success did not vary with initial vs. recurrent fistula repair: 71/100 (71 %) vs. 46/61 (75 %), $p=0.6$ (Waterman et al. 2002).

While a 6-month interval after urethroplasty before fistula repair is routine, one report indicated topical application of n-butyl cyanoacrylate (NBCA) was potentially successful when applied at first diagnosis of a fistula. There were 13 patients with single fistulas noted within 3 days of catheter removal or later after TIP repair. In all cases, a urethral stent was placed, the fistula site cleaned with 10 % iodopovidone, and then NBCA applied and the stent then removed. Patients with fistulas treated 6–24 months after surgery additionally had topical anesthesia to the fistula site, which was then scarified using a 27-G needle before NBCA application. At follow-up 2, 7 days, and apparently soon thereafter, if needed, NBCA was again applied if the fistula persisted for a total of one to seven applications. Success with >1.5 years follow-up was noted in 7/13 (54 %) and was similar for early vs. late treatment (4/6 vs. 3/7, $p=0.6$), fistulas < vs. >2 mm (5/7 vs. 2/6, $p=0.$), after one vs. multiple applications (3/3 vs. 4/10, $p=0.2$), and for subcoronal, distal shaft, and midshaft locations (Prestipino et al. 2011).

Glans Dehiscence

Glans dehiscence, defined as complete separation of the glans wings, occurred in significantly more patients after proximal or reoperative (15 %) than primary distal TIP (4 %).

Recurrent glans dehiscence occurred in 27 % of reoperative TIP glansplasties and over 50 % of third glansplasties.

A report comprising prospectively collected data in 641 consecutive patients after primary distal and proximal and reoperative TIP reported glans dehiscence in 32 (3.8 %), 4 % after distal and 15 % after proximal and reoperative surgeries. Multivariable analysis found that primary proximal and reoperative TIP had greater odds for glans dehiscence than distal TIP (proximal OR 4.38 [95 % CI 1.94–9.42]; reoperative TIP OR 3.95 [95 % CI 1.66–8.72]). Other potential factors, including age and glansplasty suture (chromic vs. polyglactin), did not predict this complication. Review of other published results indicated similar occurrence of glans dehiscence after glansplasty in either 1 or 2 layers, using 5–0, 6–0, or 7–0 sutures of polyglecaprone, polydioxanone, or polyglactin (Snodgrass et al. 2011).

Another report from the same institution described outcomes for reoperations specifically for repair of glans dehiscence. Most primary and secondary glansplasties used one-layer subepithelial 6–0 polyglactin suture, usually a total of three stitches from the meatus to the corona. Of 618 primary distal and proximal TIP repairs, 29 with glans dehiscence had reoperative glansplasty, of which recurrent dehiscence developed in 7/26 (27 %) with follow-up. Another 100 patients had primary repair elsewhere and presented with glans dehiscence, with recurrent dehiscence occurring in 11/85 (13 %) with follow-up, which was not significantly different, $p=0.13$. A total of 11 boys had a third glansplasty, with recurrent dehiscence in 5/8 (63 %) with follow-up (Snodgrass et al. 2012).

Meatal Stenosis

There is no published, generally accepted definition for meatal stenosis.

The author considers meatal caliber <8 Fr in an asymptomatic patient potential stenosis.

Systematic literature review found meatal stenosis reported in 3 % of patients after distal TIP and 0.7 % following Mathieu.

A large series of consecutive patients undergoing distal TIP reported no meatal stenosis.

We found no reports of outcomes following treatment of meatal stenosis after hypospadias repair.

A systematic literature review of primary distal hypospadias repairs published from 1990 to 2009 included 23 papers, with 1,872 TIP patients in 15 case series and 1,496 Mathieu repairs in 10 series. Reported meatal stenosis occurred in 3 % TIP and 0.7 % Mathieu, $p<0.001$, the authors noting that this diagnosis could vary from center to center because it is subjective (Wilkinson et al. 2012).

Prevention

Analysis in 426 consecutive boys undergoing distal TIP hypospadias repair by one surgeon, with 279/426 (65 %) having calibration, uroflowometry, and/or urethroscopy postoperatively, reported no case of meatal stenosis (meatal caliber <8 Fr). Technical details emphasized to avoid stenosis included:

- UP incision to near the corpora cavernosa so that the plate is sufficiently wide.
- Tubularization of the UP not extending distally beyond the midglans (approximately 3 mm from the glans junction), leaving an oval, not rounded, opening.
- Not suturing the neourethra to glans wings, which allows UP tubularization to stop below the external neomeatus without leaving a glanular hypospadias (Snodgrass et al. 2010).

Treatment

Few reports discuss treatment for meatal stenosis and subsequent outcomes. Early postoperative narrowing could represent transient edema and require no therapy. If stenosis occurs due to vascular insufficiency, it is unlikely dilations will achieve a long-term stable meatus. Meatotomy is an option, but we found no articles describing its use and outcomes after hypospadias repair.

One report stated that four of the initial seven distal TIP cases developed fistulas 2 weeks after surgery, attributed to meatal stenosis (which was not defined). Meatal dilations were done, a stent replaced for 5 days, and then daily dilation (size not stated) was done for 3 months. The fistulas all closed. Follow-up was not described to determine if meatal stenosis recurred (Elbakry 1999).

Strictures

Systematic literature review reported no case of neourethra stricture after distal TIP.

Dissection of the UP and urethra from the corpora cavernosa with proximal TIP repair resulted in increased strictures, all symptomatic, over proximal TIP without these maneuvers (17 % vs. 0 %) in one report, but not another.

A retrospective study reported that all post-hypospadias repair strictures diagnosed in a 6-year period presented with symptoms.

The literature review by Wilkinson et al. (2012) mentioned above also reported occurrence of neourethral stricture after TIP and Mathieu repairs for primary distal hypospadias: 0/758 TIP and 2/302 Mathieu, $p=0.08$.

A report using prospectively collected data from consecutive proximal TIP operated by a single surgeon analyzed 75 patients, of which 29 had the UP and urethra mobilized from the corpora cavernosa to facilitate straightening the VC. Neourethra strictures ranging from 1 mm to 1 cm in length occurred in 5/29 (17 %) vs. 0/46, $p=0.02$. The strictures were all symptomatic, with UTI and/or urinary retention, and were diagnosed at 6 weeks–1.5 years postoperatively (Snodgrass et al. 2012).

In contrast, a retrospective review that included 32 patients with UP plus urethra mobilization/UP tubularization with ($n=20$) and without ($n=12$) dorsal incision reported no strictures during a mean 24 months' (6 months–3 years) follow-up (Bhat 2007).

A retrospective review identified stricture repair in 38 patients during a 6-year period. All patients presented with symptoms, predominantly "difficulty voiding/decreased stream" in 22 (58 %), with none detected by uroflowometry without complaints. Prior repairs included "Duplay or King tube" ($n = 14$), tubularized ($n = 9$) or onlay ($n = 1$) preputial flaps, Mathieu ($n = 3$), and tubularized or onlay grafts ($n = 10$), with 23 (61 %) originally having proximal hypospadias. Location and length of the strictures was not stated (Duel et al. 1998).

Another retrospective study found 73 cases of urethral stricture after hypospadias repair over a 10-year period ending in 2007. Presenting complaints, if any, were not described, nor was stricture length or location. Prior urethroplasties were UP tubularizations with ($n = 29$) or without ($n = 5$) incisions (47 %), meatal advancement ($n = 5$, 7 %), two-stage repairs ($n = 21$, 29 %), flap repairs ($n = 10$, 14 %), or tubularized grafts ($n = 3$, 4 %). Of these, 46 (63 %) were described as glanular to subcoronal, but means to distinguish meatal stenosis from glanular stricture were not described (Gargollo et al. 2011).

Treatment

A prospective study limited DIVU to strictures <1 cm after hypospadias repair, reporting success with 2-year follow-up in 56 %. Failure was predicted by prior tubularized grafts or flaps and prior DIVU.

A retrospective review of oral mucosal inlay graft for hypospadias strictures reported success in 92 %, with the remainder forming recurrent stricture at the proximal junction to the native urethra.

One prospective study of 72 patients with strictures <1 cm found technique in prior hypospadias repair influenced response to DIVU, with urethrotomy successful at 2-year follow-up in 2/18 tubularized flaps and 0/32 tubularized grafts, vs. 8/11 onlay flaps and 7/11 urethral plate tubularizations, $p < 0.05$. Of 32 recurrent strictures, 12 still <1 cm underwent repeat DIVU and all failed. This report also found that adjunctive urethral dilation after DIVU did not improve outcomes over DIVU alone. Failure of DIVU should not be treated with second DIVU, but should instead prompt open urethroplasty (Husmann and Rathbun 2006).

A retrospective review of 53 patients, mean age 12 ± 7 years (3–34), with inlay graft reoperation reported that the indication for surgery was stricture in 37. Mean length of the graft for the entire cohort was 5 ± 2 cm (3–7.5), preferentially harvested from lower lip. With follow-up a mean 23 ± 10 months (12–30), 3/37 (8 %) developed recurrent stricture at the proximal junction to the native urethra (Ye et al. 2008).

Diverticula

Diverticula are more common following flap repairs than UP tubularizations, and can occur in the absence of distal obstruction.

Retrospective review was done of a single surgeon experience with 130 proximal hypospadias repairs between 1991 and 2004. Operations used included 72 (55 %) one-stage preputial flaps (36 tubularized and 36 onlay), and 58 (45 %) staged repairs (18 Belt-Fuque and 40 Bracka grafts). Mean follow-up was 16 years (6–19), and mean age of patients at last evaluation was 15 years (7–27). Assessments used during follow-up and frequency of follow-up evaluations were not stated. A diverticulum (ventral ballooning and post-void dribbling) was diagnosed in 5 cases, all after preputial flaps, for an incidence of 5/72 (7 %). None of these were diagnosed with simultaneous distal stenosis, and all occurred before puberty at a mean of 7 years (3–8) after surgery. There were no recurrences after diverticulum repair with follow-up a mean of 9 years (5–15). "Proximal" hypospadias was not defined, nor was original meatal location; it is noteworthy that only 20 (15 %) patients had VC, and all needed only dorsal plication for correction, which implies less "severe" hypospadias (Vallasciani et al. 2012), in press.

A retrospective review of 58 onlay vs. 74 tubularized preputial flaps by one surgeon found overall complications in approximately one-third of patients in both groups, but diverticula only after tubularized flaps [9/74 (12 %), $p = 0.016$] (Wiener et al. 1997). However, multivariable analysis was not done to take into account the significant differences in severity of the hypospadias defect between these two cohorts.

Another retrospective review concerning repair of hypospadias complications in 123 patients included diverticula in 13, only 1 with associated neourethra obstruction. Prior repairs included seven onlay and five tubularized preputial flaps and one bladder mucosa tubularized graft (Snyder et al. 2005).

Literature review did not find reports of diverticula after TIP (Snodgrass 2011).

Treatment

Recurrence or need for additional surgery after excision has been reported in two retrospective series in 8 and 11 %.

Repair by Snyder et al. (2005) mentioned above included excision and "multilayered closure," with 1/13 (8 %) recurring during follow-up a mean of 24 months. Two other cases developed fistulas.

Another retrospective review of hypospadias complications included 22 diverticula, of which 18 were repaired. Each was considered to have distal obstruction and diverticula tissue was used in correction. Otherwise, surgical technique was not described, and follow-up was not stated. Two out of 18 (11 %) subsequently had additional surgery (Secrest et al. 1993).

Reoperations

TIP

Reoperative TIP can be done when the UP is not grossly scarred, despite prior midline incision, with complications reported in from 12 to 30 % of patients (Table 9.3). Use of a barrier flap has been shown to reduce fistulas.

Analysis of prospectively collected data in 69 consecutive patients having a mean of 1.1 (1–3) prior operations reported indications for reoperation were repair dehiscence ($n = 63$), coronal fistulas ($n = 3$), meatal stenosis ($n = 2$), and post-onlay diverticulum ($n = 1$). Of these, 62 originally had distal, 4 midshaft, and 3 proximal hypospadias. Complications occurred in 12 (19 %) of 63 patients with follow-up a mean of 6 months (1–53). Initially, a barrier flap was not created to cover the neourethra, and 5 of these 10 patients developed fistulas vs. 2 in the next 51 in which either a dartos or tunica vaginalis flap was used, $p = 0.008$ (flap use was not recorded in two). Glans dehiscence occurred in six patients, including one who also had a fistula. Of 55 patients in whom the prior surgical technique was known, complications occurred in 7/35 with prior UP incision vs. 5/20 without prior incision, $p = 0.74$ (Snodgrass et al. 2009).

A retrospective analysis reported 30 reoperative TIP in boys at mean age 4 years following a mean 1.6 failed repairs (1–3). The meatus was distal in 19, midshaft in 8, and proximal in 3. Urethroplasty included subepithelial closure using 5–0 or 6–0 polyglactin covered by a dartos flap. All were followed for 1 year, and then recontacted for additional review at ≥4 years. Complications occurred in nine (30 %) patients; there were six fistulas, with five also having meatal stenosis, and three meatal stenoses. Factors that appeared to increase likelihood for complications included more than one prior operation and midshaft -proximal meatus, but multivariable analysis was not done (Ziada et al. 2006).

Another retrospective review included 40 TIP reoperations for patients with fistulas ($n = 14$) or dehiscence ($n = 26$), using 7–0 polyglactin rapide and either dartos or tunica vaginalis barrier coverage. The number of prior surgeries was not stated. During follow-up a mean of 42 months (for a larger series including primary repairs), complications developed in five (12.5 %)—three fistulas, one meatal stenosis, and one urethral stricture (Riccabona et al. 2003).

Buccal Inlay

If the UP has been excised but an unscarred skin strip remains as a neo-plate, dorsal incision with buccal inlay grafting resembles TIP repair.

One prospective and two retrospective reviews reported 15 % complication rates in patients with a mean of two to four prior operations (Table 9.4).

Prospective data were reported from 16 consecutive buccal inlay patients following a mean

Table 9.3 Reoperative TIP outcomes

			Meatus			Indications									Complications				
Author	No. pts.	Mean (range) Surgeries	D	M	P	F	MS	Stx	GD	D	VC	No. pts. f/u	Mean f/u (mos)	No. pts. complications	F	MS	Stx	GD	D
(Riccabona et al. 2003)	40	NS	NS	NS	NS	14	–	–	26	–	–	40	42	5 (12.5 %)	3	1	1	0	0
(Ziada et al. 2006)	30	1.6 (1–3)	19	8	3	13	–	–	–	–	0	30	NS (≤60)	7 (23 %)	6	8	–	–	–
Snodgrass 2009	69	1.1 (1–3)	62	4	3	3	2	–	63	1	–	63	6.4 (1–53)	12 (19 %)	7	0	0	6	0

F fistula, *MS* meatal stenosis, *Stx* stenosis, *GD* glans dehiscence, *D* diverticulum, *VC* ventral curvature, *NS* not stated

Table 9.4 Inlay graft reoperations

			Meatus			Indications								Complications				
Author	No. pts.	Mean (range) prior surgeries	D	M	P	F	MS	Stx	GD	D	No. pts. f/u	Mean f/u (mos)	No. pts. complications	F	MS	Stx	GD	D
(Schwentner et al. 2006)	31	4(1–18)	13	–	18	–	–	–	NS	–	31	31	5 (16 %)	1	0	4	0	–
(Ye et al. 2008)	53	2(1–6)	–	–	–	–	–	37	16	–	53	23	8 (15 %)	5	–	3	–	0
Snodgrass 2009	16	2(1–9)	10	3	3	–	1	–	15	1[a]	13	5	2 (15 %)	1	0	0	1	0

F fistula, *MS* meatal stenosis, *Stx* stenosis, *GD* glans dehiscence, *D* diverticulum, *VC* ventral curvature, *NS* not stated

[a]One patient had both meatal stenosis and a urethral diverticulum

of 1.9 (1–9) prior operations. The meatus was distal in ten, midshaft in three, and proximal in three cases. Complications developed in 2/13 (15 %) with follow-up, comprising one glans dehiscence and one fistula despite a dartos flap (Snodgrass et al. 2009).

The retrospective study by Ye et al. (2008) mentioned above reviewed 53 patients, mean age 12 years (3–34), with inlay graft reoperation for stricture in 37 and dehiscence in 16. The mean number of prior repairs was two (1–6). Mean length of the graft was 5 ± 2 cm (3–7.5), preferentially harvested from lower lip. With follow-up a mean 23 ± 10 months (12–30), complications developed in eight (15 %)—five fistulas and three recurrent strictures at the proximal junction to the urethra (Ye et al. 2008).

Another retrospective review included 31 patients, mean age 14 years (15 months–26 years), who failed a mean of four prior repairs (1–18) and presented with a variety of complications, including fistulas, strictures, diverticula, and dehiscence (numbers not stated). Grafts were harvested from prepuce ($n = 15$), penile skin ($n = 12$), or groin skin ($n = 4$) with mean length of 4 cm (1–15). At mean follow-up of 30 months (8–66), complications occurred in five (16 %)—four strictures at the proximal junction and one fistula (Schwentner et al. 2006).

Two-Stage Buccal Grafting

Case series of patients having failed a mean of four or five hypospadias repairs report first-stage complications needing an additional grafting procedure before urethroplasty in ≤13 %.

Second-stage urethroplasty complications occurred in approximately 38 % of patients (Table 9.5).

Lip grafts are thinner than cheek grafts and have a significantly smaller likelihood for glans dehiscence.

Systematic literature review regarding donor site morbidity (not limited to hypospadias surgery) reported complications in 4 % of adults.

Prospective data were reported from 48 consecutive patients with a mean of four (1–20) prior operations who underwent two-stage oral mucosa graft reoperation. These included 9 distal, 6 midshaft, and 33 proximal hypospadias cases, requiring reoperation for wound dehiscence ($n = 27$), VC ($n = 13$), stricture ($n = 6$), meatal stenosis ($n = 6$) with BXO in two, fistula and dehiscence ($n = 6$), and hair in the urethra ($n = 1$). Focal ($n = 4$) or complete ($n = 1$) graft complications (10 %) required patching in a separate stage before urethroplasty. Second-stage urethroplasty complications occurred in 17/45 (38 %) with follow-up, mostly glans dehiscence when cheek rather than lip was used in the glans (8/25 vs. 0/17, $p = 0.01$), fistulas ($n = 7$), and meatal stenosis ($n = 2$), with no strictures or diverticulum (Snodgrass et al. 2009).

A retrospective series of 100 patients failing an average of five (3–16) prior operations included 21 with distal, 40 with midshaft, and 37 with proximal hypospadias. Graft donor sites included prepuce ($n = 39$) (considered the optimal source since prepuce is thinner than either skin from other sites or oral mucosa), oral mucosa ($n = 34$), post-auricular ($n = 22$,) or from the upper arm ($n = 5$). Partial graft loss occurred in seven, requiring regrafting before second-stage urethroplasty in two. Total number of patients with complications was not reported, but urethroplasty complications included fistulas ($n = 9$), strictures ($n = 6$), persistent hypospadias ($n = 6$), and persistent curvature ($n = 4$) (Gill and Hameed 2011).

Another retrospective case series reported 30 patients undergoing two-stage oral mucosa grafting (mean number of failed prior repairs not stated), of which there were 5 distal, 12 midshaft, and 13 proximal hypospadias cases. Indications for reoperation were not stated, although nine had BXO. Regrafting was required before second-stage tubularization in four (13 %). Urethroplasty complications occurred in 11 (37 %), comprising meatal stenosis ($n = 5$), fistulas ($n = 3$), and glans dehiscence ($n = 3$) (Leslie et al. 2011).

Donor site morbidity for buccal tissue harvest (not specific to hypospadias surgery) was determined by systematic literature review to occur in 4 % of adult patients, with no differences in overall complications between cheek vs. lip harvest sites (Markiewicz et al. 2008).

Table 9.5 Two-stage graft reoperations

			Meatus			Indications							Graft							Urethroplasty complications					
Author	No. pts.	Mean (range) surgeries	D	M	P	F	MS	Stx	GD	D	VC	BXO	P	O	Other skin	No. pts. graft reop	No. pts. f/u	Meanf/u (mos)	No. pts. complications	F	MS	Stx	GD	D	VC
Snodgrass 2009	48	4.3 (1–20)	9	6	33	6	6	7	27	–	13	2	0	48	0	5 (10 %)	45	8	17 (38 %)	7	2	0	8	0	–
(Gill & Hameed 2011)	100	5 (3–16)	21	40	37	82	–	33	98	–	88	–	39	34	27	2 (2 %)	100	NS (>1 year)	NS	9	–	6	–	–	4
(Leslie et al. 2011)	30	NS	5	12	13	–	NS	–	–	–	–	9	0	30	0	4 (13 %)	30	25	11 (37 %)	3	5		3		

F fistula, *MS* meatal stenosis, *Stx* stenosis, *GD* glans dehiscence, *D* diverticulum, *VC* ventral curvature, *NS* not stated

Table 9.6 Reoperative skin flaps

Series	No. of patients	Mean no. prior repairs	Mean follow-up in months	Complication rate (%)	Complications F	MS	Stx	GD	D	VC	Failure
(Jayanthi et al. 1994)	28[a]	1 in 30, 2–6 in 14	NS	8 (29)	2	1	1	–	–	–	4
(Emir and Erol 2003)	55[a]	1.4 (1–3)	3	16 (29)	14	–	–	2	–	–	–
(Bar-Yosef et al. 2005)	34[a]	1.6 (1–3)	29	9 (26)	5	2	–	–	–	–	2
(Jayanthi et al. 1994)	16[b]	–	NS	9 (56)	4	–	2	–	–	–	4
(Emir and Erol 2003)	33[c]	1.5 (1–3)	NS	16 (48)	14	–	–	2	–	–	–
(Patel et al. 2005)	11[c]	2 (1–5)	24.5	6 (55)	5	–	–	–	1	1	–

F fistula, *MS* meatal stenosis, *Stx* stenosis, *GD* glans dehiscence, *D* diverticulum, *VC* ventral curvature, *NS* not stated
[a]Mathieu flip-flap
[b]Tube or onlay flap
[c]Onlay

Skin Flaps

Several retrospective series report Mathieu reoperations after a mean of approximately 1.5 prior repairs, with subsequent complications in over 25 % (Table 9.6).

Reoperative tubularized or onlay flaps were reported to have complications in over 50 % in two small case series.

A retrospective review of cases from 1986 to 1992 found 39 reoperations, 25 after one failed repair and 14 after two to six operations. Reoperation was done by Mathieu in 28 and skin flap in 16 (8 tubularized, 8 onlay). Follow-up was a mean of 17 months (0.5–60), with complications developing in 8/28 Mathieu (29 %) and 9/16 (56 %) island flaps (Jayanthi et al. 1994).

Another retrospective evaluation concerned Mathieu reoperations performed in 55 patients during a 20-year period for large fistulas or glans dehiscence after a mean of 1.4 prior operations (1–3). Mean follow-up was 3 months (1–8), with complications noted in 16 (29 %), fistulas in 14, and dehiscence in 2 (Emir and Erol 2003).

A third retrospective study reported 34 reoperative Mathieu procedures after a mean of 1.5 (1–3) failures. With mean follow-up of 29 months (1–84), complications occurred in nine (26 %), including fistulas and two meatal stenoses (Bar-Yosef et al. 2005).

Another retrospective review reported 11 reoperations after a mean of 2 (1–5) prior hypospadias repairs using onlay flap. During mean follow-up of 24 months, complications occurred in six (55 %), including six fistulas, one diverticulum, and one flap contracture with persistent VC (Patel et al. 2005).

Adult Outcomes After Prepubertal Repair

A systematic literature review pooled data from 20 studies reporting outcomes in patients operated at <6 years of age using a variety of surgical techniques who had follow-up at >14 years of age:

- ***Urinary Function*: Patients reported obstructive voiding symptoms, spraying, and deviated stream significantly more than controls, and had decreased Q_{max} on uroflowometry.**
- ***Sexual Function*: Erectile dysfunction, problems with ejaculation and overall decreased sexual satisfaction were reported by significantly more patients than controls.**
- ***Appearance*: Patients, especially those with proximal hypospadias, were less satisfied with genital appearance than controls.**

Two studies reported long-term follow-up in men after childhood repair using various preputial flaps, finding that 8 and 17 % had complications occurring after last childhood follow-up.

One study of men after Denis Browne repair leaving the meatus a mean of 1 cm below the glans tip found that 100 % who were not satisfied with surgical outcomes desired additional surgery, and another 50 % who expressed greater satisfaction with their surgery but still wanted additional surgery.

A systematic literature review through 2010 concerned outcomes in men after childhood hypospadias repair, and set inclusion criteria to designate surgery before age 6 years and follow-up at >14 years of age. Twenty studies with a total of 1,069 patients were analyzed. Mean number of operations was 2.7 (1–20); proximal hypospadias outcomes were available for 180 patients. Operative techniques included procedures not commonly used today, such as Ombredanne, Denis-Browne, van der Muelen, and Cecil-Culp, as well as the more recent MAGPI, Mathieu, onlay, and tubularized preputial flaps and Byar's flaps. Assessments and findings are presented here.

Urinary Function

Symptoms

Patients reported obstructive symptoms (77/217 [35.5 %] vs. 30/196 [15 %], $p<0.01$); spraying (245/818 [30 %] vs. 17/231 [7 %], $p<0.01$); and deviated stream (69/267 [26 %] vs. 9/81 [11 %], $p<0.01$) more often than controls. Post-void dribbling and sitting to void did not significantly vary, and were reported by 104/351 (30 %) and 15/174 (9 %) patients. Patients with proximal hypospadias reported spraying more often than those with distal repairs (46/106 [43 %] vs. 245/818 [30 %]).

Uroflowometry

Q_{max} was significantly less in patients than controls (mean 24 cc/s vs. 30 cc/s, $p<0.01$), as was Q_{max} less than 2 SD (36/265 [13.5 %] vs. 4/138 [3 %]). Patients with proximal hypospadias had significantly lower Q_{max} (mean 21 cc/s) than did those with distal hypospadias.

Sexual Function

Erectile Dysfunction

This complaint was not defined, but it was reported significantly more often in patients than age-matched controls (30/156 [19 %] vs. 3/249 [1 %], $p<0.01$).

Ejaculation

Ejaculation problems, including milking semen and poor force, were significantly more common in patients than controls (99/385 [26 %] vs. 0/48, $p<0.01$).

Sexual Satisfaction

Patients were less satisfied with sexual function than controls (153/188 [81 %] vs. 235/252 [93 %], $p<0.01$). Mean frequency of intercourse per month did not vary (5.8 vs. 6.4).

Cosmesis

There was no difference in concern for abnormal appearance in patients vs. controls (approximately 33 %), but patients were more likely dissatisfied with that appearance (143/493 [29 %] vs. 24/581 [4 %]). Patients with proximal hypospadias were even more dissatisfied with penile appearance than those with distal hypospadias (25/46 [54 %] vs. 143/493 [29 %]).

The authors commented that pooling data from studies with various methodological designs, heterogenous data, and small patient numbers is a weak method for comparisons (Rynja et al. 2011).

Sexual function was reported in a study of men after Denis Browne repair by one surgeon vs. age matched controls. Four hundred patients were eligible for inclusion after uncomplicated (i.e., no reoperations) midshaft or proximal hypospadias surgery (mean age 4.5 years, range 3–7) and current age ≥21 years. Non-validated questionnaires were mailed to all these and to another 150 age-matched controls (means for selection not stated). Of the patient questionnaires, 167 were returned with no address, and of the remaining 233, 104 (45 %) responded; of 150 control questionnaires, 63 (42 %) responded. Mean age of patients and controls was 32 years. The meatus was reported by patients to be a mean of 1 cm from the tip of the glans, and 79 % stated that the urinary stream was deviated. Sixty-three percent reported no VC, while 5 % had "major" curvature. Patients were significantly less satisfied with their genital appearance vs. controls, yet reported significantly higher sexual satisfaction. Overall satisfaction with surgical results was 7 on a 10-point scale, but there were 12 patients (12 %) who marked <5, with median score 3 (2–3) that was significantly less than patients scoring ≥5. This subgroup of patients also scored significantly lower than the others on satisfaction with genital appearance, regular sexual activity, and sexual satisfaction. All these dissatisfied patients responded that they wished to have additional surgery, vs. 50 % of those whose scoring satisfaction with surgery was higher (Kiss et al. 2011).

Sexual function was compared in 57 patients previously operated for hypospadias (34 distal, 9 midshaft, 14 proximal, techniques used not stated) randomly selected from 130 cases repaired between 1985 and 1990 who were >18 years of age, and 60 age-matched controls (means of selection not described). Questionnaires (non-validated) were mailed, and 37 patients, mean age 28 ± 6 years, and 39 controls, mean age 26 ± 5 years, responded. These patients had been operated at mean age of 11 ± 9 years of age, with a mean of 4 (1–17) operations. On a scale of 1–5, satisfaction with surgical outcomes was rated a mean of 3.9 ± 0.8. The following observations were reported:

- Patients and controls similarly reported good-quality erections.
- Both cohorts reported similar prevalence of penile curvature (40 %), although in patients this was usually ventral while controls described more lateral bending.
- 13/37 (35 %) patients reported ejaculation problems, including weakness and need to milk the ejaculate vs. no reported problems by controls.
- There was no difference in cohorts regarding either sexual inhibitions or relationships, and there was similar body image satisfaction (approximately 85 % satisfied).
- Mean total sexual partners was lower in patients vs. controls (5 vs. 7, $p = 0.02$), and mean frequency of intercourse during 1 month was also less for patients (4 ± 4 vs. 7 ± 6, $p = 0.04$).
- Fewer patients reported being "completely satisfied" with their sex life than controls (51 % vs. 77 %, $p = -0.03$) (Bubanj et al. 2004).

Late complications were reported in another study, mentioned above, that evaluated patients who underwent tubularized and onlay preputial flap repair by one surgeon for proximal hypospadias between 1981 and 1992. Of 125 patients, medical information could only be retrieved for 73, of which 49 could be contacted for follow-up ≥10 years postoperatively and 30 agreed to examination. These patients had been operated at mean age 17 months (8–74) with tubularized repair in 14 and onlay in 16, and follow-up was a mean of 14 years later (12–21). New complications were found in 5/30 (17 %)—two fistulas and three meatal stenoses (Patel et al. 2004).

Late complications were also reported by a study that contacted all 44 patients who underwent second-stage preputial flap repair (Belt-Fuque) by one surgeon between 1985 and 1993, of which 25 could be restudied a mean of 13 years (11–17) later, and another 2 responded to questionnaires. Meatal location was midshaft in 14, penoscrotal in 9, and perineal in 4. Following initial repair, complications developed in 13 (48 %) of these participants, but at late follow-up, none had additional problems. Another two (8 %) had new complications—one fistula and one stricture (Lam et al. 2005).

References

AAP (American Academy of Pediatrics. Pediatrics). Timing of elective surgery on the genitalia of male children with particular reference to the risks, benefits, and psychological effects of surgery and anesthesia. Pediatrics. 1996;97(4):590–4.

Allen JS, Summers JL, Wilkerson JE. Meatal calibration of newborn boys. J Urol. 1972;107(3):498.

Almodhen F, Alzahrani A, Jednak R, Capolicchio JP, El Sherbiny MT. Nonstented tubularized incised plate urethroplasty with Y-to-I spongioplasty in non-toilet trained children. Can Urol Assoc J. 2008; 2(2): 110–4.

Andersson M, Doroszkiewicz M, Arfwidsson C, Abrahamsson K, Holmdahl G. Hypospadias repair with tubularized incised plate: does the obstructive flow pattern resolve spontaneously? J Pediatr Urol. 2011;7(4):441–5.

Aoki K, Fujimoto K, Yoshida K, Hirao Y, Ueoka K. One-stage repair of severe hypospadias using modified tubularized transverse preputial island flap with V-incision suture. J Pediatr Urol. 2008; 4(6):438–41.

Badawy H, Morsi H. Long-term followup of dermal grafts for repair of severe penile curvature. J Urol. 2008;180(4 Suppl):1842–5.

Bar-Yosef Y, Binyamini J, Matzkin H, Ben-Chaim J. Midline dorsal plication technique for penile curvature repair. J Urol. 2004;172(4 Pt 1):1368–9.

Bar-Yosef Y, Binyamini J, Matzkin H, Ben-Chaim J. Salvage Mathieu urethroplasty: reuse of local tissue in failed hypospadias repair. Urology. 2005;65(6):1212–5.

Bhat A. Extended urethral mobilization in incised plate urethroplasty for severe hypospadias: a variation in technique to improve chordee correction. J Urol. 2007;178(3 Pt 1):1031–5.

Braga LH, Pippi Salle JL, Dave S, Bagli DJ, Lorenzo AJ, Khoury AE. Outcome analysis of severe chordee correction using tunica vaginalis as a flap in boys with proximal hypospadias. J Urol. 2007a;178(4 Pt 2): 1693–7. discussion 7.

Braga LH, Pippi Salle JL, Lorenzo AJ, Skeldon S, Dave S, Farhat WA, et al. Comparative analysis of tubularized incised plate versus onlay island flap urethroplasty for penoscrotal hypospadias. J Urol. 2007b;178(4 Pt 1): 1451–6. discussion 6–7.

Braga LH, Lorenzo AJ, Bagli DJ, Dave S, Eeg K, Farhat WA, et al. Ventral penile lengthening versus dorsal plication for severe ventral curvature in children with proximal hypospadias. J Urol. 2008;180(4 Suppl):1743–7. discussion 7–8.

Bubanj TB, Perovic SV, Milicevic RM, Jovcic SB, Marjanovic ZO, Djordjevic MM. Sexual behavior and sexual function of adults after hypospadias surgery: a comparative study. J Urol. 2004;171(5):1876–9.

Bush NC, Holzer M, Zhang S, Snodgrass W. Age does not impact risk for urethroplasty complications after tubularized incised plate repair of hypospadias in prepubertal boys. J Pediatr Urol. 2012 in press; doi:10.1016/j.jpurol.2012.03.014

Caesar RE, Caldamone AA. The use of free grafts for correcting penile chordee. J Urol. 2000;164(5):1691–3.

Calzolari E, Contiero MR, Roncarati E, Mattiuz PL, Volpato S. Aetiological factors in hypospadias. J Med Genet. 1986;23(4):333–7.

Chalapathi G, Rao KL, Chowdhary SK, Narasimhan KL, Samujh R, Mahajan JK. Testosterone therapy in microphallic hypospadias: topical or parenteral? J Pediatr Surg. 2003;38(2):221–3.

Cheng EY, Kropp BP, Pope JC, Brock JW. 3rd Proximal division of the urethral plate in staged hypospadias repair. J Urol. 2003;170(4 Pt 2):1580–3. discussion 4.

Chertin B, Koulikov D, Fridmans A, Farkas A. Dorsal tunica albuginea plication to correct congenital and acquired penile curvature: a long-term follow-up. BJU Int. 2004;93(3):379–81.

Chuang JH, Shieh CS. Two-layer versus one-layer closure in transverse island flap repair of posterior hypospadias. J Pediatr Surg. 1995;30(5):739–42.

Cox MJ, Coplen DE, Austin PF. The incidence of disorders of sexual differentiation and chromosomal abnormalities of cryptorchidism and hypospadias stratified by meatal location. J Urol. 2008;180(6):2649–52; discussion 52.

Dajusta D, Bush N, Snodgrass W. Glans penis width in patients with hypospadias compared to health controls. Boston, MA: American Academy of Pediatrics; 2011.

Davits RJ, van den Aker ES, Scholtmeijer RJ, de Muinck Keizer-Schrama SM, Nijman RJ. Effect of parenteral testosterone therapy on penile development in boys with hypospadias. Br J Urol. 1993;71(5):593–5.

de Mattos e Silva E, Gorduza DB, Catti M, Valmalle AF, Demede D, Hameury F, et al. Outcome of severe hypospadias repair using three different techniques. J Pediatr Urol. 2009;5(3):205–11. discussion 12–4.

DeCastro BJ, Costabile RA, McMann LP, Peterson AC. Oral ketoconazole for prevention of postoperative penile erection: a placebo controlled, randomized, double-blind trial. J Urol. 2008;179(5):1930–2.

Duel BP, Barthold JS, Gonzalez R. Management of urethral strictures after hypospadias repair. J Urol. 1998;160(1):170–1.

Eassa W, Jednak R, Capolicchio JP, Brzezinski A, El-Sherbiny M. Risk factors for re-operation following tubularized incised plate urethroplasty: a comprehensive analysis. Urology. 2011;77(3):716–20.

Elbakry A. Tubularized-incised urethral plate urethroplasty: is regular dilatation necessary for success? BJU Int. 1999;84(6):683–8.

Elganainy EO, Abdelsalam YM, Gadelmoula MM, Shalaby MM. Combined Mathieu and Snodgrass urethroplasty for hypospadias repair: a prospective randomized study. Int J Urol. 2010;17(7):661–5.

El-Hout Y, Braga LH, Pippi Salle JL, Moore K, Bagli DJ, Lorenzo AJ. Assessment of urethral plate appearance through digital photography: do pediatric urologists agree in their visual impressions of the urethral plate in children with hypospadias? J Pediatr Urol. 2010;6(3):294–300.

Elicevik M, Tireli G, Sander S. Tubularized incised plate urethroplasty: 5 years' experience. Eur Urol. 2004;46(5): 655–9. discussion 9.

Elmore JM, Kirsch AJ, Scherz HC, Smith EA. Small intestinal submucosa for corporeal body grafting in severe hypospadias requiring division of the urethral plate. J Urol. 2007;178(4 Pt 2):1698–701. discussion 701.

El-Sherbiny MT. Tubularized incised plate repair of distal hypospadias in toilet-trained children: should a stent be left? BJU Int. 2003;92(9):1003–5.

Emir L, Erol D. Mathieu urethroplasty as a salvage procedure: 20-year experience. J Urol. 2003;169(6):2325–6. author reply 6–7.

Ferro F, Zaccara A, Spagnoli A, Lucchetti MC, Capitanucci ML, Villa M. Skin graft for two-stage treatment of severe hypospadias: back to the future? J Urol. 2002;168(4 Pt 2):1730–3. discussion 3.

Friedman T, Shalom A, Hoshen G, Brodovsky S, Tieder M, Westreich M. Detection and incidence of anomalies associated with hypospadias. Pediatr Nephrol. 2008;23(10):1809–16.

Friedrich MG, Evans D, Noldus J, Huland H. The correction of penile curvature with the Essed-Schroder technique: a long-term follow-up assessing functional aspects and quality of life. BJU Int. 2000;86(9):1034–8.

Gargollo PC, Cai AW, Borer JG, Retik AB. Management of recurrent urethral strictures after hypospadias repair: is there a role for repeat dilation or endoscopic incision? J Pediatr Urol. 2011;7(1):34–8.

Gearhart JP, Jeffs RD. The use of parenteral testosterone therapy in genital reconstructive surgery. J Urol. 1987;138(4 Pt 2):1077–8.

Gershbaum MD, Stock JA, Hanna MK. A case for two-stage repair of perineoscrotal hypospadias with severe chordee. J Urol. 2002;168(4 Pt 2):1727–8. discussion 9.

Ghanem MA, Nijman RJ. Outcome analysis of tubularized incised urethral plate using dorsal dartos flap for proximal penile hypospadias repair. J Pediatr Urol. 2011;6(5):477–80.

Gill NA, Hameed A. Management of hypospadias cripples with two-staged Bracka's technique. J Plast Reconstr Aesthet Surg. 2011;64(1):91–6.

Gopal SC, Gangopadhyay AN, Mohan TV, Upadhyaya VD, Pandey A, Upadhyaya A, et al. Use of fibrin glue in preventing urethrocutaneous fistula after hypospadias repair. J Pediatr Surg. 2008;43(10):1869–72.

Granberg C, Bush N, Snodgrass W. Objective criteria for preoperative testosterone use before proximal hypospadias repair: evidence for androgen resistance. American Academy of Pediatrics National Conference and Exhibition; New Orleans, LA2012.

Guarino N, Vallasciani SA, Marrocco G. A new suture material for hypospadias surgery: a comparative study. J Urol. 2009;181(3):1318–22. discussion 22–3.

Hammouda HM, El-Ghoneimi A, Bagli DJ, McLorie GA, Khoury AE. Tubularized incised plate repair: functional outcome after intermediate followup. J Urol. 2003;169(1):331–3. discussion 3.

Hayashi Y, Kojima Y, Nakane A, Maruyama T, Kohri K. Can a slit-like meatus be achieved with the V-incision sutured meatoplasty for onlay island flap hypospadias repair? BJU Int. 2007;99(6):1479–82.

Holland AJ, Smith GH. Effect of the depth and width of the urethral plate on tubularized incised plate urethroplasty. J Urol. 2000;164(2):489–91.

Husmann DA, Rathbun SR. Long-term followup of visual internal urethrotomy for management of short (less than 1 cm) penile urethral strictures following hypospadias repair. J Urol. 2006;176(4 Pt 2):1738–41.

Jayanthi VR, McLorie GA, Khoury AE, Churchill BM. Can previously relocated penile skin be successfully used for salvage hypospadias repair? J Urol. 1994;152(2 Pt 2):740–3. discussion 3.

Jayanthi VR, McLorie GA, Khoury AE, Churchill BM. Functional characteristics of the reconstructed neourethra after island flap urethroplasty. J Urol. 1995;153(5):1657–9.

Kaefer M, Diamond D, Hendren WH, Vemulapalli S, Bauer SB, Peters CA, et al. The incidence of intersexuality in children with cryptorchidism and hypospadias: stratification based on gonadal palpability and meatal position. J Urol. 1999;162(3 Pt 2):1003-6; discussion 6–7.

Kajbafzadeh AM, Arshadi H, Payabvash S, Salmasi AH, Najjaran-Tousi V, Sahebpor AR. Proximal hypospadias with severe chordee: single stage repair using corporeal tunica vaginalis free graft. J Urol. 2007;178(3 Pt 1):1036–42. discussion 42.

Kaya C, Kucuk E, Ilktac A, Ozturk M, Karaman MI. Value of urinary flow patterns in the follow-up of children who underwent Snodgrass operation. Urol Int. 2007;78(3):245–8.

Kaya C, Bektic J, Radmayr C, Schwentner C, Bartsch G, Oswald J. The efficacy of dihydrotestosterone transdermal gel before primary hypospadias surgery: a prospective, controlled, randomized study. J Urol. 2008;179(2):684–8.

Kiss A, Sulya B, Szasz AM, Romics I, Kelemen Z, Toth J, et al. Long-term psychological and sexual outcomes of severe penile hypospadias repair. J Sex Med. 2011;8(5):1529–39.

Korvald C, Stubberud K. High odds for freedom from early complications after tubularized incised-plate urethroplasty in 1-year-old versus 5-year-old boys. J Pediatr Urol. 2008;4(6):452–6.

Lam PN, Greenfield SP, Williot P. Two-stage repair in infancy for severe hypospadias with chordee: long-term results after puberty. J Urol. 2005;174(4 Pt 2):1567–72. discussion 72.

Leslie B, Lorenzo AJ, Figueroa V, Moore K, Farhat WA, Bagli DJ, et al. Critical outcome analysis of staged buccal mucosa graft urethroplasty for prior failed hypospadias repair in children. J Urol. 2011;185(3):1077–82.

Litvak AS, Morris Jr JA, McRoberts JW. Normal size of the urethral meatus in boys. J Urol. 1976;115(6):736–7.

Luo CC, Lin JN, Chiu CH, Lo FS. Use of parenteral testosterone prior to hypospadias surgery. Pediatr Surg Int. 2003;19(1–2):82–4.

Lutzker LG, Kogan SJ, Levitt SB. Is routine intravenous urography indicated in patients with hypospadias? Pediatrics. 1977;59(4):630–3.

Markiewicz MR, DeSantis JL, Margarone 3rd JE, Pogrel MA, Chuang SK. Morbidity associated with oral mucosa harvest for urological reconstruction: an overview. J Oral Maxillofac Surg. 2008;66(4):739–44.

McAleer IM, Kaplan GW. Is routine karyotyping necessary in the evaluation of hypospadias and cryptorchidism? J Urol. 2001;165(6 Pt 1):2029–31; discussion 31–2.
McLorie G, Joyner B, Herz D, McCallum J, Bagli D, Merguerian P, et al. A prospective randomized clinical trial to evaluate methods of postoperative care of hypospadias. J Urol. 2001;165(5):1669–72.
Meir DB, Livne PM. Is prophylactic antimicrobial treatment necessary after hypospadias repair? J Urol. 2004;171(6 Pt 2):2621–2.
Moore CC. The role of routine radiographic screening of boys with hypospadias: a prospective study. J Pediatr Surg. 1990;25(3):339–41.
Moreno-Garcia M, Miranda EB. Chromosomal anomalies in cryptorchidism and hypospadias. J Urol. 2002; 168(5):2170–2; discussion 2.
Nerli RB, Koura A, Prabha V, Reddy M. Comparison of topical versus parenteral testosterone in children with microphallic hypospadias. Pediatr Surg Int. 2009; 25(1):57–9.
Olsen LH, Grothe I, Rawashdeh YF, Jorgensen TM. Urinary flow patterns in infants with distal hypospadias. J Pediatr Urol. 2011;7(4):428–32.
Orkiszewski M, Madej J. The meatal/urethral width in healthy uncircumcised boys. J Pediatr Urol. 2010;6(2): 130–3.
Oswald J, Korner I, Riccabona M. Comparison of the perimeatal-based flap (Mathieu) and the tubularized incised-plate urethroplasty (Snodgrass) in primary distal hypospadias. BJU Int. 2000;85(6):725–7.
Patel RP, Shukla AR, Snyder 3rd HM. The island tube and island onlay hypospadias repairs offer excellent long-term outcomes: a 14-year followup. J Urol. 2004;172(4 Pt 2):1717–9. discussion 9.
Patel RP, Shukla AR, Leone NT, Carr MC, Canning DA. Split onlay skin flap for the salvage hypospadias repair. J Urol. 2005;173(5):1718–20.
Perlmutter AD, Montgomery BT, Steinhardt GF. Tunica vaginalis free graft for the correction of chordee. J Urol. 1985;134(2):311–3.
Perlmutter AE, Morabito R, Tarry WF. Impact of patient age on distal hypospadias repair: a surgical perspective. Urology. 2006;68(3):648–51.
Pope JCI, Kropp BP, McLaughlin KP, Adams MC, Rink RC, Keating MA, et al. Penile orthoplasty using dermal grafts in the outpatient setting. Urology. 1996; 48(1):124–7.
Powell CR, McAleer I, Alagiri M, Kaplan GW. Comparison of flaps versus grafts in proximal hypospadias surgery. J Urol. 2000;163(4):1286–8. discussion 8–9.
Prestipino M, Bertozzi M, Nardi N, Appignani A. Outpatient department repair of urethrocutaneous fistulae using n-butyl-cyanoacrylate (NBCA): a single-centre experience. BJU Int. 2011;108(9):1514–7.
Riccabona M, Oswald J, Koen M, Beckers G, Schrey A, Lusuardi L. Comprehensive analysis of six years experience in tubularised incised plate urethroplasty and its extended application in primary and secondary hypospadias repair. Eur Urol. 2003;44(6):714–9.
Ritchey ML, Ribbeck M. Successful use of tunica vaginalis grafts for treatment of severe penile chordee in children. J Urol. 2003;170(4 Pt 2):1574–6. discussion 6.
Rynja SP, de Jong TP, Bosch JL, de Kort LM. Functional, cosmetic and psychosexual results in adult men who underwent hypospadias correction in childhood. J Pediatr Urol. 2011;7(5):504–15.
Santangelo K, Rushton HG, Belman AB. Outcome analysis of simple and complex urethrocutaneous fistula closure using a de-epithelialized or full thickness skin advancement flap for coverage. J Urol. 2003;170 (4 Pt 2):1589–92. discussion 92.
Sarhan O, Saad M, Helmy T, Hafez A. Effect of suturing technique and urethral plate characteristics on complication rate following hypospadias repair: a prospective randomized study. J Urol. 2009;182(2):682–5. discussion 5–6.
Savanelli A, Esposito C, Settimi A. A prospective randomized comparative study on the use of ventral subcutaneous flap to prevent fistulas in the Snodgrass repair for distal hypospadias. World J Urol. 2007;25(6): 641–5.
Scarpa M, Castagnetti M, Musi L, Rigamonti W. Is objective assessment of cosmetic results after distal hypospadias repair superior to subjective assessment? J Pediatr Urol. 2009;5(2):110–3.
Schnack TH, Zdravkovic S, Myrup C, Westergaard T, Christensen K, Wohlfahrt J, et al. Familial aggregation of hypospadias: a cohort study. Am J Epidemiol. 2008; 167(3):251–6.
Schwentner C, Gozzi C, Lunacek A, Rehder P, Bartsch G, Oswald J, et al. Interim outcome of the single stage dorsal inlay skin graft for complex hypospadias reoperations. J Urol. 2006;175(5):1872–6. discsussion 6–7.
Secrest CL, Jordan GH, Winslow BH, Horton CE, McCraw JB, Gilbert DA, et al. Repair of the complications of hypospadias surgery. J Urol. 1993;150(5 Pt 1):1415–8.
Shankar KR, Losty PD, Hopper M, Wong L, Rickwood AM. Outcome of hypospadias fistula repair. BJU Int. 2002;89(1):103–5.
Shukla AR, Patel RP, Canning DA. The two-stage hypospadias repair. is it a misnomer? J Urol. 2004;172 (4 Pt 2):1714–6. discussion 6.
Snodgrass WT. Tubularized incised plate hypospadias repair: indications, technique, and complications. Urology. 1999;54(1):6–11.
Snodgrass W. Hypospadias. In: Wein AJ, editor. Campbell-Walsh Urology. 10th ed. Philadelphia: Elsevier; 2011. p. 3503–36.
Snodgrass W, Bush N. Tubularized incised plate proximal hypospadias repair: continued evolution and extended applications. J Pediatr Urol. 2011;7(1):2–9.
Snodgrass W, Prieto J. Straightening ventral curvature while preserving the urethral plate in proximal hypospadias repair. J Urol. 2009;182(4 Suppl):1720–5.

Snodgrass W, Ziada A, Yucel S, Gupta A. Comparison of outcomes of tubularized incised plate hypospadias repair and circumcision: a questionnaire-based survey of parents and surgeon. J Pediatr Urol. 2008;4(4): 250–4.

Snodgrass WT, Bush N, Cost N. Algorithm for comprehensive approach to hypospadias reoperation using 3 techniques. J Urol. 2009;182(6):2885–91.

Snodgrass WT, Bush N, Cost N. Tubularized incised plate hypospadias repair for distal hypospadias. J Pediatr Urol. 2010;6(4):408–13.

Snodgrass W, Cost N, Nakonezny PA, Bush N. Analysis of risk factors for glans dehiscence after tubularized incised plate hypospadias repair. J Urol. 2011;185(5): 1845–9.

Snodgrass W, Villanueva C, Bush N. Outcomes of reoperations for glans dehiscence in prepubertal boys with hypospadias. New Orleans, LA: American Academy of Pediatrics National Conference and Exhibition; 2012.

Snyder CL, Evangelidis A, Snyder RP, Ostlie DJ, Gatti JM, Murphy JP. Management of urethral diverticulum complicating hypospadias repair. J Pediatr Urol. 2005;1(2):81–3.

Soergel TM, Cain MP, Kaefer M, Gitlin J, Casale AJ, Davis MM, et al. Complications of small intestinal submucosa for corporal body grafting for proximal hypospadias. J Urol. 2003;170(4 Pt 2):1577–8. 8–9.

Springer A, Subramaniam R. Split dorsal dartos flap transposed ventrally as a bed for preputial skin graft in primary staged hypospadias repair. Urology. 2012; 79(4):939–42.

Stoll C, Alembik Y, Roth MP, Dott B. Genetic and environmental factors in hypospadias. J Med Genet. 1990;27(9):559–63.

Thiounn N, Missirliu A, Zerbib M, Larrouy M, Dje K, Flam T, et al. Corporeal plication for surgical correction of penile curvature. Experience with 60 patients. Eur Urol. 1998;33(4):401–4.

Ulman I, Erikci V, Avanoglu A, Gokdemir A. The effect of suturing technique and material on complication rate following hypospadias repair. Eur J Pediatr Surg. 1997;7(3):156–7.

Vallasciani S, Berrettini A, Nanni L, Manzoni G, Marrocco G. Observational retrospective study on acquired megalourethra after primary proximal hypospadias repair and its recurrence after tapering. J Pediatr Urol. 2012 in press; doi:10.1016/j.jpurol.2012.05.005.

van der Horst C, Martinez Portillo FJ, Seif C, Melchior D, Stubinger H, Alken P, et al. [Quality of life after surgical correction of penile deviation with the Schroeder-Essed plication]. Aktuelle Urol. 2003; 34(2):109–14.

Van Savage JG, Palanca LG, Slaughenhoupt BL. A prospective randomized trial of dressings versus no dressings for hypospadias repair. J Urol. 2000;164 (3 Pt 2):981–3.

Ververidis M, Dickson AP, Gough DC. An objective assessment of the results of hypospadias surgery. BJU Int. 2005;96(1):135–9.

Villanueva C, Bush N, Snodgrass W. Duration of follow-up to identify urethral complications after TIP hypospadias repair. New Orleans, LA: American Academy of Pediatrics National Conference and Exhibition; 2012.

Waterman BJ, Renschler T, Cartwright PC, Snow BW, DeVries CR. Variables in successful repair of urethrocutaneous fistula after hypospadias surgery. J Urol. 2002;168(2):726–30. discussion 9–30.

Weber DM, Schonbucher VB, Gobet R, Gerber A, Landolt MA. Is there an ideal age for hypospadias repair? A pilot study. J Pediatr Urol. 2009;5(5):345–50.

Weiser AC, Franco I, Herz DB, Silver RI, Reda EF. Single layered small intestinal ubmucosa in the repair of severe chordee and complicated hypospadias. J Urol. 2003;170(4 Pt 2):1593–5. disussion 5.

Wiener JS, Sutherland RW, Roth DR, Gonzales Jr ET. Comparison of onlay and tubularized island flaps of inner preputial skin for the repair of proximal hypospadias. J Urol. 1997;158(3 Pt 2):1172–4.

Wilkinson DJ, Farrelly P, Kenny SE. Outcomes in distal hypospadias: a systematic review of the Mathieu and tubularized incised plate repairs. J Pediatr Urol. 2012;8(3):307–12.

Wolffenbuttel KP, Wondergem N, Hoefnagels JJ, Dieleman GC, Pel JJ, Passchier BT, et al. Abnormal urine flow in boys with distal hypospadias before and after correction. J Urol. 2006;176(4 Pt 2):1733–6. discussion 6–7.

Wood HM, Kay R, Angermeier KW, Ross JH. Timing of the presentation of urethrocutaneous fistulas after hypospadias repair in pediatric patients. J Urol. 2008;180(4 Suppl):1753–6.

Yamaguchi T, Kitada S, Osada Y. Chromosomal anomalies in cryptorchidism and hypospadias. Urol Int. 1991;47(2):60–3.

Yang S, Hsieh C, Chen Y, Chen S. Normal size of the urethral meatus in uncircumcised boys. J Urol ROC. 2001;12(1):20–3.

Ye WJ, Ping P, Liu YD, Li Z, Huang YR. Single stage dorsal inlay buccal mucosal graft with tubularized incised urethral plate technique for hypospadias reoperations. Asian J Androl. 2008;10(4):682–6.

Ziada AM, Morsi H, Aref A, Elsaied W. Tubularized incised plate (TIP) in previously operated (redo) hypospadias. J Pediatr Urol. 2006;2(5):409–14.

Phimosis, Meatal Stenosis, and BXO

10

Patricio C. Gargollo

The primary aim in diagnosis and treatment of phimosis and meatal stenosis is relief of symptoms.

The primary aim in diagnosis and treatment of balanitis xerotica obliterans (BXO) is to avoid urethral stricture from progressive disease.

A secondary aim for circumcision is to reduce likelihood for sexually transmitted disease in adults.

Evidence for these aims:

- **Our review found no study reporting the incidence of symptomatic phimosis.**
- **The normal foreskin does not fully retract at birth, but persistent failure to retract occurs in <10 % of teens.**
- **RCTs demonstrate betamethasone ointment is more effective than placebo to achieve partial or complete retraction, but placebo is also effective in up to 45 % of cases.**
- **Our review found no definition for meatal stenosis.**
- **One study of boys with deflected urinary stream undergoing meatotomy reported that symptoms improved and mean Q_{max} increased.**
- **There is poor evidence that meatotomy is indicated for a small-appearing meatus, dysuria, or incontinence.**
- **BXO involvement of glans and meatus clinically resolves in most patients within 2 years of circumcision.**

P.C. Gargollo, M.D. (✉)
Department of Pediatric Urology, University of Texas Southwestern Medical Center and Children's Medical Center Dallas, 1935 Medical District Drive, MS F4.04, Dallas, TX 75235, USA
e-mail: patricio.gargollo@childrens.com

Phimosis

Prevalence and Natural History

The foreskin normally does not fully retract at birth. Two studies by pediatricians reported that phimosis persisted in <10 % of boys after age 3 years. By age 16, the foreskin did not fully retract in 1 %.

Phimosis is normal at birth, with subsequent retractability over time reported in several series:

- Observations were made by a pediatrician in 100 newborns, 200 boys to age 5 years, and 200 aged 5–13, noting the foreskin was fully retractable in 4 % at birth, 20 % at 6 months, 50 % at 1 year, and 90 % at ≥3 years (Gairdner 1949).
- Another pediatrician reported the state of the foreskin in 9,545 boys 6–17 years of age, finding phimosis overall in 4 %, decreasing from 8 % at age 6 years to 1 % in those 16 years of age (Oster 1968).
- Foreskin status was recorded in 10,421 Chinese boys presenting to a children's hospital, excluding urology clinic patients. All newborns had non-retractable foreskin, vs. 7 % of males 11–18 years of age (Yang et al. 2009).
- Natural history of the prepuce was deduced from a sample of 600 Japanese boys 0–15

W.T. Snodgrass (ed.), *Pediatric Urology: Evidence for Optimal Patient Management*,
DOI 10.1007/978-1-4614-6910-0_10, © Springer Science+Business Media New York 2013

years of age presenting to pediatric surgical and urologic clinics (reasons for examination not stated) over a 1-year period. Status of the prepuce was categorized into five types:

- No retraction.
- Exposure of urethral meatus.
- Exposure of 50 % of glans.
- Exposure of glans to above the corona at site of (inner) preputial adhesion.
- Exposure of entire glans.

Before 6 months of age, no boy in this sample had type 5 complete retraction, and after 11 years of age, no boy had type 1 no retraction (Kayaba et al. 1996).

Medical Therapy

Because phimosis spontaneously corrects, therapy should be limited to boys with related symptoms.

We found no population-based study describing incidence of symptoms in uncircumcised boys.

One study using uroflowometry and PVR reported no differences in boys with phimosis and ballooning during voiding compared to those without ballooning.

A study compared uroflow, PVR, and renal US in 32 consecutive boys, mean age 7 years, with phimosis, of which 18 had ballooning during voiding. Renal US was normal in all, there was no difference in mean Q_{max} (15 cc/s), and no difference in mean PVR (3.5–6 cc) in those with vs. without ballooning (Babu et al. 2004).

Steroids for Primary Phimosis

Two RCTs reported that betamethasone significantly improved retraction vs. placebo:

- **Neither described indications for therapy.**
- **Success defined as retraction exposing more than one-third of the glans occurred in 86 % steroid vs. 44 % placebo patients.**
- **Success defined as full retraction occurred in 55 % steroid vs. 30 % placebo.**
- **Recurrent phimosis developed in ≤15 %.**

A double-blinded RCT tested 0.1 % betamethasone cream vs. aqueous cream (placebo) in 137 boys, mean age 7 years (3–15), on a waiting list for circumcision (indications, including symptoms, not described). Retractability of the prepuce was graded as follows:

1. Full retraction
2. Full retraction but tight behind the glans
3. Exposure of more than one-third of glans
4. Exposure of less than one-third of glans
5. Pinhole opening
6. No retraction

All patients had grades 4–6. Treatment was retraction to extent possible without causing pain or skin fissure with cream application twice daily for 4 weeks. The primary endpoint was grade 3 or less, and all patients not improved to this extent were treated with betamethasone for another 4 weeks. Assessment was done by a different doctor than the one that prescribed therapy; compliance was assessed by examining the tube of cream at follow-up. It was not stated if phimosis grade was equivalent between groups. At 4 weeks, 49/66 (74 %) betamethasone vs. 31/71 (44 %) placebo patients were considered cured, $p<0.01$. Of 57 not responding who completed four subsequent weeks of betamethasone, 43 (75 %) were cured. Therefore, 118/137 (86 %) had retractability to expose one-third of the glans or greater with steroid treatment. Retraction was then recommended "several times a day," with follow-up at 18 months. Of the 118, 92 returned, with 13 (14 %) having recurrence of phimosis described as "minor." Response by phimosis grade was not reported (Lund et al. 2005).

Another double-blinded RCT used the five-point phimosis grading scale by Kayaba described above:

1. No retraction (58 % patients)
2. Exposure of urethral meatus (19 %)
3. Exposure of 50 % of glans (21 %)
4. Exposure of glans to above the corona (2 %)
5. Exposure of entire glans

One hundred ninety-five boys, mean age 5 years (3–10), were randomized to four groups: (1) 0.2 % betamethasone plus hyaluronidase, (2) 0.2 % betamethasone, (3) 0.1 % betamethasone, and (4) placebo. Indications for treatment were not stated. There was no difference between groups based on age or phimosis grade. Treatment was retraction with cream application twice daily for 60 days; success was defined as grade 5, total retraction. Success occurred in 57 %, 59 %, and 48 % of groups 1 through 3 (no significant differences) vs. 29 % placebo, $p<0.001$. Success by phimosis grade was 54 % grades 1 and 2, and 33 % grade 3. Follow-up was done at 240 days in successful cases (instructions for retraction, if any, not stated). Recurrence (not defined) was reported in 2 % (Nascimento et al. 2011).

A prospective study evaluated 260 boys, mean age 34 months (3–168), with "symptomatic phimosis" described as 42 % with ballooning and 16 % with balanoposthitis, but also 13 % UTI, and others with itching, "straining," dysuria, and smegma. Phimosis was graded as follows:

1. Full retraction (including limitation by inner preputial–glans adhesions)
2. Full retraction, tight behind glans
3. Meatus visible
4. Slight retraction, meatus and glans not visible
5. No retraction

Treatment was done using 0.05 % betamethasone 2×/daily until phimosis resolved, followed by "daily hygiene" (not described). Success was ≤ grade 2. Reassessment was done at 1, 2, and 4 weeks and 6 months. At 1 week, 72 %, and by 4 weeks, 91 % had success, which was similar for grades 3–5 phimosis. At 6 months, 25 (9 %) had recurrence (Reddy et al. 2012).

Steroids for Secondary Phimosis

One study reported betamethasone for secondary phimosis after neonatal circumcision completely exposed the glans in 64 % of patients.

One retrospective study concerned newborns referred within 1 month of circumcision with a "trapped penis" from secondary phimosis, identifying 14 patients. Treatment was 0.05 % betamethasone 3×/daily for 3 weeks. Complete exposure of the glans occurred in nine (64 %), complete exposure with a persistent cicatrix was noted in another two who were also undergoing a vertical relaxing incision, and the remaining three had no improvement, leading to reoperation. Follow-up after medical therapy was 3–6 months without secondary treatment (Palmer et al. 2005).

Neonatal Circumcision

Anesthesia

Ring block was found to be significantly better than dorsal nerve block or EMLA for newborn circumcision.

Cochrane review of RCTs comparing pain interventions with no treatment or placebo during neonatal circumcision reported the following:

- Fourteen trials with 592 newborns compared dorsal nerve block to no treatment/placebo, finding significantly lower heart rate, decreased time crying, and increased O_2 saturation with nerve block.
- Six trials with 200 newborns found that EMLA significantly reduced heart rate and time crying vs. placebo.
- Three trials with 139 newborns compared nerve block to EMLA, reporting significantly lower heart rate and pain scores with nerve block (Brady-Fryer et al. 2004).

Fifty-four full-term newborns had Gomco circumcision done in a double-blinded placebo controlled trial testing EMLA, dorsal nerve block, and ring block. Blocks used 1 % lidocaine. Primary outcomes were heart rate and cry, which were significantly greater in the placebo group than in all three treatment groups. The ring block was more effective than EMLA or dorsal nerve block, since the latter were not effective during foreskin separation from the glans or dorsal slit (Lander et al. 1997).

Gomco and Plastibell

One review found wound separation more common with Gomco circumcision and infection more common after Plastibell circumcision.

One retrospective review of Plastibell outcomes stated that malposition of the ring occurred in 0.5 %.

One study reported greater complications when Gomco was used in 6-month-old infants than in newborns.

Review of 5,521 newborn circumcisions performed from 1963 to 1972 before nursery discharge was done by medical students, residents, or faculty physicians. Gomco was used in 48 %, and Plastibell in 52 %, with hemorrhage (requiring "special efforts to stem blood flow") in 59 (1 %), infection in 23 (0.4 %), wound separation in 9 (0.2 %), excess skin removal in 2 (0.04 %), and Plastibell too tight in 7 (0.1 %): an overall incidence of 100 (2 %) complications. There was no difference in hemorrhage, but wound separation was significantly more common with Gomco; infection was more likely using the Plastibell (Gee and Ansell 1976).

Plastibell neonatal circumcision was done in 3,000 boys from 2004 to 2008 by urologists or pediatricians. Complications occurred in 1 %, including hemorrhage in 8, "inappropriate penile appearance" (apparently excessive residual skin or tags) in 12, and "malposition of the ring" in 14 (Simforoosh et al. 2012).

Gomco circumcision was done in 98 neonates, mean age 17 days (4–30), and 32 infants, mean age 6.5 months (3–8.5), the latter using general anesthesia. During the initial 30 postoperative days, there were no complications in neonatal procedures, vs. 12 (30 %) infant circumcisions. All complications were bleeding, which required fulguration or suturing (Horowitz and Gershbein 2001).

Mogen Clamp

One report from Israel, where the Mogen clamp is commonly used by ritual circumcisers, found one case of partial glans amputation from a presumed 19,478 procedures.

A review of complications after newborn circumcision in Israel, most done by certified ritual circumcisers who use the Mogen clamp, estimated a rate of 0.3 % based on assessment of 66 cases from 19,478 male births. These included hemorrhage in 16, wound infection in 2, and partial glans amputation in 1. Late complications were excessive skin in 38 and shortage of skin in 4 (Ben Chaim et al. 2005).

Circumcision with Bleeding Disorders

Interventions to reduce bleeding from circumcision in hemophiliacs include preoperative factor replacement and tranexamic acid, intraoperative fibrin glue, and postoperative factor replacement for up to 7 days.

Bleeding despite these preventative measures occurred in 4–24 % of patients.

Bleeding was reported as late as 8 days after circumcision.

Literature review found six studies published from 1992 and 2004 with 163 hemophiliac patients undergoing circumcision. Factor replacement therapy was used in five, antifibrinolytics alone were used in one, and postoperative replacement was continued for 2–8 days. Bleeding complications were reported in up to 50 % (Hermans et al. 2009).

As part of a prospective trial, 25 hemophiliac boys, median age 20 months (7–34), who had either no or "minimal" exposure to factor VIII, received factor VIII and tranexamic acid infusion and then underwent circumcision. The wound was dressed with a gelatin sponge absorbable hemostatic agent and Vaseline gauze removed at ≤7 days. Patients were discharged home within 6 h of circumcision. Bleeding occurred in one patient (4 %) on the eighth postoperative day (Elalfy et al. 2012).

A retrospective review found 48 children with bleeding disorders who had circumcision, including 24 with hemophilia A, 5 with hemophilia B, and 15 with von Willebrand disease. Overall, bleeding complications occurred in 11 (23 %):

- The bleeding disorder was known preoperatively in 21 (44 %), with circumcision done at ≤6 weeks in 16. Of these 21, 12 had factor replacement before surgery, but 3 still had bleeding complications, including transfusion in 2.
- The bleeding disorder was not known in 27, of which 25 were circumcised at ≤6 weeks. "Oozing" occurred in 8 (30 %), but none required transfusion.
- Bleeding in the 11 patients occurred immediately in 9, within hours in 1, and 2 weeks later in 1 (with known disease and factor replacement) (Rodriguez et al. 2010).

Another retrospective review reported on the Izmir protocol, which was done for 50 boys, mean age 9 years (1–16), with known hemophilia. These children had oral tranexamic acid beginning 1 day preoperatively and continuing for 7 days, factor infusion to achieve ≥90 % levels 1 h preoperatively, fibrin glue applied subepithelially and over the incision line, and postoperative factor infusions every 12 h for 48 h. Postoperative bleeding occurred in three (6 %) (Yilmaz et al. 2010).

Comparison of the Izmir protocol was made to patients treated earlier using factor replacement for up to 7 days without fibrin glue in a retrospective analysis. Bleeding complications developed in 6/20 circumcised with longer factor replacement and no fibrin glue vs. 7/37 (19 %) following the Izmir plan, $p=0.5$, indicating that the Izmir protocol was as effective as traditional longer-duration factor replacement (Sasmaz et al. 2012).

Circumcision with Aspirin Therapy for Heart Disease

Our review found no report concerning circumcision in children with congenital heart disease taking aspirin.

Early Complications

Systematic review found early complications after circumcision in 1.5 % of neonates and 6 % of children >1 year of age.

A systematic review was done regarding reported complications (excluding residual excess skin) after circumcision, finding the following:

- Sixteen prospective studies of neonates and infants from 12 countries, median frequency of complications was 1.5 % (0–16 %)
- Ten prospective studies of boys ≥1 year of age from ten countries, median frequency of complications was 6 % (2–14 %) (Weiss et al. 2010).

A review was done using the Comprehensive Hospital Abstract Reporting System to estimate complications following 130,475 newborn circumcision over a 9-year period ending in 1996. Recorded diagnoses potentially indicating circumcision complication (bleeding, suture laceration, wound-penis, etc.) were found in 287 (0.2 %), or 1 of every 476 newborn circumcisions (Christakis et al. 2000).

Late Complications

Excess residual skin and meatal stenosis are the most commonly reported late complications from circumcision.

One report defining excess skin as covering ≥50 % of the glans with downward compression of the penopubic junction reported occurrence in an estimated 0.2 %.

Meatal stenosis occurred in <1 % after newborn circumcision in two studies, neither of which defined criteria for the diagnosis.

A cross-sectional study evaluated 3,125 circumcised boys aged 6–12 years in Iran, with most (71 %) having the procedure after age 2 years and only 3 % done as neonates. These operations had been done by surgeons/urologists (32 %), primary care physicians (19 %) or paramedical personnel (6 %), and traditional circumcisers (44 %). Ninety-three had a normal examination; the most common complications diagnosed were excessive residual skin (not defined) in 4 %, and excessive removed skin, meatal stenosis (not defined), granuloma, penile rotation, and chordee in ≤1 % each. Significantly fewer complications occurred after circumcisions performed by urologists/surgeons (4 %) than by primary physicians (10 %) or traditional circumcisers (8 %) (Yegane et al. 2006).

The prospective study by Simforoosh et al. (2012) mentioned above reported meatal stenosis (not defined) was diagnosed in 11 (0.4 %) at 15-month follow-up, with all undergoing meatotomy.

A review of newborn circumcisions in Israel defined excess residual skin as covering ≥50 % of the glans while pressure was applied at the penopubic base to control for pre-pubic fat. By these criteria, 38 cases were diagnosed at four medical centers, which had a total of 19,478 male births, for a rate of 0.2 %, assuming all patients with this complication returned for follow-up (Ben Chaim et al. 2005).

A retrospective review was done for patients referred to a pediatric surgical service for circumcision revision. Between 1995 and 1999, 56 boys, 6 weeks to 11 years of age, had reoperation, all stated to have excessive residual skin (not defined); 29 (52 %) also had penile adhesions (not defined), and 8 (14 %) had phimosis. The authors stated that "because dissatisfaction with the circumcision already had been expressed by the parent or primary care physician, we revised all referred children" (Brisson et al. 2002).

Secondary Phimosis

One study reported that secondary phimosis developed in 3 % following newborn Gomco circumcision.

Treatment using either betamethasone or mechanical stretching of the phimotic ring was reported successful in 64–100 % of cases.

The study by Palmer et al. (2005) described above found that treatment using 0.05 % betamethasone applied 3×/daily for 3 weeks resolved secondary phimosis in 9/14 (64 %) infants referred within 1 month of circumcision. Follow-up after medical therapy was 3–6 months without secondary treatment (Palmer et al. 2005).

From a total of 521 infant (median age 2 months, 2 weeks–4 months) Gomco circumcisions, 15 (3 %) developed secondary phimosis. Another 13 with this complication were referred, and these 28 infants had nerve block performed and dilation of the phimotic ring using a hemostat to deliver the concealed glans. With follow-up of 1 month, three (11 %) had recurrence treated with repeat glans delivery from below the phimotic ring. No circumcision revisions were done (Blalock et al. 2003).

Medical Benefits

AAP Policy Statement, 2012

The AAP circumcision task force recently updated 1999 recommendations stating that "the health benefits of newborn circumcision outweigh the risks and that the procedure's benefits justify access to this procedure for families that choose it. Specific benefits include prevention of UTI, penile cancer, and transmission of some sexually transmitted infections, including HIV."

UTI Reduction

See Chap. 1.

Reduced Disease Transmission in Adults

HIV

Three RCTs conducted in young-adult African males reported a 50 % reduction in HIV infection with circumcision during follow-up ≤2 years.

A RCT in South Africa included 3,274 men randomized to circumcision or control with follow-up to 21 months scheduled. The trial was stopped at mean follow-up of 18 months after interim analysis found 20 HIV infections in circumcision men vs. 49 in controls, RR 0.4 (95 % CI 0.2–0.7). This represented a 60 % risk reduction (Auvert et al. 2005).

A RCT was conducted in Kenya, mostly within a tribal group with a circumcision prevalence of approximately 10 % and an HIV prevalence of 18 % males and 25 % females. Two thousand seven hundred eighty-four uncircumcised HIV-negative males, mean age 20 years, were randomly assigned to circumcision or control groups with follow-up HIV testing to 24 months postoperatively. At 2 years, 2 % of circumcised and 4 % of uncircumcised males were HIV-positive, $p = 0.006$; RR in circumcised men was 0.5 (95 % CI 0.3–0.8), corresponding to a risk reduction of 53 %. The trial was stopped early, when interim analysis showed these results (Bailey et al. 2007).

A similar study was conducted in Uganda in 4,996 uncircumcised men aged 15–49 years, which also showed circumcision efficacy of 51 % (95 % CI 16–72) for HIV avoidance (Gray et al. 2007).

HPV

HPV prevalence is less in circumcised men. One meta-analysis found that circumcision did not reduce risk for acquiring HPV.

Meta-analysis was done on 21 studies with 8,046 circumcised and 6,336 uncircumcised males, with circumcision associated with significantly reduced odds for genital HPV, OR 0.6 (95 % CI 0.4–0.8) (Albero et al. 2012).

A systematic literature review and meta-analysis was done regarding impact of circumcision on human papillomavirus transmission, which included 21 studies (two RCTs, both conducted in Africa) with 8,046 circumcised and 6,336 uncircumcised men. Reported findings included the following:

- Circumcision reduced odds for genital HPV prevalence (OR 0.57 [95 % CI 0.42–0.77]).
- Circumcision did not reduce risk for genital HPV acquisition (summary effect 1.01 [95 % CI 0.66–1.53]) (Albero et al. 2012).

Other STDs

Circumcision did not reduce gonorrhea, chlamydia, or syphilis infections in the RCTs described above for HIV. There was reduced risk for herpes simplex virus type 2 infection.

The Kenyan RCT described above to determine circumcision impact on HIV seroconversion also evaluated risk for *Neisseria gonorrhea*, *Chlamydia trachomatis*, or *Trichomonas vaginalis* infection in circumcised vs. control males. Circumcision did not reduce risk for these nonulcerative sexually transmitted infections (Mehta et al. 2009).

The Ugandan RCT also studied circumcision impact on prevention of herpes simplex virus type 2 (HSV-2), human papillomavirus (HPV), and syphilis, reporting no reduction for syphilis, but reduced HSV-2 (8 % vs. 10 %, HR 0.7 [95 % CI 0.6–0.9], $p=0.008$) and HPV (18 % vs. 28 %, RR 0.65 [95 % CI 0.5–0.9], $p=0.009$) (Tobian et al. 2009).

Meatal Stenosis

Diagnosis

Our review found no definition for meatal stenosis.

One study in which 90 % of patients had a deflected urinary stream reported that Q_{max} was >5 cc/s in cases, and that mean Q_{max} was greater after meatotomy.

A retrospective study of meatal stenosis identified 50 patients with the condition, 34 symptomatic and 16 without symptoms (criteria for diagnosis not stated). All had newborn or neonatal circumcision. Meatotomy in symptomatic cases was done at mean age 4 years for "poor stream" (36 %), dysuria (30 %), straining (14 %), retention (not defined) (8 %), dribbling (6 %), and bedwetting (19 %) (all with other additional symptoms). All these complaints were said to be relieved at follow-up 1–3 months later. Asymptomatic patients also had meatotomy (Upadhyay et al. 1998).

Another retrospective study found 120 males, mean age 2.5 years (3 months–6 years), diagnosed with meatal stenosis based on a pinhole meatus and inability to pass a 6-Fr catheter. Twenty-seven percent had no symptoms, while 33 % had a deflected and smaller urinary stream and 35 % had dysuria. US done in all cases reported no obstructive uropathy (Mahmoudi 2005).

Evaluation in 132 males aged 5–10 years old with a history of neonatal circumcision referred to a surgical clinic without urinary complaints included meatal calibration with a 5-Fr catheter. In 27 (20 %), the catheter would not pass, and 25 of these had decreased-caliber stream and prolonged voiding (uroflowometry not reported). Three had bilateral hydronephrosis and bladder thickening and UD showed "obstructed bladder outlet." Results of meatotomy were not described except to state residual urine persisted in these three cases while others had improvement (means to assess not stated) (Joudi et al. 2011).

A retrospective study was done in 22 boys, mean age 8 years (4–13), diagnosed with meatal stenosis, for deflected urinary stream ($n=20$, 91 %), frequency ($n=9$, 41 %), dysuria ($n=6$, 27 %), or after UTI ($n=2$, 9 %). Uroflowometry was done pre- and post-meatotomy (by 6 weeks); the authors reported a significant increase in Q_{max} from mean 10 cc/s to a mean of 16 cc/s, $p=0.001$. Flow patterns were plateau in 16 pre-meatotomy, with persistence in 6 (37.5 %) after meatotomy. Mean PVR decreased from 19 to 14 cc, $p=0.01$. It is noteworthy that Q_{max} was >5 cc/s in all patients before meatotomy. All symptoms resolved without recurrence in a mean of 12 months (6–28) (VanderBrink et al. 2008).

Prevalence

One study of consecutive males reported that while meatal stenosis (meatal opening ≤2 mm with symptoms) only occurred in circumcised boys, there was no significant difference vs. uncircumcised boys.

A study included 1,100 consecutive males ≤18 years of age undergoing physical examination by a single pediatrician from 1995 to 2001. Diagnosis of meatal stenosis was made on the basis of symptoms ("dysuria, voiding complaints, stream abnormalities, abdominal discomfort") and meatal opening ≤2 mm. Ninety-one (8 %) were not circumcised. Meatal stenosis was diagnosed only in circumcised boys, overall in 3 % (95 % CI 1.76–3.79 %), and with increased incidence in prepubertal boys >3 years of age (7 % [95 % CI 4.48–10.10 %]). However, there was no significant difference in circumcised vs. uncircumcised males overall or in patients >3 years, OR with circumcision 3.5 (95 % CI 0.62–infinity). The author commented that the study had sufficient subjects to have an 80 % chance of detecting an 8 % difference in meatal stenosis rates (Van Howe 2006).

The prospective study by Simforoosh et al. (2012) mentioned above reported that meatal stenosis (not defined) was diagnosed in 11 (0.4 %) at 15-month follow-up, with all undergoing meatotomy.

A retrospective study was done in 117 patients undergoing circumcision at median age approximately 5 years in a single clinic in 1976, for recurrent balanitis in 45, preputial scarring in 25, ballooning of the prepuce during voiding in 41, and asymptomatic phimosis in 6. Follow-up included determination of the width of the meatus at 3 months. Thirteen (11 %) were diagnosed as having "stricture" of the meatus that required meatotomy, but criteria for that determination, related symptoms, and results were not described. A questionnaire was answered by 92 patients 5 years later in which 4 % stated that they had a "thin jet at voiding"(Stenram et al. 1986).

Eighteen hundred schoolboys aged 6–10 years were examined by "spreading the meatus," with 578 (32 %) considered to have meatal stenosis on the basis of a "pinpoint or just slightly larger" opening. The authors admitted that these were "astounding" results (Allen and Summers 1974).

Meatotomy

One study reported that office meatotomy using EMLA was effective, with only 5 % experiencing discomfort.

Fifty-eight boys, mean age 4 years (20 months–10 years), had office meatotomy using EMLA topical ointment applied 60 min before the procedure. Oral midazolam was used in two. During meatotomy, three (5 %) were described as having "some discomfort." Follow-up in 57 was ≥3 months, with one (2 %) partial recurrence (Cartwright et al. 1996).

Balanitis Xerotica Obliterans

Diagnosis

BXO is clinically suspected in secondary phimosis and/or from a white sclerotic ring at the tip of the prepuce.

BXO is suspected when a previously retractile prepuce becomes nonretractile, typically with a white sclerotic ring at the tip of the foreskin. Pathologic examination demonstrates atrophy of the epidermis, loss of rete pegs, and inflammatory cell infiltration in the dermal-epidermal junction.

Incidence

Three studies reported BXO in from 10 to 40 % of consecutive boys undergoing circumcision.

During a 10-year period ending 2001, 1,178 consecutive boys, mean age 7 years (2–16), were referred to a urology clinic in Hungary for phimosis, excluding an unknown number wanting circumcision for "cultural or social" reasons. Neither symptoms nor clinical findings (white sclerotic ring) were described. All patients had circumcision with pathologic examination of the specimen. BXO was diagnosed pathologically in 471 (40 %) boys, mean age 9 years with youngest 2 years old. Ninety-three percent of these with BXO had secondary phimosis, vs. 32 % of patients without BXO (Kiss et al. 2005).

Another study involved 100 consecutive boys, mean age 6 years (1–17), undergoing circumcision in Switzerland (indications not described). BXO was diagnosed histologically in 10 (10 %) after being suspected preoperatively in 12 (Meuli et al. 1994).

After encountering a child with BXO, the next 100 consecutive foreskins removed in an Australian hospital at parent's request ($n=35$), for phimosis ($n=38$), or for balanitis or during hypospadias repair and other "miscellaneous conditions" were histrologically examined. BXO was described in nine (9 %); age of these children and whether the condition was suspected clinically was not stated (Bale et al. 1987).

Medical Treatment

Topical Steroids

One trial reported that BXO phimosis improved with steroid ointment, but histologic changes persisted.

A double-blinded RCT compared 0.05 % mometasone furoate vs. placebo in 40 boys, mean age 9 years (5–15), with phimosis due to BXO on the basis of "typical macroscopic findings" (not described). Ointment was applied 1x daily for 5 weeks, then prepuce retraction was scored and circumcision performed. Phimosis was graded 1–4 (complete retraction vs. no retraction). Those with steroid had a significant improvement from mean 3.4 ± 0.15 to 2.9 ± 0.2 (better in 7 and unchanged in 10) vs. placebo, with decreased retraction from mean 3 ± 0.2 to 3.4 ± 0.2 (worse in 5 and unchanged in 11). The authors did not state if any steroid-treated child had clinical resolution of phimosis, and apparently all had histologic confirmation of BXO despite steroid treatment (Kiss et al. 2001).

Tacrolimus

One study reported that tacrolimus applied to the glans and meatus effective to resolve BXO after circumcision, but without an untreated control group.

Tacrolimus ointment, 0.1 %, was applied to the glans and meatus 2×/daily for 3 weeks beginning 3 weeks after circumcision in 20 boys, mean age 10 years (5–16), with BXO. Of these, 11 only had the lesion apparent in the prepuce, while another 3 had visible glans, 4 had visible meatal involvement, and 2 had both glans and meatal involvement. All visible signs disappeared with 3 weeks treatment, with 1 (11 %) recurrence in 6 months on the glans successfully retreated with 6-month subsequent follow-up. Of the 11 patients treated without known residual disease 1 (9 %) recurred at the meatus at 8 months and responded to retreatment for 3 weeks with subsequent 8-month follow-up. The authors admitted that circumcision alone can be effective for clearing visible glans and meatal lesions (Ebert et al. 2008).

Circumcision

BXO involving the glans and meatus was reported in two studies to resolve or improve within 2 years after circumcision.

In 231/471 (49 %) boys with BXO reported by Kiss et al. (2005) above, the glans also had whitish discoloration that resolved spontaneously in all cases within 2 years after circumcision. Seven (2 %) had meatal involvement treated with meatotomy at circumcision. Outcome in these was not specifically stated (Kiss et al. 2005).

Of the ten confirmed cases of preputial BXO in the series reported by Meuli et al. (1994) above, seven had "characteristic glans lesions" (not defined) but none had meatal stenosis. These resolved in five and improved in the other two at 5-year follow-up after circumcision.

A retrospective review found 300 patients with BXO "limited to the foreskin or glans," of which 287 (96 %) had circumcision as the sole therapy. In the others, meatotomy was done in five, oral mucosa graft urethroplasty in four, and excision of BXO from the glans with skin grafting in four. Of the 287 with only circumcision, persistence of BXO was noted in 11 (4 %), involving the glans in 5 or spreading to the urethra in 6. Treatment with topical clobetasol was not effective for glans involvement (duration of use not stated). Length of follow-up was not stated (Depasquale et al. 2000).

References

Albero G, Castellsague X, Giuliano AR, Bosch FX. Male circumcision and genital human papillomavirus: a systematic review and meta-analysis. Sex Transm Dis. 2012;39(2):104–13.

Allen JS, Summers JL. Meatal stenosis in children. J Urol. 1974;112(4):526–7.

Auvert B, Taljaard D, Lagarde E, Sobngwi-Tambekou J, Sitta R, Puren A. Randomized, controlled intervention trial of male circumcision for reduction of HIV infection risk: the ANRS 1265 Trial. PLoS Med. 2005; 2(11):e298.

Babu R, Harrison SK, Hutton KA. Ballooning of the foreskin and physiological phimosis: is there any objective evidence of obstructed voiding? BJU Int. 2004;94(3):384–7.

Bailey RC, Moses S, Parker CB, Agot K, Maclean I, Krieger JN, et al. Male circumcision for HIV prevention in young men in Kisumu, Kenya: a randomised controlled trial. Lancet. 2007;369(9562):643–56.

Bale PM, Lochhead A, Martin HC, Gollow I. Balanitis xerotica obliterans in children. Pediatr Pathol. 1987;7(5–6):617–27.

Ben Chaim J, Livne PM, Binyamini J, Hardak B, Ben-Meir D, Mor Y. Complications of circumcision in Israel: a one year multicenter survey. Isr Med Assoc J. 2005;7(6):368–70.

Blalock HJ, Vemulakonda V, Ritchey ML, Ribbeck M. Outpatient management of phimosis following newborn circumcision. J Urol. 2003;169(6):2332–4.

Brady-Fryer B, Wiebe N, Lander JA. Pain relief for neonatal circumcision. Cochrane Database Syst Rev (Online). 2004(4):CD004217.

Brisson PA, Patel HI, Feins NR. Revision of circumcision in children: report of 56 cases. J Pediatr Surg. 2002;37(9):1343–6.

Cartwright PC, Snow BW, McNees DC. Urethral meatotomy in the office using topical EMLA cream for anesthesia. J Urol. 1996;156(2 Pt 2):857–8. discussion 8–9.

Christakis DA, Harvey E, Zerr DM, Feudtner C, Wright JA, Connell FA. A trade-off analysis of routine newborn circumcision. Pediatrics. 2000;105(1 Pt 3):246–9.

Depasquale I, Park AJ, Bracka A. The treatment of balanitis xerotica obliterans. BJU Int. 2000;86(4):459–65.

Ebert AK, Rosch WH, Vogt T. Safety and tolerability of adjuvant topical tacrolimus treatment in boys with lichen sclerosus: a prospective phase 2 study. Eur Urol. 2008;54(4):932–7.

Elalfy MS, Elbarbary NS, Eldebeiky MS, El Danasoury AS. Risk of bleeding and inhibitor development after circumcision of previously untreated or minimally treated severe hemophilia a children. Pediatr Hematol Oncol. 2012;29(5):485–93.

Gairdner D. The fate of the foreskin, a study of circumcision. Br Med J. 1949;2(4642):1433–7. illust.

Gee WF, Ansell JS. Neonatal circumcision: a ten-year overview: with comparison of the gomco clamp and the plastibell device. Pediatrics. 1976;58(6):824–7.

Gray RH, Kigozi G, Serwadda D, Makumbi F, Watya S, Nalugoda F, et al. Male circumcision for HIV prevention in men in Rakai, Uganda: a randomised trial. Lancet. 2007;369(9562):657–66.

Hermans C, Altisent C, Batorova A, Chambost H, De Moerloose P, Karafoulidou A, et al. Replacement therapy for invasive procedures in patients with haemophilia: literature review, European survey and recommendations. Haemophilia. 2009;15(3):639–58.

Horowitz M, Gershbein AB. Gomco circumcision: when is it safe? J Pediatr Surg. 2001;36(7):1047–9.

Joudi M, Fathi M, Hiradfar M. Incidence of asymptomatic meatal stenosis in children following neonatal circumcision. J Pediatr Urol. 2011;7(5):526–8.

Kayaba H, Tamura H, Kitajima S, Fujiwara Y, Kato T. Analysis of shape and retractability of the prepuce in 603 Japanese boys. J Urol. 1996;156(5):1813–5.

Kiss A, Csontai A, Pirot L, Nyirady P, Merksz M, Kiraly L. The response of balanitis xerotica obliterans to local steroid application compared with placebo in children. J Urol. 2001;165(1):219–20.

Kiss A, Kiraly L, Kutasy B, Merksz M. High incidence of balanitis xerotica obliterans in boys with phimosis: prospective 10-year study. Pediatr Dermatol. 2005; 22(4):305–8.

Lander J, Brady-Fryer B, Metcalfe JB, Nazarali S, Muttitt S. Comparison of ring block, dorsal penile nerve block, and topical anesthesia for neonatal circumcision: a randomized controlled trial. JAMA. 1997;278(24):2157–62.

Lund L, Wai KH, Mui LM, Yeung CK. An 18-month follow-up study after randomized treatment of phimosis in boys with topical steroid versus placebo. Scand J Urol Nephrol. 2005;39(1):78–81.

Mahmoudi H. Evaluation of meatal stenosis following neonatal circumcision. Urol J. 2005;2(2):86–8.

Mehta SD, Moses S, Agot K, Parker C, Ndinya-Achola JO, Maclean I, et al. Adult male circumcision does not reduce the risk of incident Neisseria gonorrhoeae, Chlamydia trachomatis, or Trichomonas vaginalis infection: results from a randomized, controlled trial in Kenya. J Infect Dis. 2009;200(3):370–8.

Meuli M, Briner J, Hanimann B, Sacher P. Lichen sclerosus et atrophicus causing phimosis in boys: a prospective study with 5-year followup after complete circumcision. J Urol. 1994;152(3):987–9.

Nascimento FJ, Pereira RF, Silva 2nd JL, Tavares A, Pompeo AC. Topical betamethasone and hyaluronidase in the treatment of phimosis in boys: a double-blind, randomized, placebo-controlled trial. Int Braz J Urol. 2011;37(3):314–9.

Oster J. Further fate of the foreskin. Incidence of preputial adhesions, phimosis, and smegma among Danish schoolboys. Arch Dis Child. 1968;43(228):200–3.

Palmer JS, Elder JS, Palmer LS. The use of betamethasone to manage the trapped penis following neonatal circumcision. J Urol. 2005;174(4 Pt 2):1577–8.
Reddy S, Jain V, Dubey M, Deshpande P, Singal AK. Local steroid therapy as the first-line treatment for boys with symptomatic phimosis—a long-term prospective study. Acta Paediatr. 2012;101(3):e130–3.
Rodriguez V, Titapiwatanakun R, Moir C, Schmidt KA, Pruthi RK. To circumcise or not to circumcise? Circumcision in patients with bleeding disorders. Haemophilia. 2010;16(2):272–6.
Sasmaz I, Antmen B, Leblebisatan G, Sahin Karagun B, Kilinc Y, Tuncer R. Circumcision and complications in patients with haemophilia in southern part of Turkey: Cukurova experience. Haemophilia. 2012; 18(3):426–30.
Simforoosh N, Tabibi A, Khalili SA, Soltani MH, Afjehi A, Aalami F, et al. Neonatal circumcision reduces the incidence of asymptomatic urinary tract infection: a large prospective study with long-term follow-up using Plastibell. J Pediatr Urol. 2012;8(3):320–3.
Stenram A, Malmfors G, Okmian L. Circumcision for phimosis: a follow-up study. Scand J Urol Nephrol. 1986;20(2):89–92.
Tobian AA, Serwadda D, Quinn TC, Kigozi G, Gravitt PE, Laeyendecker O, et al. Male circumcision for the prevention of HSV-2 and HPV infections and syphilis. N Engl J Med. 2009;360(13):1298–309.
Upadhyay V, Hammodat HM, Pease PW. Post circumcision meatal stenosis: 12 years' experience. N Z Med J. 1998;111(1060):57–8.
Van Howe RS. Incidence of meatal stenosis following neonatal circumcision in a primary care setting. Clin Pediatr (Phila). 2006;45(1):49–54.
VanderBrink BA, Gitlin J, Palmer LS. Uroflowmetry parameters before and after meatoplasty for primary symptomatic meatal stenosis in children. J Urol. 2008;179(6):2403–6. discussion 6.
Weiss HA, Larke N, Halperin D, Schenker I. Complications of circumcision in male neonates, infants and children: a systematic review. BMC Urol. 2010;10:2.
Yang C, Liu X, Wei GH. Foreskin development in 10 421 Chinese boys aged 0–18 years. World J Pediatr. 2009;5(4):312–5.
Yegane RA, Kheirollahi AR, Salehi NA, Bashashati M, Khoshdel JA, Ahmadi M. Late complications of circumcision in Iran. Pediatr Surg Int. 2006;22(5):442–5.
Yilmaz D, Akin M, Ay Y, Balkan C, Celik A, Ergun O, et al. A single centre experience in circumcision of haemophilia patients: Izmir protocol. Haemophilia. 2010;16(6):888–91.

11 Ureteropelvic Junction Obstruction

Warren T. Snodgrass and Patricio C. Gargollo

The primary goal in diagnosing and treating ureteropelvic junction obstruction (UPJO) is to prevent ipsilateral renal function loss.

Secondary goals are to minimize associated comorbidities, including the following:

1. **fUTI.**
2. **Pain.**
3. **Hematuria.**
4. **Urolithiasis.**

Summary of evidence for these aims:

- **Extent of hydronephrosis (HN) by either SFU grade or anterior-posterior (AP) diameter does not correlate with renal function.**
- **To our knowledge, no study demonstrates that prolonged drainage determined by T1/2, appearance of the curve, or other measurement correlates with renal function or predicts future renal function loss.**
- **Most patients have <10 % change in ipsilateral renal function after pyeloplasty.**
- **Zero to 39 % of patients observed without surgery have ipsilateral function loss variously described as >5 %, >10 %, or <40 %, but following pyeloplasty, final ipsilateral renal function loss is 0–6 %.**
- **No RCT shows benefit for surgery over observation to preserve ipsilateral renal function.**
- **Two studies reported resolution of renal colic after surgery. No studies were found documenting impact of pyeloplasty on recurrent UTI, hematuria, or renal stone formation.**

Threshold for Postnatal Evaluation of Prenatal Hydronephrosis

There is no consensus on the threshold of antenatal HN that should prompt postnatal imaging, no agreement on timing for postnatal imaging, and uncertainty as to the significance of some potentially pathologic findings, such as VUR.

Meta-analysis reports that likelihood for pathologic findings increases with the extent of antenatal HN, based on AP diameter. Increased risk for any pathology (UPJO, VUR, PUV, ureteral obstruction, other), based on third-trimester AP diameter, was as follows:

- **≤9 mm, 12 % (95 % CI 4.5–28).**
- **10–15 mm, 45 % (95 % CI 25.3–66.6).**
- **15 mm, 88 % (95 % CI 53.7–98.0).**

Risk was greatest for UPJO, 5 % for AP ≤9 mm, 17 % for AP 10–15 mm, and 54 % for AP >15 mm.

One prospective study reported a third-trimester antenatal AP diameter of 15 mm discriminated obstruction in 80 % of fetuses with 73 %/82 % sensitivity/specificity.

W.T. Snodgrass, M.D. (✉) • P.C. Gargollo, M.D.
Department of Pediatric Urology, University of Texas Southwestern Medical Center and Children's Medical Center Dallas, 1935 Medical District Drive, MS F4.04, Dallas, TX 75235, USA
e-mail: warren.snodgrass@childrens.com; patricio.gargollo@childrens.com

W.T. Snodgrass (ed.), *Pediatric Urology: Evidence for Optimal Patient Management*,
DOI 10.1007/978-1-4614-6910-0_11,

VUR risk is approximately 16 %, regardless of extent of antenatal HN or if postnatal US is normal (*see* Chap. 2).

A meta-analysis screened 1,645 articles on antenatal HN from 1966 to 2005 to determine if the extent of dilation is associated with postnatal outcome. Only 17 case series met criteria, from which a dataset of 1,308 subjects was derived. A summary (simplified here) defined classification of antenatal dilation based on AP diameter in the third-trimester as "mild" ≤9 mm, "moderate" 9–15 mm, and "severe" ≥15 mm. Postnatal pathologies were defined as UPJ, VUR, PUV, ureteral obstruction (ureterocele, ectopic ureter, megaureter), and "other" (multicystic dysplastic kidney, PBS, hydrometrocolpos, bladder agenesis). Overall risk for any of these pathologies increased by increasing extent of antenatal HN:

- ≤9 mm (n=587), 12 % (95 % CI 4.5–28).
- 9–15 mm (n=235), 45 % (95 % CI 25.3–66.6).
- ≥15 mm (n=94), 88 % (95 % CI 53.7–98.0).

Considering specific pathologic categories, risks were highest for UPJ: mild, 5 % (95 % CI 2.0–11.9); moderate, 17 % (95 % CI 7.6–33.9); and severe, 54 % (95 % CI 21.7–83.6). Only VUR showed no significant trend for increasing risk of occurrence with increasing degree of antenatal HN (Lee et al. 2006).

A prospective study defined antenatal HN by third-trimester AP diameter ≥7 mm, resulting in postnatal US at 3–4 weeks of age, "subsequent" VCUG, and diuretic MAG-3 renography for those with SFU grades 3–4 postnatal HN. Pyeloplasty was indicated by differential renal function loss >10 % and <40 % function and/or progressive HN on serial US. Of 257 infants, obstruction was diagnosed in 62 (24 %) with mean antenatal AP diameter 22.3 ± 12.1 mm. ROC analysis determined that an antenatal AP diameter threshold of 15 mm discriminated obstruction in 80 % of fetuses with 73 % sensitivity and 82 % specificity (Coplen et al. 2006).

The meta-analysis performed by the 2010 AUA Reflux Guidelines Panel to determine risk for VUR in newborns with antenatal HN considered 34 studies in which mean percentage of newborns/infants screened by cystography was 78 % (11–100 %). VUR occurred in a mean of 16 % (7–35 %) of those with cystography. VUR in the non-dilated kidney comprised 25 % of detected cases. Extent of antenatal HN did not predict VUR likelihood. VUR grade was approximately 1/3 each for grades I-II, grade III, and grades IV-V (Skoog et al. 2010).

Timing of Postnatal Imaging

A single study reported that 38 % of renal units in newborns with prenatal HN >8 mm had increased dilation on US done at ≥7 days compared to US done at ≤48 h after birth.

One guideline recommended initial nuclear renography at 1 month of age.

Timing of Ultrasound

One prospective study of 21 newborns (37 kidneys) that defined prenatal HN as AP diameter >8 mm at ≥33 weeks obtained postnatal US within 48 h of birth and again at 7–10 days. Of the 37 renal units, 5 showed no HN on either postnatal US and in another 10 there was no change in HN observed between studies. An increase in HN was noted in 14/37 (38 %), of which 8 increased to grade 3. The grade decreased in 8 (22 %), but only 1 of these had initial grade ≥3 that decreased to grade 1 (Wiener and O'Hara 2002).

Timing of Nuclear Renography

Guidelines issued by the Pediatric Committee of the European Association of Nuclear Medicine recommend 1 month of age for the initial renogram, based on expert opinion (Gordon et al. 2011).

Impact of Technical Factors in Nuclear Renography

Renography provides information on individual kidney percentage function and drainage, both of which are potentially impacted by various technical factors.

One study reported a 5 % difference in two common methods used to subtract background nonrenal activity when determining differential renal function.

Another study of MAG-3 renograms found >5 % variation between the two common methods used to calculate renal function in 25 % of patients <1 year of age versus 10 % in those >1 year of age.

Many factors potentially influence observed drainage after furosemide, resulting in a recommendation by one guideline panel that renogram drainage not be used as an indication for pyeloplasty.

One retrospective study of hydronephrotic kidneys otherwise considered stable found variation in drainage depending on technique used and on serial diuretic renograms, also concluding drainage should not be used as the indication for surgery.

Estimates of Differential Renal Function

Prospective analysis was performed in 8 kidneys with right HN, 17 with left HN, and 9 with bilateral HN as well as in 14 without HN using MAG-3 renography to determine effect of background non-renal activity on differential function measured by two methods: subrenal or perirenal. A significant mean difference in differential renal function of 4.8 % (−7 to +25, SD 5.3) was observed, with the perirenal background correction method considered superior to accurately report renal function (Caglar et al. 2008).

Three hundred ninety-four MAG-3 renograms in children with unilateral HN were reprocessed to calculate differential renal function by two methods—the "integral" versus the Rutland/Patlak plot analysis. For the entire review, the mean difference was −0.8 % (range −21.0–16.9 %, SD 3.9 %). There was a greater spread in differential renal function between these techniques in children <1 year of age, with disparity >5 % in 25 % versus 10 % in those >1 year ($p < 0.0005$). The greatest differences occurred in renograms performed at 0–3 months (Ozcan et al. 2006).

Drainage After Furosemide

The Pediatric Committee of the European Association of Nuclear Medicine reviewed expert opinion regarding confounding factors in the interpretation of radionuclide clearance. These include patient hydration, bladder fullness, supine positioning, reduced ipsilateral renal function (which reduces tracer extraction from the circulation, slows filling of the dilated renal pelvis, and potentially reduces diuretic response), and variable renal pelvic size (despite similar SFU grades of HN). They concluded that qualitative assessment of the renogram curve may be sufficient to reduce concerns for obstruction when:

- There is a short time to maximum tracer activity and a rapidly descending curve with nearly complete renal drainage.
- There is delayed time to maximum activity and delayed emptying followed by prompt washout with furosemide.
- There is delayed uptake and delayed excretion despite furosemide, but rapid clearance on a post-micturation view (if continuous bladder drainage is not used).

Conversely, a continuously rising activity curve despite these maneuvers was said to increase concern for obstructed emptying. The panel cautioned T1/2 is an empiric determination, variable by the initial and final activity points chosen.

Because of several variables potentially impacting drainage, the panel concluded that reduced drainage alone is not an indication for surgery (Gordon et al. 2011).

A retrospective review included 24 children with prenatally detected unilateral HN meeting the following criteria: AP renal pelvis diameter >15 and <45 mm at age 2–4 weeks, no increase in AP diameter >9 mm during minimum 2-year follow-up, and minimum of three diuretic renograms without variation in renal function >5 % (all had function >40 %). Bladder catheters were not used, and data acquisition was done supine, with post-void views after standing for 5 min. Drainage was analyzed using pelvic excretion efficiency and half-time. Half-time was prolonged in 68 % of kidneys with HN, while it was delayed in 80 % by pelvic excretion efficiency before voiding and

44 % after voiding. Using pelvic excretion efficiency, 71 % showed variation in the pattern of drainage on serial studies despite other evidence that the HN was stable (Amarante et al. 2003).

Supranormal Renal Function

Supranormal function defined as >55 % was found by one study to vary depending on the means used to calculate renal function.

Three studies report supranormal function in approximately 5 % of renograms.

Renography 1 year after pyeloplasty in seven kidneys with supranormal function found four with persistent function >55 %, one with 53 %, and the other two to have <45 % in one study.

Prospective evaluation of 48 neonates with unilateral prenatal HN ≥5 mm AP diameter that included MAG-3 diuretic renography at 1 month reported 4 (8 %) with ipsilateral renal function ≥55 % (Moon et al. 2003). Background subtraction method was not stated, but it was described similar to the integral technique.

The study by Ozcan et al. (2006) mentioned above analyzing MAG-3 renograms using two techniques for differential renal function (integral vs. Rutland/Patlak methods) reported that supranormal function defined as >55 % was found less often using the Rutland/Patlak plot analysis, and that only 5 % of 394 renograms maintained supranormal function when both methods were used.

A retrospective database review identified 72 children with antenatal HN who underwent MAG-3 renography and Cr-EDTA glomerular clearance. Differential renal function by renography was determined using the integral method. Absolute function for each kidney was expressed in mL/min/1.72 m^2/kidney, with values <40 mL/min/1.72 m^2 and values >70 mL/min/1.72 m^2 considered abnormal. Abnormal differential function ≥50 % was found in 4/72 patients over 1 year of age, all involving the left kidney. All had absolute split renal function within the normal range as defined, while in three patients the contralateral sonographically normal kidney had ≤40 mL/min/1.72 m^2, leading to the conclusion that supranormal function is infrequent and may indicate borderline contralateral hypofunction (Maenhout et al. 2005).

Another retrospective review included seven patients with ipsilateral function ≥55 % and normal contralateral kidney by ultrasound, reporting that at 1 year after pyeloplasty, renal function remained >55 % in four and decreased to 38, 44, and 53 % in the other three (Song et al. 2007a).

Etiologies of UPJO

Data from three retrospective reviews of pyeloplasty cases indicate that most prenatally detected UPJO are due to intrinsic narrowing, and less commonly from either high ureteral insertion or crossing vessels.

Older children presenting with symptoms have a greater prevalence of crossing vessels.

A retrospective review of over 1,000 pyeloplasties reported fibroepithelial polyps in 0.5 %.

A retrospective review of 98 consecutive children, median age 1 year (5 days–16 years), undergoing pyeloplasty between 1986 and 1992 reported the etiology was an intrinsic anomaly of the UPJ in 78 %, high ureteral insertion in 11 %, and crossing vessels in 11 % (Salem et al. 1995).

A retrospective review of pyeloplasty for symptomatic UPJO between 1986 and 1999 included 38 children, mean age 8 years, finding crossing vessels in 22 (58 %), intrinsic anomalies of the UPJ in 10 (26 %), high ureteral insertion in 2 (5 %), and fibroepithelial polyps in 2 (5 %) (Cain et al. 2001).

Another retrospective review reported intrinsic narrowing versus crossing vessels in 54 prenatally detected and 30 symptomatic children undergoing pyeloplasty at mean age 3.5±7 months versus 6±3 years. Crossing vessels were encountered in 6/54 (11 %) and 12/30 (40 %), $p=0.004$ (Calisti et al. 2003).

A retrospective review of 1,710 pyeloplasties over a 35-year period identified 9 (0.5 %) cases with fibroepithelial polyp as the cause of UPJO. Patients ranged in age from 6 weeks to 9 years. The diagnosis was made preoperatively in two, as a filling defect seen on IVP or antegrade nephrostography. Follow-up after dismembered pyeloplasty was a mean 44 months (1–135) with no known recurrence or new polyp occurrence (Adey et al. 2003).

Outcomes of Observational Management for Prenatally Detected UPJO

Kaplan-Meier curves showing time for resolution of SFU grades 3 and 4 HN have not been reported.

Four series reported resolution (decrease to SFU grades 0–1 HN) occurring in from 0 to 66 % SFU grade 3 and 0–14 % grade 4 kidneys during mean follow-up that ranged from 15 to 142 months (Table 11.1).

Indications for pyeloplasty are not standardized. Reported reasons include progressive HN, initial or acquired decreased ipsilateral renal function and/or drainage, failure to resolve HN, and symptoms (pain, UTI, stones).

Pyeloplasty rates in four series for SFU grades 3 and 4 kidneys varied, in part by differing indications for surgery, but ranged from 11 to 70 % of grade 3 and 29–100 % of grade 4 kidneys (Table 11.2).

Table 11.1 Spontaneous resolution (to SFU grades 0–1 HN) in renal units with prenatally detected SFU grades 3 and 4 HN

Authors	Mean f/u	SFU grade 3	SFU grade 4
Bajpai	39 m	6/9 (66 %)	0/11 (0 %)
Onen	54 m	11/19 (58 %)	1/19 (5 %)
Karnak	15 m	17/50 (34 %)	3/21 (14 %)
Yang	142 m	0/122 (0 %)	0/69 (0 %)

Risk for renal function decrease during observation is unclear, given that timing of initial and follow-up renography, and definition of significant functional loss are not standardized. Reported rates of renal function decrease in observed units range from 1 to 25 %, with persistent differential renal function decrease in 0–6 %.

UTI has been reported in from 2 to 31 % of infants with UPJO during observation in retrospective studies. Two studies had similar infection rates, one using antibiotic prophylaxis and the other not. No RCT has tested antibiotic prophylaxis in children with UPJO.

Renal colic has rarely been reported in patients with prenatally detected UPJO during observation.

Spontaneous Resolution of SFU 1 and 2 HN

A retrospective review reported outcomes in 56 SFU grade 1 and 51 SFU grade 2 kidneys after prenatal detection. During follow-up at a mean of 15 months (1.5–142, median 12), spontaneous resolution occurred in 34 (61 %) and 33 (65 %), with none progressing to a higher grade or having surgery (Karnak et al. 2009).

Another retrospective study of prenatally detected HN reported follow-up a mean of 142 months with resolution in 250/273 (92 %) SFU grade 1 and 25/165 (15 %) with SFU grade 2 HN, at mean of 13 months (2 weeks–6 years). All others were stable or improved, except for progression to SFU grades 3 or 4 that occurred in 21 (13 %) with SFU grade 2 (time to progression not stated) (Yang et al. 2010).

Table 11.2 Pyeloplasty after initial observation for prenatally detected SFU grade 3 and 4 HN kidneys

				Indications			
Authors	Mean time to surgery	SFU 3	SFU 4	Progressive HN	Function loss	Symptoms	Recovery of function loss post-pyeloplasty
Onen	6.5 m	2/19 (11 %)	11/19 (58 %)	11 (29 %)	5 (14 %)	–	5/5 (100 %)
Karnak	15 m	4/50 (8 %)	6/21 (29 %)	NS	1 (1 %)	NS	NS
Hafez	7 m	10/33 (30 %)	6/11 (55 %)	16 (36 %)	11 (25 %)	–	5/11 (45 %)
Yang	6–20 m	85/122 (70 %)	69/69 (100 %)	85 (55 %)	60 (39 %)	NS	"all"

NS not stated

Spontaneous Resolution of SFU 3 and 4 HN

Initial observation was done in 15 infants with prenatally detected HN evaluated at 4–12 weeks of age with US and DTPA renography. SFU grade 3 HN occurred in 9 and grade 4 in 11 renal units (bilateral in 5). Initial ipsilateral differential function was ≥35 % in all kidneys (mean 46.5, 35–65). By mean follow-up of 39 months (8–60), 6/9 grade 3 kidneys resolved HN and 3 decreased to grade 2. In contrast, of 11 grade 4 renal units, none improved to grades 0 to 1, 1 decreased to grade 2, 6 showed no change, and 4 were operated (Bajpai and Chandrasekharam 2002).

Nineteen neonates with bilateral SFU grades 3 ($n=19$) and 4 HN ($n=19$) were initially observed regardless of differential function, T1/2 or HN grade. All had normal global renal function by serum creatinine. Indications for pyeloplasty were decreased differential function >10 % and/or progressive HN (means for determining progression and number of US required for this diagnosis were not stated). During mean follow-up of 54 months (14–187), resolution to SFU grades 0–1 HN occurred in 1/19 (5 %) grade 4 kidneys and 11/19 (58 %) grade 3 kidneys. Improvement to SFU grade 2 occurred in 3/19 (16 %) grade 4 and 6/19 (32 %) grade 3 kidneys. Pyeloplasty was done in 11/19 (58 %) grade 4 and 2/19 (11 %) grade 3 kidneys, discussed below (Onen et al. 2002).

Another series utilizing a standardized protocol reported outcomes in 71 SFU grades 3 and 4 kidneys during observation for 15 ± 14 months. Renography was done at 1 month of age, and those with ipsilateral differential renal function <40 % underwent immediate pyeloplasty, leaving 50 SFU grade 3 and 21 SFU grade 4 kidneys observed. HN resolution occurred in 20/71 (28 %), comprising 17/50 (34 %) grade 3 and 3/21 (14 %) grade 4 kidneys (Karnak et al. 2009).

The study by Yang et al. (2010) mentioned above included 122 neonates with SFU grade 3 and 69 with SFU grade 4 HN after prenatal detection. During follow-up a mean of 142 months, none resolved. Thirty percent with SFU 3 were stable or improved, while the other 70 % progressed to grade 4. Those with initial grade 4 were all said to have no improvement, with 50 % having surgery at a median 6 months and the others at 20 months.

Pyeloplasty

Twenty-four neonates with bilateral SFU grades 3 ($n=19$) and 4 HN ($n=19$) were initially observed regardless of differential function, T1/2, or HN grade, as discussed above (Onen et al. 2002). All had normal global renal function by serum creatinine. Indications for pyeloplasty were decreased differential function >10 % and/ or progressive HN. At mean age 6.5 months (2–22), pyeloplasty was done in 11/19 (58 %) SFU grade 4 and 2/19 (11 %) grade 3 kidneys for progressive HN ($n=8$), decreased function ($n=2$), or both ($n=3$). Of these patients, 11 had SFU grade 4 HN and the changes on renal US that defined progressive HN warranting pyeloplasty were not described.

The series by Karnak et al. (2009) described above performed immediate pyeloplasty in infants with differential renal function <40 % or prolonged T1/2, which comprised no SFU grade 3 and 20/41(49 %) with grade 4 HN. With subsequent conservative management for 15 ± 14 months (1.5–142), 4/50 (8 %) SFU grade 3 and 6/21 (29 %) SFU grade 4 kidneys had pyeloplasty for persistently prolonged T1/2, increased HN, pain, or UTI (none of these indications were further described). Only one kidney had decreased differential renal function, the extent and the postoperative outcome of which were not stated.

An observation protocol for unilateral prenatally detected HN included 33 SFU grade 3 and 11 grade 4 renal units, with differential renal function <40 % in 18 (42 %) and T1/2 >20 min in 23 (53 %). Indications for surgery were increasing HN on two ultrasounds (the second within 2–4 weeks) or UTI. At mean follow-up of 38 months (23–52), 16 (36 %) underwent pyeloplasty (10/33 [30 %] grade 3; 6/11 [55 %] grade 4) at mean age of 7 months (3–12) (Hafez et al. 2002). Extent of increased AP diameter or parenchymal thinning used to define progression in grade 4 kidneys was not described.

Pyeloplasty was done in 70 and 100 % of SFU grade 3 and 4 patients reported by Yang et al. (2010). Indications were progression of HN from grade 3 to 4 or failure of grade 4 to improve on 2 US (at 3 and 6 months) and "very poor" drainage. Together there were 154 pyeloplasties, with approximately half those with grade 3 and 4 having surgery at a median of 6 months and the other half at median 20 months.

A study of patients with prenatally detected HN, defined by AP diameter rather than SFU grade, observed those with function >40 % on DTPA renography obtained at 1 month of age regardless of washout times or curves or extent of postnatal HN. There were 100 renal units (number of unilateral vs. bilateral cases was not stated) that were observed for at least 1 to ≥6 years (mean, median of observation were not stated). Of these, 23 (23 %) underwent pyeloplasty for decreased function to <40 % ($n = 14$), UTI ($n = 3$), pain ($n = 1$), concentrating defect in a solitary kidney creating polyuria ($n = 1$), and noncompliance with follow-up ($n = 4$). Operations occurred during the first year in 5, second in 7, third in 7, fifth in 2, and sixth in 2. AP diameter was <12 mm in 34 and >12 mm in 66 during US at 1 month of age, and all 23 pyeloplasties derived from the cohort with >12 mm (23/66 [35 %]) (Ransley et al. 1990). The mean and range of AP diameters for those <12 and >12 mm were not stated. The extent of renal function loss resulting in pyeloplasty was not described. Spontaneous resolution rates and time intervals were not reported.

Risk for Renal Function Loss

As discussed above, Onen et al. (2002) reported 5/38 (14 %) bilateral SFU grades 3 and 4 kidneys had functional decrease of greater than 10 % during observation at follow-up a mean of 6.5 months (2–22). Recovery of function occurred in all five after pyeloplasty. Actual function changes in these renal units were not described.

Karnak et al. (2009) observed 71 kidneys with SFU grades 3 and 4 HN with differential renal function ≥40 %, operating on only 1 (1 %) for decreased renal function to <40 % during follow-up a mean of 15 months.

Decreased renal function to <40 % (or >5 % for those with initial function <40 %) was observed by Yang et al. (2010) in13/165 (8 %) with SFU grade 2, 47/122 (39 %) with SFU grade 3, and 35/67 (52 %) with SFU grade 4 HN. Following pyeloplasty, the authors stated there was "no persistent deterioration of renal function," but rather demonstrated significant improvement.

Hafez et al. (2002) obtained initial DTPA renography at 4–6 weeks of age for 45 patients with SFU grades 3 and 4 kidneys, repeated only in the 16 with subsequent progressive HN leading to pyeloplasty. In these 16, mean baseline renal function was 32 % (8–54), and the decrease was to a mean 23 % (8–39), with 9/16 (56 %) having >5 % loss. DTPA 3 months after pyeloplasty was a mean of 30 % (10–48), with improvement in 14 and stable function in 2.

A retrospective analysis of 272 patients (SFU grade not stated) was done, identifying 44 (16 %) patients (35 with SFU grades 3 and 4) undergoing pyeloplasty for differential renal functional loss. Patients were initially observed after DTPA or MAG-3 renography at 6–8 weeks of age, and had pyeloplasty for decreased ipsilateral function of >5 % (mean 8 ± 2 %), which occurred at a mean of 8 ± 1 months. Mean initial differential renal function in SFU grade 3 kidneys was 38 %, which decreased to a mean of 30 % but then improved postoperatively to mean of 39 %. For SFU grade 4 kidneys, initial renal function was a mean of 34 %, decreasing to 26 % and improving after surgery to 32 % (Chertin et al. 2002).

Ransley et al. (1990) did not use SFU grading, but reported that 23/66 (35 %) kidneys with AP diameter >12 mm and initial DTPA differential renal function ≥40 % at 1 month of age eventually had pyeloplasty. Of these, 14/66 (21 %) had preoperative decreased function to <40 % (actual changes not reported). Five of 14 (36 %) had complete functional return after surgery, while 4 improved, 3 remained unchanged, and 1 deteriorated further (data were not shown).

Risk for UTI

A retrospective study reviewed charts of 56 newborns (45 males) having SFU grades 3 ($n=9$) and 4 ($n=47$) HN that was detected prenatally, with DTPA renography demonstrating T1/2 >20 min. Exclusion included any grade of VUR. No antibiotic prophylaxis was used. UTI was defined as "symptomatic infection with a positive urine culture." At mean follow-up of 26.7 months (1–122), UTI occurred in one (2 %) patient (Roth et al. 2009).

Another retrospective review studied 64 males and 11 females with SFU grades 3 ($n=37$) and 4 ($n=38$) HN from UPJO and "obstructive washout pattern" with T1/2 >20 min to determine UTI occurrence during the first year of life. UTI was only defined for those hospitalized (number not stated) with febrile illness having "positive urine culture and bacteruria or pyuria ≥5WBCs/HPF." No male was circumcised, and patients were not given antibiotic prophylaxis. UTI occurred in 23/75 (31 %) patients, with no difference between males and females or those with SFU grades 3 versus 4 HN. However, it was not clear if patients were all identified by HN or if some presented with fUTI and were then found to have HN (Song et al. 2007b).

A retrospective analysis of fUTI risk in 192 infants (125 males, none circumcised) with prenatal HN included patients with no uropathy, UPJO, VUR, and megaureters. Bagged urines were used for specimens in infants. Antibiotic prophylaxis (cephalexin 2× months, then trimethoprim) was used in all 53 with UPJO. During median follow-up, for the entire series of 24 months (IQ range 12–39), UTI occurred in 13/53 (25 %) (Coelho et al. 2008).

Other Symptoms

Symptoms are an uncommon cause for pyeloplasty in prenatally detected HN. Bajpai and Chandrasekharam (2002) reported that none of their 15 patients with SFU grades 3,4 HN were symptomatic at either presentation or follow-up to a mean of 36 months (8–60). Ransley et al. (1990) followed 100 kidneys with antenatal HN for 1 to more than 6 years and stated that pain occurred in one child, leading to pyeloplasty. Coplen et al. (2006) performed pyeloplasty on 62 children for antenatally detected HN, with only 2 having colic at age 6 years.

Our review found no reports concerning hematuria and stone incidence in prenatally detected HN. There are case reports of hypertension improving after pyeloplasty or nephrectomy for UPJO.

Postnatally Detected UPJO

UPJO not diagnosed antenatally presents with symptoms such as renal colic/abdominal pain, abdominal mass, hematuria, or UTI, or without symptoms as a coincidental finding.

Two studies reported pain resolution in all cases following pyeloplasty for renal colic.

Dietl's Crisis

Prospective evaluation was performed in 18 consecutive children, mean age 7.5 years (4–15), presenting during a 6-year period ending in 2004 with abdominal pain and found to have HN during the acute episode that resolved when asymptomatic. Symptoms were recurrent in 15/18 beginning a mean of 8 months (2–24) before diagnosis, and included flank pain in 14 and periumbilical/epigastric or diffuse abdominal pain in 8. Sixteen had vomiting. Symptoms resolved within 2 days. Renal US during the acute episode reported SFU grades 3 and 4 HN, that decreased to grades 1 and 2 in 16 when non-symptomatic. DTPA diuretic renography was obtained in 17 within 3 days of symptoms, finding ipsilateral renal function a mean of 35 % (10–55), with "obstructive patterns and prolonged washout" in 15, and an "equivocal pattern" in the other 2. At pyeloplasty in 17 cases (1 lost to follow-up), intrinsic obstruction was found in 6, extrinsic factors in 9 ("kinked ureter" in 6, high insertion in 2, crossing vessels in 1), and a fibroepithelial polyp in 2. During follow-up a mean of 3.6 years (4 months–7 years), there was no recurrent flank/abdominal pain (Tsai et al. 2006).

A retrospective review was done to identify children evaluated for UPJO over a 3-year period ending 2001, reporting 8/122 (7 %) had Dietl's crisis at mean age 12 years (5–19). All had recurrent abdominal pain with nausea and vomiting for ≥1 year. Ipsilateral renal function ranged from 36 to 66 % (excluding one with a solitary kidney). Surgery resolved symptoms in all patients at follow-up (time not stated) (Alagiri and Polepalle 2006).

Other Presentations

A retrospective review of all unilateral pyeloplasties done between 1990 and 1997 identified 21 children who presented at a mean age of 7 years (9 months–18 years) with pain ($n=11$), UTI ($n=8$), or as an incidental finding in 2. All had SFU grades 3,4 HN with mean preoperative differential function of 39 % (10–58 %) and T1/2 >20 min (McAleer and Kaplan 1999).

Another retrospective review of 95 consecutive pyeloplasties done from 1986 to 1992 reported presentation other than prenatal detection in 71 (75 %). UPJO was an incidental finding in 21 (30 %). The remaining patients had symptoms, including abdominal pain ($n=17$, 24 %), UTI ($n=14$, 20 %), mass (10, 14 %),and gross hematuria ($n=9$, 13 %) (Salem et al. 1995).

Management of UPJO with Ipsilateral Differential Function <10 %

Two retrospective series reported symptomatic UPJO with differential function <10 % initially managed by nephrostomy for 4–6 weeks. Improved function to a mean ≥30 % occurred in 70 and 100 %.

Only one series reported nephrostomy drainage for function <10 % in prenatally detected (asymptomatic) UPJO in nine kidneys; only two had improved function (19 and 41 %).

A series of symptomatic patients, mean age 5 years (2 months–11 years), included 17 (8 prenatally detected) with SFU grade 4 HN and differential function less than 10 % with DTPA renography, all initially treated with a percutaneous nephrostomy for 4 weeks with subsequent repeat renography. Of these, 12 (71 %) had second renogram function >10 % (mean 29±3 %) resulting in pyeloplasty, while the other 5 were unchanged and so had nephrectomy. At mean follow-up of 2.3±1.3 years, renal function was 31±13 % after pyeloplasty (Gupta et al. 2001).

Another retrospective review found 12 patients among a group of 58 with UPJO presenting at mean age 4.7 years (35 days–11 years) with renal function less than 10 %. Nephrostomy drainage was done preoperatively for 4–6 weeks followed by pyeloplasty in all cases. Repeat preoperative renography showed improvement to 20–25 % function in all patients, and 6 months after surgery all had 30–35 % function (Aziz et al. 2002).

Nine kidneys with prenatally detected HN had function <10 % by DTPA renography at 1 month of age. Nephrostomy tubes were placed for 3 weeks with repeat renography and nephrectomy if function remained <10 %. Of the nine, six had nephrectomy and three pyeloplasty, with postoperative function at 1 year of 10, 19, and 41 % (Ransley et al. 1990).

Management of Bilateral UPJO

The prospective series by Onen et al. (2002) discussed above included 19 neonates with bilateral SFU grades 3 ($n=19$) and 4 HN ($n=19$) who were initially observed regardless of individual kidney differential function, T1/2, or HN grade. All had normal global renal function by serum creatinine. Indications for pyeloplasty were decreased differential function >10 % and/or progressive HN. At mean 6.5 months (2–22), pyeloplasty was done in 13/48 (27 %) kidneys, 8 for increasing HN, 2 for decreased function, and 3 for both. These operations occurred in nine patients (37.5 %), and were bilateral in four and unilateral in five. At follow-up of 54 months (14–187), resolution to SFU grades 0–1 HN occurred in 12/48 (25 %). The five with renal functional loss >10 % before surgery were stated to have full recovery (data were not shown).

A retrospective study included 13 children with prenatal HN and postnatal bilateral SFU grades 3 and 4 UPJO. All had initial surgery on one kidney (with greatest HN or least renal function) at mean 3 months (1–11). The other kidney was scheduled for pyeloplasty in 2 months, but in five (39 %) cases the HN improved sufficiently to not operate. At final follow-up at a mean 37 months (5–84), residual dilation ≥SFU grade 3 persisted in 4/21 (19 %) operated kidneys and 1/5 (20 %) not operated (Kim et al. 2010).

Laparoscopic Pyeloplasty (With or Without Robotic Assistance)

Surgical Outcomes

There was no difference in reported surgical success rates or complications between open, laparoscopic, and robotic pyeloplasty.

Laparoscopic surgery was associated with greater double-J stent use.

Meta-analysis found operative times less with open surgery, and hospitalization less with laparoscopic and robotic surgery.

A meta-analysis compared open to laparoscopic pyeloplasty, as reported by nine studies with 7,334 open and 694 laparoscopic surgeries, finding:

- No difference in reported success rates, OR 1.8 (95 % CI 0.7–4).
- No difference in complications, OR 0.8 (95 % CI 0.5–1.3).
- Significantly shorter operative times for open surgery, WMD 59 (95 % CI 41–77).
- Significantly shorter hospital stay with laparoscopic repair, WMD –0.4 (95 % CI –0.8–0.03).

In the articles reviewed there was also significantly greater use of double-J stents in laparoscopic patients (Mei et al. 2011).

Meta-analysis compared robotic versus laparoscopic pyeloplasty on the basis of eight articles and 326 patients, reporting:

- No difference in reported success rates, OR 1.3 (95 % CI 0.5–3.5).
- No difference in complications, OR 0.7 (95 % CI 0.3–1.6).
- No difference in operative times, WMD –10 min (95 % CI –25–3).
- Significantly shorter hospitalization with robotic surgery, WMD –0.5 d (95 % CI –0.6–0.4) (Braga et al. 2009).

A RCT compared open (performed by four surgeons) versus transperitoneal laparoscopic (one surgeon) pyeloplasty, excluding children less than 1 year of age. Enrollment was offered to 77 patients with 39 accepting. Mean age was similar at 7.5 years. All were stented postoperatively for 6 weeks, laparoscopic patients with a double-J stent; open-stent type was not stated. Postoperative pain control was standardized for all patients, using no regional blocks, bupivacaine in all incisions, scheduled IV ketorolac, and narcotics as needed. There was no difference between open and laparoscopic surgery regarding success 95 % versus 100 % (described as "no symptoms, normal T1/2, and improved HN"), mean operative time 130 versus 151 min, mean hospitalization 29 versus 36 h, or narcotic use 4 versus 5 doses (Penn et al. 2010).

Cosmesis

Two studies using patient questionnaires reported increased satisfaction with incisions from robotic versus open renal surgery.

A validated questionnaire used to determine patient satisfaction in children (Glasgow Children's Benefit Inventory) was mailed to all undergoing open or robotic pyeloplasty over a 2-year period. Additional non-validated questions were added to specifically distinguish between the two surgical procedures. Of 69 open and 48 robotic cases, responses were obtained from 68 to 72 %. All reaching statistical significance favored robotic surgery, including speed of return to normal activities and the incision scar (Freilich et al. 2010).

Twelve patients underwent HIdES (hidden incision endoscopic surgery) renal surgery, in which all port sites are hidden either in the umbilicus or below the bikini line, and their parents expressed their satisfaction with the cosmetic outcome 3 months postoperatively using questions from the validated Patient Scar Assessment Scale. They also compared patient results to photos taken 3 months after flank incision and laparoscopy for renal surgery using traditional port placement using the validated Wound Evaluation Scale, Manchester Scar Scale, and Patient Scar Assessment Scale. Mean patient and parent scores were significantly better for HIdES than either open or laparoscopic incisions (Gargollo 2011).

Imaging Changes After Pyeloplasty

Pyeloplasty outcomes are determined by residual HN, renal function and drainage, and symptoms.

In one study of consecutive patients considered to have surgical success, mean HN decreased a statistically insignificant 1 grade (SFU 3–2), differential renal function remained the same mean 46 %, and only drainage significantly improved 1 year postoperatively.

Three retrospective studies described changes in renal US after pyeloplasty, one reporting resolution to SFU grade 0 or 1 HN in 20 % and to ≤SFU grade 2 in 64 %; the other two reported mean changes in HN that were unchanged in one and reduced in the other.

A systematic review of published literature concerning renal function after pyeloplasty reported studies that generally had poor scientific quality, with heterogeneous indications for surgery and follow-up imaging. Conclusions regarding impact of pyeloplasty on differential renal function were as follows:

- **No preoperative parameter, including SFU grade or AP diameter, percent renal function, or drainage pattern predicted postoperative renal functional outcomes.**
- **Renal functional change with immediate pyeloplasty in antenatally detected cases was −1 to +14 %.**
- **Functional improvement after surgery was a maximum average of 2.5 % (−1.6 to 9) in antenatally detected HN and 5 % (−0.9 to 14) in postnatally detected HN.**
- **There was a mean loss of 3–7.5 % of renal function on final postoperative renography in observed patients with preoperative decrease in renal function from baseline.**
- **Approximately half the kidneys with <20 % differential function preoperatively showed improved function, varying from ≥+5 % to function >35 %.**

Two retrospective studies described pre- and post-pyeloplasty renogram drainage, one reporting 98 % had T1/2 <20 min after surgery, and the other finding improved clearance from a mean 15 to 66 % 20 min after furosemide.

Ultrasonography

A retrospective review included 47 kidneys, 21 grade 3 and 26 grade 4 HN, that had pyeloplasty. Initial postoperative US was done at 1 month in 36, showing the same or increased HN in 33. With mean follow-up at 4 years (2–9), resolution to SFU grades 0,1 was observed in only 9/47 (19 %) kidneys. Improvement to SFU grade 2 or less occurred in 12/26 (46 %) grade 4 kidneys, and in 18/21 (86 %) grade 3 kidneys (Amling et al. 1996).

Preoperative versus 12-month postoperative renal ultrasounds were compared in 70 consecutive children undergoing laparoscopic pyeloplasty at mean age 20.5 months (1–178). All were reported to have decreased HN after surgery, although the mean difference of SFU 2.9±0.08 to 2±0.1 was not significant ($p=0.6$) (Szavay et al. 2010).

A retrospective study reported HN as AP pelvic diameters in 54 consecutive patients with prenatally detected HN that underwent pyeloplasty. Postoperative US done between 6 and 12 months showed significant improvement from mean 29±10 mm to 14±5 mm (p value not stated) (Calisti et al. 2003).

Differential Renal Function

A systematic literature review retrieved a total of 704 articles, from which 36 were analyzed regarding functional renal outcomes after unilateral pyeloplasty. Heterogeneity of isotope used, surgical indications, follow-up protocols, and means for data reporting precluded meta-analysis. The 36 reports were characterized by the authors as low-quality RCT ($n=2$), individual cohort studies ($n=8$), or surgical case series ($n=26$). Results of their descriptive analysis were as follows:

1. Six studies reported mean change in final renal function in antenatally detected patients after pyeloplasty between −1.6 and 9 %; six studies reported the mean change in postnatally detected cases was −0.9 to 14 %.
2. Mean percent change in final renal functional outcomes for antenatally detected HN undergoing immediate pyeloplasty was −1 to 14 % in six studies.
3. Six studies found neither AP diameter nor SFU grade nor parenchymal thickness predicted postoperative renal functional outcome, while two studies that reported drainage pattern did not predict post-pyeloplasty renal functional outcomes.
4. Four studies with 60 patients reported mean final functional outcomes in antenatally detected HN who had a decrease from their initial renogram during observation. Initial/final preoperative differential renal function and postoperative renal function was 45 % (40–50)/30.5 % (16–41) and 37.5 % (25–47); 45 % (42–48)/33 % (28–41) and 42 % (38–46); 49 % (45–50)/37 % (35–39) and 45 % (41–50); 48 %/42 % and 44 %. Based on these data, mean final decrease in renal function ranged from −3 to −7.5 %.
5. Nine studies had data regarding renal units with <20 % function, comprising a total of 88 kidneys, of which 30/59 (51 %) had improvement after pyeloplasty variously reported as an increase in function of >5 % or differential renal function >35 %. Two studies with a total of 29 patients reported mean data, with preoperative function <20 % and postoperative mean function 19 % (14–25) and 19.5 % (±8), respectively (Castagnetti et al. 2008).

Our review found three additional studies not included by Castagnetti et al.

The analysis of 70 consecutive children mean age 20.5 months (1–178) undergoing laparoscopic pyeloplasty mentioned above reported mean differential renal function on MAG-3 renography was 46 ± 12 % preoperatively, versus 46 ± 13 % 3 months and 46 ± 15 % 1 year postoperatively, $p>0.05$ (Szavay et al. 2010). There was median follow-up at 24 months (1–48), with the number of patients undergoing postoperative renography not stated.

Retrospective review of 137 consecutive pyeloplasties done between 1994 and 2003 identified 102 patients with preoperative and postoperative renography. Median age at surgery was 6 months (15 days–150 months) and postoperative follow-up was a median 36 months (6 months–10 years). Mean preoperative renal function for the entire cohort was 35 % versus postoperative mean of 41 % ($p<0.001$). Sixty-seven of 109 (61.5 %) kidneys had ≥5 % increased postoperative function, 30 (27.5 %) were unchanged, and 12 (11 %) had >5 % decreased function, including 3 with failed repairs (Sheu et al. 2006).

Another retrospective review found 27 kidneys with SFU grades 3 and 4 UPJO in children <1 year of age who had pyeloplasty for differential function < 40 % and/or impaired drainage with flat or rising curve. Mean preoperative/postoperative renal function was 37 %/38 %. Another 21 kidneys were initially observed and had subsequent pyeloplasty for function loss >5 % or "worsening drainage" (not defined) at mean 1.4 years after initial presentation. Mean preoperative/postoperative renal function was 46 % (19–60)/44 % (18–65) (Ross et al. 2011).

Diuretic Renography Drainage

A retrospective review defined surgical success as washout time <20 min on diuretic MAG-3 renography in 127 patients with preoperative T1/2 >20 min. All but two (2 %) had postoperative T1/2 <20 min by 3–12 months. One of these with increasing T1/2 had reoperative pyeloplasty and subsequent improvement to <20 min (Pohl et al. 2001).

Drainage on MAG-3 diuretic renography was evaluated preoperatively and 1 year postoperatively in the 70 consecutive children, mean age

20.5 months (1–178), undergoing laparoscopic pyeloplasty by Szavay et al. (2010) mentioned above. Clearance was reported as decreased radionuclide activity 20 min after furosemide. All patients had improved clearance, which was significant for the entire cohort from a mean 14.7 ± 15.8 % to 66.9 ± 16.5 %, $p < 0.0001$.

Symptoms After Pyeloplasty

Resolution of colic was reported in all patients with post-pyeloplasty follow-up in two studies.

Our review found no reports concerning post-pyeloplasty UTI or hematuria.

A prospective study reported outcomes in 39 children, mean age 7 years (1–17), undergoing pyeloplasty, of which 29 (74 %) had renal colic. With mean postoperative follow-up approximately 8 months (1–32), none of 27 assessed reported colic (Penn et al. 2010).

Another prospective study included 18 children a mean age 7.5 years (4–15) diagnosed with UPJO during Dietl's crisis. Symptoms were recurrent in 15/18 beginning a mean of 8 months (2–24) before diagnosis, and included flank pain in 14 and periumbilical/epigastric or diffuse abdominal pain in 8. Sixteen had vomiting. During follow-up after pyeloplasty a mean of 3.6 years (4 months–7 years), there were no further episodes of renal colic/abdominal pain (Tsai et al. 2006).

Failed Pyeloplasty

Retrospective reviews of management for failed pyeloplasty generally have defined failure as symptoms and/or persistent or increasing HN and/or impaired drainage. Success after re-intervention generally has been defined as absence of symptoms, stable or decreased HN, or improved drainage, usually without reporting actual findings.

Reoperative pyeloplasty (open or robotic) had success reported as 90–100 %.

Endopyelotomy was considered successful in 40–95 %.

Incidence and Pathophysiology

Three series reported failure of ≤7 % dismembered pyeloplasties, diagnosed in two at means of 13 and 26 months after primary repair.

Diagnosis of recurrent UPJO was made by various combinations of symptoms (pain, UTI) and imaging (HN, "delayed drainage").

Surgical findings at reoperation included fibrosis of the UPJ, kinks due to redundant renal pelvis or adhesions, high ureteral insertions, and crossing vessels.

A retrospective study included 105 dismembered pyeloplasties in 103 children, mean age 60 months (1–204), of which 7 (7 %) failed at mean interval of 13 months (3–38). Patients presented with pain ($n = 6$) or HN ($n = 1$), with recurrent UPJO diagnosed on the basis of appearance on IVP, CT, and/or US, and in five, renography with an "obstructive pattern." Etiology was described as persistent high ureteral insertion in two, redundant pelvis with kinking in two, and crossing vessels in two, with all said to have dense scarring (Thomas et al. 2005).

Another review of dismembered pyeloplasties found a total of 524 children were operated over an 11-year period ending in 2006, with 25 (5 %) failures presenting with increasing HN, pyelonephritis, or other symptoms (not described). Of patients undergoing reoperative pyeloplasty, findings included adhesions causing ureteral kinking in six, a redundant pelvis with kinking in one, high ureteral insertion in one, ureteral narrowing in two, and fibrosis at the UPJ in six (Braga et al. 2007).

Analysis of 590 dismembered pyeloplasties in 562 patients at mean age 3.5 years reported 18 (3 %) had recurrent UPJO diagnosed a mean of 26 months (7–48) postoperatively. Of these, 14 (78 %) had pain; all had persistent or increased HN, and mean ipsilateral renal function was 21 % (10–39) versus 30.5 % (20–48) before pyeloplasty. Findings at reoperation included crossing vessels in one, redundant renal pelvis in three, and fibrosis of the UPJ in all (Helmy et al. 2009).

Reoperative Pyeloplasty

Three series reported success in 90–100 % with reoperative pyeloplasty.

Open reoperation was done in 12 patients age 5 months to 22 years after failed pyeloplasty. Procedures included a renal pelvic flap in three, dismembered pyeloplasty in seven, and nephrectomy in two. With mean follow-up of 26 months, 9 of 10 with repair were considered to have good results, variously described as "improving or resolved HN and/or good washout," while 1 had repeat obstruction and nephrectomy (Lim and Walker 1996).

Sixteen patients had antegrade or retrograde pyelography and open reoperative pyeloplasty in another review: 2 with an "atretic ureter" had a renal pelvic spiral flap, 3 had ureterocalicostomy, and 11 had repeat dismembered pyeloplasty. All had postoperative nephrostomy and 14 of 16 also had a transanastomic stent. During follow-up at a mean of 46 months (3–90), 11 of 12 with decreased function improved (data not shown). Gravity drip nephrostogram 2–3 weeks postoperatively was said to show "good drainage" in all cases. The authors reported 100 % success (Rohrmann et al. 1997).

Of the 18 patients undergoing reoperation reported by Helmy et al. (2009) discussed above, repeat dismembered pyeloplasty was done in 14, ureterocalicostomy in 2, and nephrectomy in 2 (function <12 %). During follow-up a mean of 25 months (8–41), the authors considered all outcomes a success, with no loss (or improvement) of renal function, increased HN, or symptoms (interval for postoperative assessments was not stated; data were not shown) (Helmy et al. 2009).

Robotic Reoperative Pyeloplasty

One report completed planned robotic repair in 94 %, with radiologic improvement in 88 and 100 % relief of symptoms.

Sixteen children mean age 6 years (12 months–15 years) had failed open pyeloplasty ($n=12$), robotic pyeloplasty ($n=2$), ureterocalicostomy in a horseshoe kidney ($n=1$), and failed robotic vessel hitch ($n=1$). Mean interval to diagnosis of failure was 21 months (range not stated), and was determined due to SFU grades 3 and 4 HN and T1/2 >20 min. Mean function was 39 % (8–61). Robotic pyeloplasty was done in 13 and ureterocalicostomy in 3, with 1 open conversion (in the horseshoe kidney). Mean follow-up was 15 months. Decrease in HN ≥1 grade occurred in 14 (88 %), from a mean 3.8 to 1.7. Only four had renography, with "improved T1/2 and stable to improved function" (data not shown). All were asymptomatic (Lindgren et al. 2012).

Endopyelotomy

Endopyelotomy was reported successful in from approximately 80 to 95 % of cases.

One retrospective comparison of reoperative pyeloplasty versus endopyelotomy found reoperation significantly more successful, 100 % versus 39 %.

Results of 11 percutaneous endopyelotomies for failed dismembered pyeloplasty in 10 children, median age 7 years (range not stated), were reviewed. Diagnosis of recurrent UPJO was done based on Whitaker tests, diuretic renograms, or nephrostograms (criteria not stated). Median interval from primary surgery to endopyelotomy was 7.5 months (2–54). After endopyelotomy, nephrostomy drainage was done for 48 h and a 4.6- to 7-Fr double-J stent for 6 weeks. Success was defined as "normalization or improvement of renogram washout time," stable ipsilateral renal function, decreased HN, and no symptoms. One patient with an obliterated UPJ converted to open surgery, with endopyelotomy considered successful in 7/9 (78 %) at mean follow-up 6 years (2–10). One had repeat endopyelotomy at 4 years follow-up (Capolicchio et al. 1997).

Another retrospective series included nine percutaneous endopyelotomies for failed dismembered ($n=8$) or flap ($n=1$ with horseshoe kidney) pyeloplasty in 9 children, mean age 4 years (3 months–12 years). All were referrals with stents or nephrostomies, and all had a stenotic segment <2 cm. Internal stents were used postoperatively in all cases for 4–6 weeks.

There was mean follow-up of 59 months (16–110), with all having "improved drainage on US or renography" (data not shown). One patient remained symptomatic with intermittent flank pain, for success in eight (89 %) by the author's criteria (Figenshau et al. 1996).

A third retrospective study had 31 endopyelotomies in children median age 6.5 years for failed pyeloplasty diagnosed at median interval of 4 months (1–186). Failure was defined by imaging (not further described) or recurrent flank pain. Seventy-one percent were antegrade and the remainder retrograde incisions. Success was defined as no symptoms and "improved features" on US, CT, renography, or IVP. By these criteria, the authors considered 29 (94 %) successful during median follow-up 61 months (1–204) (Kim et al. 2012).

Retrograde endopyelotomy ($n=18$) was compared to reoperative pyeloplasty ($n=12$) or ureterocalicostomy ($n=2$) in a retrospective study of children median age 6.5 years with failed dismembered UPJ repair. Mean follow-up was 47 and 33 months, and outcomes were determined by US, with renography only done for persistent HN or recurrent symptoms. Using these criteria, 39 % endopyelotomies versus 100 % reoperative pyeloplasties were considered successful, $p=0.002$. The stenotic segment was 4–8 mm (mean 6) in successful endopyelotomy cases versus 6–15 mm (mean 10) in failures, $p=0.002$ (Braga et al. 2007).

References

Adey GS, Vargas SO, Retik AB, Borer JG, Mandell J, Hendren WH, et al. Fibroepithelial polyps causing ureteropelvic junction obstruction in children. J Urol. 2003;169(5):1834–6.

Alagiri M, Polepalle SK. Dietl's crisis: an under-recognized clinical entity in the pediatric population. Int Braz J Urol. 2006;32(4):451–3.

Amarante J, Anderson PJ, Gordon I. Impaired drainage on diuretic renography using half-time or pelvic excretion efficiency is not a sign of obstruction in children with a prenatal diagnosis of unilateral renal pelvic dilatation. J Urol. 2003;169(5):1828–31.

Amling CL, O'Hara SM, Wiener JS, Schaeffer CS, King LR. Renal ultrasound changes after pyeloplasty in children with ureteropelvic junction obstruction: long-term outcome in 47 renal units. J Urol. 1996;156(6):2020–4.

Aziz MA, Hossain AZ, Banu T, Karim MS, Islam N, Sultana H, et al. In hydronephrosis less than 10 % kidney function is not an indication for nephrectomy in children. Eur J Pediatr Surg. 2002;12(5):304–7.

Bajpai M, Chandrasekharam VV. Nonoperative management of neonatal moderate to severe bilateral hydronephrosis. J Urol. 2002;167(2 Pt 1):662–5.

Braga LH, Lorenzo AJ, Skeldon S, Dave S, Bagli DJ, Khoury AE, et al. Failed pyeloplasty in children: comparative analysis of retrograde endopyelotomy versus redo pyeloplasty. J Urol. 2007;178(6):2571–5. discussion 5.

Braga LH, Pace K, DeMaria J, Lorenzo AJ. Systematic review and meta-analysis of robotic-assisted versus conventional laparoscopic pyeloplasty for patients with ureteropelvic junction obstruction: effect on operative time, length of hospital stay, postoperative complications, and success rate. Eur Urol. 2009;56(5):848–57.

Caglar M, Gedik GK, Karabulut E. Differential renal function estimation by dynamic renal scintigraphy: influence of background definition and radiopharmaceutical. Nucl Med Commun. 2008;29(11):1002–5.

Cain MP, Rink RC, Thomas AC, Austin PF, Kaefer M, Casale AJ. Symptomatic ureteropelvic junction obstruction in children in the era of prenatal sonography—is there a higher incidence of crossing vessels? Urology. 2001;57(2):338–41.

Calisti A, Perrotta ML, Oriolo L, Patti G, Marrocco G, Miele V. Functional outcome after pyeloplasty in children: impact of the cause of obstruction and of the mode of presentation. Eur Urol. 2003;43(6):706–10.

Capolicchio G, Homsy YL, Houle AM, Brzezinski A, Stein L, Elhilali MM. Long-term results of percutaneous endopyelotomy in the treatment of children with failed open pyeloplasty. J Urol. 1997;158(4):1534–7.

Castagnetti M, Novara G, Beniamin F, Vezzu B, Rigamonti W, Artibani W. Scintigraphic renal function after unilateral pyeloplasty in children: a systematic review. BJU Int. 2008;102(7):862–8.

Chertin B, Rolle U, Farkas A, Puri P. Does delaying pyeloplasty affect renal function in children with a prenatal diagnosis of pelvi-ureteric junction obstruction? BJU Int. 2002;90(1):72–5.

Coelho GM, Bouzada MC, Lemos GS, Pereira AK, Lima BP, Oliveira EA. Risk factors for urinary tract infection in children with prenatal renal pelvic dilatation. J Urol. 2008;179(1):284–9.

Coplen DE, Austin PF, Yan Y, Blanco VM, Dicke JM. The magnitude of fetal renal pelvic dilatation can identify obstructive postnatal hydronephrosis, and direct postnatal evaluation and management. J Urol. 2006;176(2):724–7. discussion 7.

Figenshau RS, Clayman RV, Colberg JW, Coplen DE, Soble JJ, Manley CB. Pediatric endopyelotomy: the Washington University experience. J Urol. 1996;156(6):2025–30.

Freilich DA, Penna FJ, Nelson CP, Retik AB, Nguyen HT. Parental satisfaction after open versus robot assisted laparoscopic pyeloplasty: results from modified Glasgow Children's Benefit Inventory Survey. J Urol. 2010;183(2):704–8.

Gargollo PC. Hidden incision endoscopic surgery: description of technique, parental satisfaction and applications. J Urol. 2011;185(4):1425–31.

Gordon I, Piepsz A, Sixt R. Guidelines for standard and diuretic renogram in children. Eur J Nucl Med Mol Imaging. 2011;38(6):1175–88.

Gupta DK, Chandrasekharam VV, Srinivas M, Bajpai M. Percutaneous nephrostomy in children with ureteropelvic junction obstruction and poor renal function. Urology. 2001;57(3):547–50.

Hafez AT, McLorie G, Bagli D, Khoury A. Analysis of trends on serial ultrasound for high grade neonatal hydronephrosis. J Urol. 2002;168(4 Pt 1):1518–21.

Helmy TE, Sarhan OM, Hafez AT, Elsherbiny MT, Dawaba ME, Ghali AM. Surgical management of failed pyeloplasty in children: single-center experience. J Pediatr Urol. 2009;5(2):87–9.

Karnak I, Woo LL, Shah SN, Sirajuddin A, Ross JH. Results of a practical protocol for management of prenatally detected hydronephrosis due to ureteropelvic junction obstruction. Pediatr Surg Int. 2009;25(1): 61–7.

Kim J, Hong S, Park CH, Park H, Kim KS. Management of severe bilateral ureteropelvic junction obstruction in neonates with prenatally diagnosed bilateral hydronephrosis. Korean J Urol. 2010;51(9):653–6.

Kim EH, Tanagho YS, Traxel EJ, Austin PF, Figenshau RS, Coplen DE. Endopyelotomy for pediatric ureteropelvic junction obstruction: a review of our 25-year experience. J Urol. 2012;188(4):1628–33.

Lee JH, Son CH, Lee MS, Park YS. Vesicoureteral reflux increases the risk of renal scars: a study of unilateral reflux. Pediatr Nephrol (Berlin, Germany). 2006;21(9):1281–4.

Lim DJ, Walker 3rd RD. Management of the failed pyeloplasty. J Urol. 1996;156(2 Pt 2):738–40.

Lindgren BW, Hagerty J, Meyer T, Cheng EY. Robot-assisted laparoscopic reoperative repair for failed pyeloplasty in children: a safe and highly effective treatment option. J Urol. 2012;188(3):932–7.

Maenhout A, Ham H, Ismaili K, Hall M, Dierckx RA, Piepsz A. Supranormal renal function in unilateral hydronephrosis: does it represent true hyperfunction? Pediatr Nephrol (Berlin, Germany). 2005;20(12):1762–5.

McAleer IM, Kaplan GW. Renal function before and after pyeloplasty: does it improve? J Urol. 1999;162(3 Pt 2):1041–4.

Mei H, Pu J, Yang C, Zhang H, Zheng L, Tong Q. Laparoscopic versus open pyeloplasty for ureteropelvic junction obstruction in children: a systematic review and meta-analysis. J Endourol. 2011;25(5):727–36.

Moon DH, Park YS, Jun NL, Lee SY, Kim KS, Kim JH, et al. Value of supranormal function and renogram patterns on 99mTc-mercaptoacetyltriglycine scintigraphy in relation to the extent of hydronephrosis for predicting ureteropelvic junction obstruction in the newborn. J Nucl Med. 2003;44(5):725–31.

Onen A, Jayanthi VR, Koff SA. Long-term followup of prenatally detected severe bilateral newborn hydronephrosis initially managed nonoperatively. J Urol. 2002;168(3):1118–20.

Ozcan Z, Anderson PJ, Gordon I. Robustness of estimation of differential renal function in infants and children with unilateral prenatal diagnosis of a hydronephrotic kidney on dynamic renography: how real is the supranormal kidney? Eur J Nucl Med Mol Imaging. 2006;33(6):738–44.

Penn HA, Gatti JM, Hoestje SM, DeMarco RT, Snyder CL, Murphy JP. Laparoscopic versus open pyeloplasty in children: preliminary report of a prospective randomized trial. J Urol. 2010;184(2):690–5.

Pohl HG, Rushton HG, Park JS, Belman AB, Majd M. Early diuresis renogram findings predict success following pyeloplasty. J Urol. 2001;165(6 Pt 2):2311–5.

Ransley PG, Dhillon HK, Gordon I, Duffy PG, Dillon MJ, Barratt TM. The postnatal management of hydronephrosis diagnosed by prenatal ultrasound. J Urol. 1990;144(2 Pt 2):584–7. discussion 93–4.

Rohrmann D, Snyder 3rd HM, Duckett Jr JW, Canning DA, Zderic SA. The operative management of recurrent ureteropelvic junction obstruction. J Urol. 1997; 158(3 Pt 2):1257–9.

Ross SS, Kardos S, Krill A, Bourland J, Sprague B, Majd M, et al. Observation of infants with SFU grades 3–4 hydronephrosis: worsening drainage with serial diuresis renography indicates surgical intervention and helps prevent loss of renal function. J Pediatr Urol. 2011;7(3):266–71.

Roth CC, Hubanks JM, Bright BC, Heinlen JE, Donovan BO, Kropp BP, et al. Occurrence of urinary tract infection in children with significant upper urinary tract obstruction. Urology. 2009;73(1):74–8.

Salem YH, Majd M, Rushton HG, Belman AB. Outcome analysis of pediatric pyeloplasty as a function of patient age, presentation and differential renal function. J Urol. 1995;154(5):1889–93.

Sheu JC, Koh CC, Chang PY, Wang NL, Tsai JD, Tsai TC. Ureteropelvic junction obstruction in children: 10 years' experience in one institution. Pediatr Surg Int. 2006;22(6):519–23.

Skoog SJ, Peters CA, Arant Jr BS, Copp HL, Elder JS, Hudson RG, et al. Pediatric vesicoureteral reflux guidelines panel summary report: clinical practice guidelines for screening siblings of children with vesicoureteral reflux and neonates/infants with prenatal hydronephrosis. J Urol. 2010;184(3):1145–51.

Song C, Park H, Park S, Moon KH, Kim KS. The change in renal function in the supranormal hydronephrotic kidney after pyeloplasty. BJU Int. 2007a;99(6):1483–6.

Song SH, Lee SB, Park YS, Kim KS. Is antibiotic prophylaxis necessary in infants with obstructive hydronephrosis? J Urol. 2007b;177(3):1098–101. discussion 101.

Szavay PO, Luithle T, Seitz G, Warmann SW, Haber P, Fuchs J. Functional outcome after laparoscopic dismembered pyeloplasty in children. J Pediatr Urol. 2010;6(4):359–63.

Thomas JC, DeMarco RT, Donohoe JM, Adams MC, Pope JCT, Brock 3rd JW. Management of the failed pyeloplasty: a contemporary review. J Urol. 2005;174(6): 2363–6.

Tsai JD, Huang FY, Lin CC, Tsai TC, Lee HC, Sheu JC, et al. Intermittent hydronephrosis secondary to ureteropelvic junction obstruction: clinical and imaging features. Pediatrics. 2006;117(1):139–46.

Wiener JS, O'Hara SM. Optimal timing of initial postnatal ultrasonography in newborns with prenatal hydronephrosis. J Urol. 2002;168(4 Pt 2):1826–9. discussion 9.

Yang Y, Hou Y, Niu ZB, Wang CL. Long-term follow-up and management of prenatally detected, isolated hydronephrosis. J Pediatr Surg. 2010;45(8):1701–6.

Multicystic Dysplastic Kidney

12

Patricio C. Gargollo

The primary aim in diagnosis and management of multicystic dysplastic kidney (MCDK) is preservation of contralateral renal function.

Secondary aims:

1. **Diagnosis and management of associated HTN.**
2. **To prevent malignancy.**

Summary of evidence for these goals:

Retrospective series variously define subnormal renal function as GFR <80 or 90 mL/min/1.73 m^2, or <80 % normal for age and gender.

- **A prospective registry reported all 76 children followed for 5–10 years had GFR >60 mL/min/1.73 m^2, with 43 % between 60 and 90 mL/min/1.73 m^2.**
- **A retrospective series of 36 children with similar follow-up and a normal contralateral kidney by US reported 12 % had GFR <80 mL/min/1.73 m^2.**
- **Analysis of potential hyperfiltration injury in patients with MCDK or unilateral renal agenesis versus normal controls reported that patients had mean GFR less than controls (93 ± 20 vs. 114 ± 14).**

Meta-analysis reported contralateral anomalies potentially impacting renal function, including UPJO in 5 %, ureterocele in 1 %, and PUV in 0.4 %.

Contralateral VUR, mostly grades 1–3, occurs in 20 %.

- **One study found no difference in serum creatinine for age in patients with versus without contralateral VUR.**
- **Twelve newborns with MCDK would need VCUG to detect one ureter with grades 3–5 VUR.**
- **Retrospective studies indicate that >50 % of contralateral VUR resolves by ≤2 years of age.**
- **No RCT shows benefit of antibiotic prophylaxis versus no therapy to prevent first fUTI in patients with contralateral VUR.**

Our review found no evidence that the diagnosis of VUR significantly impacts renal functional outcomes in children with MCDK, suggesting that routine cystography is not necessary.

Systematic literature review reports that the rate of HTN is 5 per 1,000, with insufficient data to state duration of follow-up needed to detect most cases. Two studies with a total of 27 patients report BP normalization in 68 and 100 % after nephrectomy.

Malignancy, including Wilms' tumor and renal cell carcinoma, has only been published as case reports, with no cohort study reporting tumor development during follow-up.

Our review found no evidence that renography demonstrating no uptake versus uptake alters prognosis or management of MCDK (i.e., impacts risk for HTN or malignancy), so nuclear

P.C. Gargollo, M.D. (✉)
Department of Pediatric Urology,
University of Texas Southwestern Medical
Center and Children's Medical Center Dallas,
1935 Medical District Drive, MS F4.04,
Dallas, TX 75235, USA
e-mail: patricio.gargollo@childrens.com

W.T. Snodgrass (ed.), *Pediatric Urology: Evidence for Optimal Patient Management*,
DOI 10.1007/978-1-4614-6910-0_12,

renal scan should be considered an optional investigation for children with this condition.

Sports-related renal injury was also reviewed to determine potential risk to a solitary functioning kidney, finding the following:

- **Injuries resulting in functional loss or nephrectomy are rare.**
- **Most injuries are reported related to American football, with an incidence of <0.7 %.**
- **Most injuries occur in children ≥12 years of age.**
- **No evidence-basis to restrict sports participation in children with a solitary kidney.**

Prevalence and Presentation

MCDK occurs in approximately 1:4,300 screened subjects, more often in males.

Eighty percent are diagnosed prenatally.

Systematic review of data from 19 studies published from 1986 to 2008 found a total of 371 patients with unilateral MCDK in 1,588,271 screened subjects, an incidence of 1 per 4,281. Fifty-nine percent were males, and 53 % involved the left kidney, both significantly increased over the expected 51 and 50 %, respectively.

Eighty-one percent of MCDK were diagnosed prenatally; the 19 % diagnosed postnatally were imaged for abdominal mass in 64 %, UTI in 7 %, and various other reasons in the remainder (Schreuder et al. 2009).

Imaging and Associated Conditions

Meta-analysis reported abnormalities of the contralateral kidney in approximately 5 % of patients, mostly UPJO.

Compensatory hypertrophy of the contralateral kidney has been reported on the initial US following birth, and occurs in >85 % with follow-up to 10 years.

Meta-analysis found contralateral VUR in 20 % of patients, over 50 % grades 1,2. Twelve VCUGs are needed to detect one ureter with grades 3–5 VUR.

Renographic activity ranging from 1 to 18 % has been reported in MCDK.

Renal US

Meta-analysis of 72 articles published between 1964 and 2008 reported:

- 21/389 (5 %) prenatally detected MCDK were not visible on US postnatally (five studies).
- 5 % UPJO, 1 % ureterocele, 0.6 % horseshoe kidney, and 0.4 % PUV (67 studies, 3,557 patients) (Schreuder et al. 2009).

A retrospective analysis reviewed US findings correlated with VCUG results in 76 consecutive newborns with antenatally diagnosed MCDK evaluated with a systematic imaging protocol. Two renal US were obtained, on day 3 and at 1 month, with abnormal findings defined as AP diameter ≥7 mm, calyceal or ureteral dilation, "pelvic or ureteral wall thickening" (not further described), absence of corticomedullary differentiation, or renal dysplasia:

- Normal US (n=61, 80 %); four (7 %) had VUR, grades 1 or 2.
- Abnormal US (n=15, 20 %); 12 (80 %) had VUR, grades 1,2 in 5; grade 3 in 4; grades 4,5 in 3.

Sensitivity, specificity, positive predictive value, and negative predictive value of two US within the first month of life to predict abnormal VCUG were 75, 95, 80, and 93 % (Ismaili et al. 2005).

Contralateral Renal Hypertrophy

Literature review by Schreuder et al. (2009) found two reports of contralateral hypertrophy at initial US soon after birth in 12/26 (46 %) and 8/33 (24 %) patients.

Retrospective review of 66 children with MCDK with US at mean age 12 months (6–18) found contralateral compensatory hypertrophy (renal length >95 % standard values) in 53 (80 %). Follow-up in 13 to ≥10 years showed all 13 had compensatory hypertrophy (Weinstein et al. 2008).

Ten-year follow-up was available in 43 patients in a MCDK registry, with compensatory hypertrophy (renal length >95 % standard values) in 35/40 (87.5 %) with lengths recorded (Aslam and Watson 2006).

VCUG

Meta-analysis by Schreuder et al. (2009) of 67 articles and 3,557 patients found VUR prevalence was 20 % in patients with MCDK, grade 1 in 16 %, grade 2 in 40 %, grade 3 in 24 %, grade 4 in 17 %, and grade 5 in 5 %. From the data, at least 12 newborns with MCDK would need VCUG to detect one ureter with grades 3–5 VUR.

Renography

Meta-analysis by Schreuder et al. (2009) reported seven published cohorts (from a total of 72 included articles) and described a total of 27/347 (8 %) patients who had ipsilateral activity ranging from 1 to18% on renography. Since most cohorts did not report the number of positive and negative renograms, the authors chose not to present a percentage from these data.

Outcomes of Observation

Five percent of prenatally detected MCDK are not visible on initial postnatal US. Disappearance on US occurs in approximately 50 % of cases by age 5 years. Increased length of MCDK has been reported during observation in 0–19 % of patients. Most contralateral VUR is grades 1–3, with spontaneous resolution in 50–80 % within 1–3 years.

Retrospective series reported routine use of antibiotic prophylaxis in patients with VUR. One study found 8 % of MCDK patients developed fUTI during median follow-up of 53 months, with no difference in those with VUR versus without VUR (or antibiotic prophylaxis).

Meta-analysis reported HTN develops in 5 per 1,000 MCDK.

Retrospective reviews concerning renal function are characterized by differing definitions of insufficiency (<90 mL or <80 mL/min/1.73 m^2 or <80 % normal GFR for age), failure to analyze all patients, and varying duration of follow-up. Percentage with renal insufficiency was ≥10 % at ≥5 years of age.

One study reported mean serum creatinine for age was similar in those with and without contralateral VUR.

No cohort study has reported malignancy arising from a MCDK.

Involution

As mentioned above, meta-analysis by Schreuder et al. (2009) included five studies reporting that 21/389 (5 %) prenatally detected MCDK were not visible on initial US postnatally.

Retrospective review of 323 children with prenatally detected MCDK managed by protocol from 1985 to 2009 reported that the MCDK was not visible on the initial postnatal US within the first weeks of life in 32 (10 %). Nonvisualization additionally occurred in 35 % of 249 by 2 years, 47 % of 180 by 5 years, and 62 % of 94 by 10 years. Likelihood for the lesion to become nondetectable by 10 years related to initial length; 21 % of those >5 cm versus 76 % <5 cm, $p<0.001$ (Hayes and Watson 2012).

A retrospective review of 31 children followed a mean of 6 years (6 months–11 years) reported that 17 (55 %) MCDK became undetectable on two follow-up US studies, 7 (23 %) had partial regression, and another 7 were unchanged. Mean time to become undetectable on US was 2.5 years (1–4) (Chiappinelli et al. 2011).

Of 66 MCDK undergoing US at mean age 12 months (6–18), 11 (17 %) were no longer visualized. Twenty-seven MCDK had follow-up ≥6 years, with 15 (56 %) no longer seen on US; 13 were followed to ≥10 years, with 9 (68 %) not visualized (Weinstein et al. 2008).

Fourteen patients with unilateral MCDK and complete cyst involution by US (mean age 13 months, 3–18) underwent laparoscopic nephrectomy. Dysplastic renal tissue was encountered in each case in remnants measuring from 1 to 3.5 cm (Luque-Mialdea et al. 2007).

Increased Size

A summary of nine articles on US changes in observed MCDK published from 1992 to 2004, noted that six reported an increase in size from 1.5 to 19 % of a total of 496 patients (Rabelo et al. 2004). The three reporting the largest percentages with increases are summarized here:

- Fifty-five patients were diagnosed with MCDK at mean age 15 weeks (0–48), all with no uptake on renography. Two hundred thirty-six renal US (mean 4, range 2–6 per patient) were obtained during a mean follow-up of 32 months (2–69). Ten (18 %) had mean increase in length of 2 cm (1.3–2.5) from an initial mean length of 4.6 cm at diagnosis. Mean initial length of those that reduced in size during follow-up was 4.5 cm (Rottenberg et al. 1997).
- Thirty-three patients with MCDK were diagnosed prenatally ($n=30$) or because of a palpable mass "afterwards." Serial US was obtained every 3 months for 2 years. During this time the MCDK became non-visualized in 7 (23 %), decreased in size (diameter) in 20 (67 %), and increased in 6 (20 %). There was no further description of these 6 patients to state when increase occurred and to what extent, whether it was a cystic or solid component that appeared to change, and what subsequently occurred (Heymans et al. 1998).
- A multicenter German study enrolled 204 children with MCDK, of which serial measurements of the largest diameter were available in 74 cases. In 48 the diameter decreased, while in 14 (19 %) it increased. Timing and extent of increase were not further described, the authors only noting that neither increase nor decrease in diameter appeared to be clinically significant (Rudnik-Schoneborn et al. 1998).

UTI/VUR

Data from a prospective registry of children with antenatally detected MCDK reported that 143 had VCUG, of which 27 (19 %) had VUR into the contralateral kidney that was grades 1–2 in 74 %, grade 3 in 22 %, and grade 5 in 1 child. Those with ≥grade 2 were prescribed trimethoprim (2 mg/kg/day) for 2 years, while other infants did not receive antibiotic therapy. During follow-up at a mean of 8 years (0.1–20), no febrile UTIs occurred; non-febrile UTI was diagnosed in 13 children without VUR and 7 with VUR on antibiotics, which was reported not significant. Repeat VCUG was not done (Aslam and Watson 2006).

Retrospective review of 75 patients with MCDK included 19 (25 %) with contralateral VUR (10 males) that was grade 1 ($n=1$), grade 2 ($n=8$), grade 3 ($n=8$), and grade 4 ($n=2$). Antibiotic prophylaxis apparently was used in all with VUR. Spontaneous resolution occurred in 13 (68 %) at median follow-up of 20 months, while one child with grade 3 VUR and a "history of breakthrough UTIs" had reimplantation. At median follow-up for the entire group at 53 months, febrile UTI occurred in six (8 %), four without and two with contralateral VUR (Miller et al. 2004).

Another retrospective review of 65 children with MCDK diagnosed contralateral VUR in 10 (15 %), 8 of which were boys. Grades were 1 ($n=2$), 2 ($n=2$), 3 ($n=2$), 4 ($n=1$), and 5 ($n=3$), and all were given antibiotic prophylaxis. During mean follow-up at 3 years (3 months–6 years), five resolved and two with grade 5 had reimplantation. None developed UTI (it was unclear if this statement applied only to those with VUR or to all patients) (Selzman and Elder 1995).

VCUG in the first month of life was obtained in all 76 newborns reported by Ismaili et al. (2005). Grade 1 VUR occurred in two ipsilateral ureters, both with bilateral reflux. VUR involving the contralateral kidney was diagnosed in 16 (21 %), comprising grade 1 ($n=2$), grade 2 ($n=7$), grade 3 ($n=4$), grade 4 ($n=1$), and grade 5 ($n=2$). Second cystograms were obtained between ages 1 and 2 years, showing only three cases to persist, one with unchanged grade 3 and both grade 5 decreased to grade 2. There was no mention of UTI.

Hypertension

A systematic review concerning MCDK managed without nephrectomy identified 29 published studies including 1,115 children with HTN reported in 6, a rate of 5.4 per 1,000. Of these studies, 14 did not report follow-up duration, and mean follow-up in the others was an average 4 years (3–5), with maximum follow-up of 13 years (Narchi 2005a).

A summary of articles not included in this review or subsequently published:

Series Reporting HTN

Retrospective review of 101 patients with MCDK with follow-up >1 year (mean 5.9±4.4 [1–18]), reported HTN in 6/86 (7 %), presumably representing those with BP measurements recorded. All were described as having contralateral renal abnormalities (Mansoor et al. 2011).

A retrospective review of 43 children followed for a mean time of 42 months (12–156) reported 2 (5 %) developed HTN, 1 diagnosed at age 4 months with spontaneous improvement at 12 months, and another diagnosed at age 5 years and associated with obesity (Rabelo et al. 2004).

Retrospective review was done in 36 patients with MCDK at 2 and 10 years, 4 (11 %) with prior nephrectomy. At 2 years 2 (6 %) and at 5 years, one (3 %) had systolic BP >95 % (Vu et al. 2008).

Ninety newborns and children with MCDK diagnosed between 1990 and 2007 identified 16 (18 %) with HTN, defined as systolic and /or diastolic pressure >95 % for age and gender. BP was measured monthly during the first 6 months of life, and those with suspected HTN were admitted to hospital for 3 days monitoring to confirm the diagnosis. Antihypertensives (nifedipine alone in 14, and two-drug therapy with nifedipine or propranolol plus captopril in 2) were prescribed pending nephrectomy. Mean age at diagnosis was 6 months (4 days–2 years) excluding one discovered at age 13 years. Reported preoperative systolic pressures ranged from 110 to 135, but records were lacking for review in six patients (Kiyak et al. 2009).

Series Without HTN

Analysis of a prospective registry of 323 children with prenatally detected MCDK who had BP measurements at ages 3, 6, and 12 months, then annually to age 5, then every other year to age 10, reported no patient with HTN related to the MCDK. Six of 94 (6 %) who were followed to 10 years had BP exceeding 95 %; 4 were found to be normal on 24-h ambulatory monitoring, 1 transient from balanitis, and 1 with mitral valve anomaly (Hayes and Watson 2012).

Retrospective review of 31 children (age not stated) reported BP determinations biannually for 2 years and then annually, with two determinations at each visit and the results averaged. During follow-up a mean of 6 years (6 months–11 years), no patient had BP >95 % for age and gender (Chiappinelli et al. 2011).

Renal Function

In 76 children with follow-up 5 ($n=7$) to 10 ($n=69$) years reported from a prospective registry of 323 children with prenatally detected MCDK mentioned above, median calculated GFR was 93 mL/min/1.73 m² (47–181). Of these, 40 (53 %) had normal calculated GFR >90 mL/min/1.73 m², 33 (43 %) had GFR 60–90 mL/min/1.73 m², and 2 had GFR >160 mL/min/1.73 m² (other not described) (Hayes and Watson 2012).

Renal function was available during chart review in 24/80 (30 %) children with MCDK at mean age 12 months (6–18), reporting calculated mean GFR of 84 mL/min/1.73 m² , which was ≥80 % normal for age and gender in all (Weinstein et al. 2008).

Retrospective review in 36 children with MCDK and a normal contralateral renal US all followed to 5 years and 16–10 years reported calculated GFR was <80 mL/min/1.73 m² in 2 (6 %) at 2 years, 4 (11 %) at 5 years, and 2 (12.5 %) at 10 years (Vu et al. 2008).

Retrospective review included data to calculate GFR in 82/101 children with MCDK at 6.5±4.7 years of age. Eight of 82 (10 %) had GFR <90 mL/min/1.73 m², of which 5 had contralateral renal abnormalities (HN, megaureter, g3 VUR, hypoplasia) and another 2 had medical renal disease (UTI with renal failure, nephrotic syndrome). GFR ranged from 15 to 86 mL/min/1.73 m² in these patients (median 78) (Mansoor et al. 2011).

Retrospective review was done concerning hyperfiltration injury in 66 children at mean age 8±5 years with either MCDK ($n=27$) or unilateral renal agenesis ($n=39$) compared to 34 normal controls at mean age 9±4 years (no difference).

Five other patients with abnormal contralateral kidney by US and/or renography were excluded. Median serum creatinine and fractional sodium excretion were significantly higher in patients, as was occurrence of microalbuminuria, which was seen in 23 % versus none in controls. Mean calculated GFR (mL/min/1.73 m^2) was significantly less in patients (93±20 vs. 114±14) (Schreuder et al. 2008).

One retrospective analysis of 75 patients diagnosed with MCDK at median age 0 months and followed a median 53 months compared mean serum creatinine in 19 (25 %) with contralateral VUR (grades 1, 2 in 47 %, grade 3 in 42 %, and grade 4 in 10.5 %) to 56 without VUR for the same age categories. There was no difference by regression analysis (Miller et al. 2004).

Malignancy

A systematic review of all published cohort studies for MCDK without nephrectomy included 26 reports and 1,041 children, none of which developed Wilms' tumor during mean follow-up (reported by 18) ranging from 1 to 6.5 years and a maximum of 23 years (Narchi 2005b).

The report from the MCDK registry by Hayes and Watson (2012) mentioned above included 323 children with prenatally detected MCDK, with 94 (29 %) undergoing US at 10 years. Nephrectomy was done in 12 patients, 11 initially before a universal observation protocol was adopted and 1 with suspected malignancy but benign pathology. Details of this case, including patient age, US findings, and pathology, were not discussed.

Several case reports detail malignancies developing from a MCDK:

- A 5-year-old girl with right MCDK diagnosed at birth presented with a palpable mass that at nephrectomy was found to include malignant rhabdoid tumor (Cui et al. 2010).
- A 5-month-old female with antenatal diagnosis of MCDK presented with a palpable mass with multifocal Wilms' tumor and nephrogenic rests (Homsy et al. 1997).
- A 3-month-old female presented with HTN and during evaluation was found to have a renal mass that consisted of MCDK and Wilms' tumor (Homsy et al. 1997).
- A 19-year-old female with a history of absent right kidney and left pyeloplasty at 6 months presented with right flank pain and was thought to have pyelonephritis of a MCDK. Subsequent nephrectomy found collecting duct carcinoma, a variant of renal cell carcinoma (Cuda et al. 2006).

A listing of additional case reports of renal cell tumors arising from MCDK in patients aged 15–68 years was included in the report by Homsy et al. (1997).

In a comment to an article, Beckwith stated that the National Wilms' Tumor Study Pathology Center had 7,500 Wilms' tumor specimens, of which 5 (0.07 %) arose from MCDK (Beckwith 1997).

Nephrectomy for Hypertension

Nephrectomy for HTN has normalized BP in 63 and 100 % of patients in two studies with a total of 27 patients.

A retrospective review of children undergoing nephrectomy for HTN included 11 MCDK, of which 7 (63 %) had normalization of BP by the first postoperative visit at a median 1.7 months. Among the entire series of 21 nephrectomies for HTN reported, contralateral renal abnormalities were diagnosed in 5/14 (36 %) with BP normalization and in 3/7 (43 %) without normalization (Schlomer et al. 2011).

All 16 patients diagnosed with HTN by Kiyak et al. (2009) mentioned above underwent nephrectomy within less than 40 days after diagnosis, and all postoperative BP were <95 % percentile, systolic pressures ranging from 80 to 105.

Sports Participation with a Solitary Kidney

Three reports indicate that American football accounts for the majority of renal injuries in children ≥12 years of age, at a rate ≤0.7 %.

Risk for renal trauma from team or individual sports participation is very small; one

study calculating the risk for renal loss showed one kidney per 2.67 million participating children per year.

Surgery for sports-related renal injuries is rare.

A review of one trauma registry found similar nephrectomy rates for injuries due to motor vehicle accidents, pedestrians being struck, and falls versus bicycling and sports.

These data do not support restrictions on sports participation in children with a solitary kidney.

Prospective data from the National Athletic Trainers' Association High School Injury Surveillance Study collected from 1995 to 1997 reported over 4.4 million athlete-exposures (one athlete participating in one game or practice) with 18 (0.07 %) kidney injuries out of a total of 23,666 injuries. None required surgery. Twelve (67 %) occurred playing football (Grinsell et al. 2012).

A study queried the National Pediatric Trauma Registry from 1990 to 1999 for recorded sports-related renal trauma in three age groups: 5–11, 12–14, and 15–18 years. Sports searched for were (team sports) American football, ice hockey, basketball, baseball, soccer, and (individual sports) rollerblading, skateboarding, skiing, sledding, and wrestling. There were 5,439 sports-related injuries, with renal injuries in 42 (0.7 %), related to football in 26 (62 %), ice hockey in 3, basketball in 5, baseball in 6, soccer in 2, and none from others searched. Most of these renal injuries occurred in children ≥12 years of age (38, 90 %). There were no resultant nephrectomies, nor injuries causing functional loss of the kidney (Wan et al. 2003a).

Another study reviewed all renal injuries reported to the National Pediatric Trauma Registry from 1995 to 2001, finding 813 patients at average age 11 years. Of these, 293 (36 %) resulted from motor vehicle collisions, 119 (15 %) from pedestrians being struck, and 107 (13 %) from falls. Bicycle injuries occurred in 92 (11 %), of which 31 related to a bicyclist being struck by a motor vehicle. Sports-related renal injuries were reported in 85 (10 %), 24 % playing football. Of sport and bicycle injuries, 74/161 (46 %) described renal injuries were hematomas without capsular disruption. Nephrectomy was done in 21/519 (4 %) children with injury due to accidents or falls versus 4/177 (2 %) related to sports or bicycling (2 to sledding, 1 skiing and 1 jet skiing), which was not significantly different, $p=0.3$ (Johnson et al. 2005).

A fourth study reviewed a regional trauma registry of a single children's hospital for 1993–2000. Sports examined included football, ice hockey, basketball, baseball, soccer, wrestling, skiing, snowboarding, sledding, bicycling, and playground play. Of 4,921 children with trauma, renal injuries occurred in 15 (0.3 %), 5 (33 %) associated with football. Renal injuries were grade 1 ($n=2$), grade 2 ($n=5$), grade 3 ($n=4$), grade 4 ($n=3$), and grade 5 ($n=1$), and occurred at mean age 13.5 ± 2.4 years. Three (20 %) injured kidneys had UPJO, and one with grade 5 injury was removed. From these data and census data from the referring region, the authors calculated there is risk for one kidney being lost per 2.67 million participating children in sports per year (Wan et al. 2003b).

All National Football League (NFL) renal injuries from 1986 to 2004 were reviewed. There were a total of 48 renal injuries, or 2.7 per season, with 42 (81 %) contusions and 6 lacerations. None required surgery, and all athletes returned to play (Brophy et al. 2008).

References

Aslam M, Watson AR. Unilateral multicystic dysplastic kidney: long term outcomes. Arch Dis Child. 2006;91(10):820–3.

Beckwith JB. New developments in the pathology of Wilms tumor. Cancer Invest. 1997;15(2):153–62.

Brophy RH, Gamradt SC, Barnes RP, Powell JW, DelPizzo JJ, Rodeo SA, et al. Kidney injuries in professional American football: implications for management of an athlete with 1 functioning kidney. Am J Sports Med. 2008;36(1):85–90.

Chiappinelli A, Savanelli A, Farina A, Settimi A. Multicystic dysplastic kidney: our experience in non-surgical management. Pediatr Surg Int. 2011;27(7):775–9.

Cuda SP, Brand TC, Thibault GP, Sutherland RS. Collecting duct carcinoma arising from multicystic dysplastic kidney disease. J Pediatr Urol. 2006; 2(5):500–2.

Cui Y, Eom M, Jung SH, Kim KJ, Jung WH. Malignant rhabdoid tumor of the kidney combined with multicystic dysplasia in a 5-year-old child. J Korean Med Sci. 2010;25(5):785–9.

Grinsell MM, Butz K, Gurka MJ, Gurka KK, Norwood V. Sport-related kidney injury among high school athletes. Pediatrics. 2012;130(1):e40–5.

Hayes WN, Watson AR. Unilateral multicystic dysplastic kidney: does initial size matter? Pediatr Nephrol (Berlin, Germany). 2012;27(8):1335–40.

Heymans C, Breysem L, Proesmans W. Multicystic kidney dysplasia: a prospective study on the natural history of the affected and the contralateral kidney. Eur J Pediatr. 1998;157(8):673–5.

Homsy YL, Anderson JH, Oudjhane K, Russo P. Wilms tumor and multicystic dysplastic kidney disease. J Urol. 1997;158(6):2256–9. discussion 9–60.

Ismaili K, Avni FE, Alexander M, Schulman C, Collier F, Hall M. Routine voiding cystourethrography is of no value in neonates with unilateral multicystic dysplastic kidney. J Pediatr. 2005;146(6):759–63.

Johnson B, Christensen C, Dirusso S, Choudhury M, Franco I. A need for reevaluation of sports participation recommendations for children with a solitary kidney. J Urol. 2005;174(2):686–9; discussion 9.

Kiyak A, Yilmaz A, Turhan P, Sander S, Aydin G, Aydogan G. Unilateral multicystic dysplastic kidney: single-center experience. Pediatr Nephrol (Berlin, Germany). 2009;24(1):99–104.

Luque-Mialdea R, Martin-Crespo R, Cebrian J, Moreno L, Carrero C, Fernandez A. Does the multicystic dysplastic kidney really involute? The role of the retroperitoneoscopic approach. J Pediatr Urol. 2007;3(1):48–52.

Mansoor O, Chandar J, Rodriguez MM, Abitbol CL, Seeherunvong W, Freundlich M, et al. Long-term risk of chronic kidney disease in unilateral multicystic dysplastic kidney. Pediatr Nephrol (Berlin, Germany). 2011;26(4):597–603.

Miller DC, Rumohr JA, Dunn RL, Bloom DA, Park JM. What is the fate of the refluxing contralateral kidney in children with multicystic dysplastic kidney? J Urol. 2004;172(4 Pt 2):1630–4.

Narchi H. Risk of hypertension with multicystic kidney disease: a systematic review. Arch Dis Child. 2005a; 90(9):921–4.

Narchi H. Risk of Wilms' tumour with multicystic kidney disease: a systematic review. Arch Dis Child. 2005b; 90(2):147–9.

Rabelo EA, Oliveira EA, Diniz JS, Silva JM, Filgueiras MT, Pezzuti IL, et al. Natural history of multicystic kidney conservatively managed: a prospective study. Pediatr Nephrol (Berlin, Germany). 2004;19(10):1102–7.

Rottenberg GT, Gordon I, De Bruyn R. The natural history of the multicystic dysplastic kidney in children. Br J Radiol. 1997;70(832):347–50.

Rudnik-Schoneborn S, John U, Deget F, Ehrich JH, Misselwitz J, Zerres K. Clinical features of unilateral multicystic renal dysplasia in children. Eur J Pediatr. 1998;157(8):666–72.

Schlomer BJ, Smith PJ, Barber TD, Baker LA. Nephrectomy for hypertension in pediatric patients with a unilateral poorly functioning kidney: a contemporary cohort. J Pediatr Urol. 2011;7(3):373–7.

Schreuder MF, Langemeijer ME, Bokenkamp A, Delemarre-Van de Waal HA, Van Wijk JA. Hypertension and microalbuminuria in children with congenital solitary kidneys. J Paediatr Child Health. 2008;44(6):363–8.

Schreuder MF, Westland R, van Wijk JA. Unilateral multicystic dysplastic kidney: a meta-analysis of observational studies on the incidence, associated urinary tract malformations and the contralateral kidney. Nephrol Dial Transplant. 2009;24(6):1810–8.

Selzman AA, Elder JS. Contralateral vesicoureteral reflux in children with a multicystic kidney. J Urol. 1995;153(4):1252–4.

Vu KH, Van Dyck M, Daniels H, Proesmans W. Renal outcome of children with one functioning kidney from birth. A study of 99 patients and a review of the literature. Eur J Pediatr. 2008;167(8):885–90.

Wan J, Corvino TF, Greenfield SP, DiScala C. Kidney and testicle injuries in team and individual sports: data from the national pediatric trauma registry. J Urol. 2003a;170(4 Pt 2):1528–32. discussion 31–2.

Wan J, Corvino TF, Greenfield SP, DiScala C. The incidence of recreational genitourinary and abdominal injuries in the Western New York pediatric population. J Urol. 2003b;170(4 Pt 2):1525–7. discussion 7.

Weinstein A, Goodman TR, Iragorri S. Simple multicystic dysplastic kidney disease: end points for subspecialty follow-up. Pediatr Nephrol (Berlin, Germany). 2008; 23(1):111–6.

13 Ureteroceles and Ectopic Ureters

Micah A. Jacobs and Warren T. Snodgrass

Primary aims in the diagnosis and treatment of ureteroceles and ectopic ureters:

1. **To prevent or reduce UTI.**
2. **To prevent renal damage.**
3. **To prevent or correct urinary incontinence.**

Postnatal Management of Prenatally Detected Ureteroceles and Ectopic Ureters

Selective Observation of Ureteroceles

Indications for surgical intervention in ureterocele are febrile UTI (fUTI) and bladder outlet obstruction.

One series managing patients by prospective protocol reported that 70 % had resolved or improved hydronephrosis (HN) and VUR, while 23 % had breakthrough UTI and 8 % developed outlet obstruction.

Retrospective series with selective observation based on various factors reported that most patients had stable or improved HN and resolved VUR, with <10 % developing breakthrough UTI and <5 % outlet obstruction.

M.A. Jacobs, M.D., M.P.H. • W.T. Snodgrass, M.D. (✉)
Department of Pediatric Urology, University of Texas Southwestern Medical Center and Children's Medical Center Dallas, 1935 Medical District Drive, MS F4.04, Dallas, TX 75235, USA
e-mail: micah.jacobs@childrens.com; warren.snodgrass@childrens.com

A prospective protocol was used to manage 13 patients with ureterocele that was duplex in 11 and single in 2 with MCDK who presented at median age 18 days. Ten were prenatally detected, and three presented with fUTI. Based on either "good" or no function (MCDK) on MAG-3 renography, drainage from the upper pole <30 min, and no bladder outlet obstruction, these patients were all observed with antibiotic prophylaxis (medication not stated). During follow-up at a median of 48 months (25–97), the ureteroceles associated with MCDK were asymptomatic. Upper pole hydronephrosis present in six resolved ($n=3$) or improved to SFU grade 2 ($n=3$), and VUR grade 3 and 4 of the lower pole present in five resolved. The other four had surgery at median 11 months, due to breakthrough UTI in 3 and progressive obstruction in 1 (Han et al. 2005).

Retrospective analysis was done in 52 children with prenatal duplex ureterocele, in which surgical intervention was generally determined by breakthrough UTI, upper pole function >10 %, lower pole obstruction, grade 4 or 5 lower pole reflux, or bladder outlet obstruction. Using these criteria, 14 were observed, eight with VUR, with median follow-up of 8 years (1.6–13). Antibiotic prophylaxis (medication not stated) was used "routinely until toilet training" or age 5, if there was VUR. No patient developed UTI, VUR resolved in 3/4 cases with cystography, and hydronephrosis was stable ($n=8$) or improved/resolved with collapse of the ureterocele ($n=6$) (Shankar et al. 2001).

W.T. Snodgrass (ed.), *Pediatric Urology: Evidence for Optimal Patient Management*,
DOI 10.1007/978-1-4614-6910-0_13, © Springer Science+Business Media New York 2013

A retrospective study found 10 newborns, six females, with prenatally detected ureteroceles who had "adequate drainage of the affected unit" without lower pole obstruction, grade 4 or 5 VUR, or bladder outlet obstruction managed with antibiotic prophylaxis (medication not stated) and observation. Six were duplex and 4 single-system ureteroceles, 1 with MCDK. During mean follow-up of 3 years, HN (initially SFU grade 3 in 2 and less in the others) resolved in six and was improved or stable in 4. VUR grade 3 into the lower pole was initially present in 4, which resolved in 2. No patient underwent repair (Direnna and Leonard 2006).

Another retrospective analysis included 40 neonates with prenatally detected ureterocele initially observed with antibiotic prophyaxis (medication not stated) with planned open surgery at 6 months (selection for observation vs. puncture was not stated, but implied these had no lower pole VUR and no bladder outlet obstruction). During observation, 3 (8 %) had UTI and 2 (5 %) had progressive ureterocele enlargement resulting in bladder outlet obstruction (Husmann et al. 2002).

UTI in Newborns

No trials compare antibiotic prophylaxis versus no treatment for newborns with prenatally diagnosed anomalies, including ureteroceles or ectopic ureters.

One small series of neonates with prenatal ureterocele reported that 53 % had UTI with no difference in those with versus without antibiotic prophylaxis.

A study in which newborns with ureteroceles with VUR were punctured and those without VUR observed found breakthrough UTI in 8 % of both groups by age 6 months.

Another series that used antibiotic prophylaxis in newborns with ureterocele or ectopic ureter without VUR reported that 42 % developed fUTI at median 3 months of age.

No trial has compared antibiotic prophylaxis versus no treatment in neonates with prenatally detected ureterocele or ectopic ureter.

Retrospective review concerned 15 neonates, 13 females, with prenatally detected ureterocele that was duplex in 14 cases and associated with VUR in 10. Of these, 10 were evaluated within the first week of life, 3 in the second, and 1 at 3 and 6 weeks each. FUTI occurred in seven (47 %) due to *E. coli* ($n=6$) and *S. aureus*, in three despite prophylactic antibiotics (medication not stated). There was no difference in UTI in those with versus without antibiotic (43 % vs. 62.5 %, $p=0.6$) (Besson et al. 2000).

Another retrospective study involved 72 neonates with prenatally detected duplex system ureteroceles all treated from birth with antibiotic prophylaxis (medication not stated). Of these, 32 had endoscopic puncture at a median age of 5 days, while the other 40 were initially observed but had open surgery at ≤6 months of age (median 3 months, 2–6). UTI occurred after puncture and before age 6 months in 3/32 (9 %) in 1 with bladder outlet obstruction from incomplete decompression, and in 3/40 (8 %) with delayed intervention (Husmann et al. 2002).

The protocol used by Han et al. (2005) described above reported that 3/11 (27 %) neonates with duplex ureteroceles selected for nonsurgical management in part because they were considered to be at low risk for infection had breakthrough UTI, despite antibiotic prophylaxis at median time 11 months.

The ten patients observed by Direnna and Leonard (2006) described above, with 6 duplex and 4 single-system ureteroceles, reported no breakthrough UTI during mean follow-up of 3 years. Antibiotic prophylaxis was used in all for a mean of 1.5 years.

Retrospective review of consecutive neonates treated with a systematic protocol included 12 prenatally detected with duplex ectopic ureter or ureterocele without VUR and initially treated with antibiotic prophylaxis (medication not stated). Five (42 %) developed breakthrough fUTI at median age 3 months (2–8), three with ectopic ureter and 2 with ureterocele (Prieto et al. 2009).

Endoscopic Management of Ureterocele

Secondary surgery after ureterocele puncture is reported more likely with extravesical ureteroceles, duplex systems, and pre-puncture VUR.

One retrospective comparison of puncture versus upper pole heminephrectomy for duplex ureterocele with no VUR reported secondary surgery more likely after puncture, mostly for new VUR.

Indications for secondary surgery often are not reported.

Systematic literature review was done to determine secondary operation rates after ureterocele puncture, reporting additional surgery was more likely with:

- Extravesical ureterocele, RR 2.8 (95 % CI 2.06–3.74).
- Duplex system, RR 3.9 (95 % CI 1.14–10.93).
- Pre-puncture VUR, RR 1.56 (95 % CI 1.24–1.96).

The authors used secondary surgery as the endpoint, but indications for both initial puncture and subsequent surgery were not always reported in reviewed articles (Byun and Merguerian 2006).

Retrospective review was done in 52 children, 42 % female, undergoing ureterocele puncture done at median age 3 months (1 month–12 years). This series dated from 1984 to 2001, and only 12 (23 %) had prenatal diagnosis, while the others presented after UTI. Ninety-two percent had ureteral duplication, and the 52 cases were classified as intravesical in 73 % and extravesical in 27 %. Antibiotic prophylaxis (not described) was used for all with VUR until resolution. Preoperative and postoperative nuclear renography was done (postoperative time interval not stated). Nonfunctioning upper poles ($n=10$) or kidneys ($n=9$) were removed. Median follow-up was 9 years (6 months–18 years):

- Poor function in the upper pole ($n=25$) did not improve, and normal to moderately impaired function did not decrease after puncture and during follow-up ("moderate" and "poor" were not defined; actual data not shown).
- No patient with poor function had pyelonephritis.
- VUR spontaneously resolved in 59 % of affected renal units; others mostly had endoscopic correction. Indication for VUR treatment was not stated.
- No patient had incontinence.
- No patient had infection after puncture (Chertin et al. 2003).

Another retrospective series included 60 children, 68 % female, with ureteroceles treated with puncture: duplex in 51 that was intravesical in 22 and extravesical in 29, and single system in nine with intravesical ureterocele. Thirty-two (52 %) presented before 3 months of age, and 31 (52 %) were prenatally detected, while 29 (48 %) had fUTI. With follow-up a mean of 20 months (4–62), 19 (32 %) had additional surgery.

- None of the nine single-system ureteroceles had additional surgery, and of four of nine with new VUR after puncture, three resolved.
- Of 51 duplex ureteroceles, 19 had secondary surgery, including seven (14 %) with "persistent VUR and infection."

Otherwise, indications for secondary surgery were not described (Hagg et al. 2000).

A third retrospective series of 28 patients with duplex ureterocele and no VUR that underwent puncture reported new VUR in 16 (57 %) and persistent obstruction in 2 (7 %). During follow-up a median of 2 years (3 months–6 years), reimplantation was done in 12 for breakthrough UTI or persistent reflux. Compared to partial nephrectomy in patients with similar preoperative findings (duplex ectopic ureterocele and no VUR), puncture was significantly more likely to result in further surgery or persisting VUR, 64 % versus 15 % (see below) (Husmann et al. 1999).

Upper Tract Surgery for Ureterocele and Ectopic Ureter

Retrospective series report secondary surgery in <20 % for VUR or symptomatic remnant upper pole stumps (see below).

In a retrospective review, 26 patients with duplex ureterocele and no VUR had partial nephrectomy as initial therapy. New lower pole VUR occurred in eight (30 %), which then resolved in 4 and led to reimplantation in 4 (15 %) due to breakthrough UTI during median follow-up of 2 years (1–4). These outcomes were compared to puncture in similar patients, and it was concluded that heminephrectomy results in fewer secondary operations (see section above) (Husmann et al. 1999).

Another review included 29 patients with 30 ureteroceles, six with VUR, who underwent upper pole heminephrectomy ($n=29$) or pyelopyelostomy and then had follow-up for a mean of 25 months (9–30). New VUR occurred in 4 and then resolved in 3, and 4 (14 %) others developed breakthrough UTI leading to lower tract surgery (Gomes et al. 2002).

An upper tract approach was used in 31 duplex systems with ectopic ureters in 30 females and one male as newborns to age 17 years. Of these, 23 systems were considered on various imaging studies (IVP, CT, nuclear renography) to have poor or no function and had heminephrectomy, while the other eight had "sufficient function to warrant salvage" (not defined) and so had high ureteroureterstomy or ureteroplyelostomy. The orifice of the ectopic ureter was identified in 19 (58 %), at the bladder neck or urethra in 15, and vagina or vestibule in 4. During follow-up a mean of 4.5 years (8 months–10 years), 3 (10 %) had fUTI leading to remnant stump removal (subsequent clinical course not described), and 1 had pain with voiding, resulting in stump removal (see below). Preoperative VUR occurred in nine (29 %), into the ipsilateral lower pole in 5 and contralateral in 4. One of these had reimplantation for "persistent reflux," while outcomes of VUR in the others were not stated (Plaire et al. 1997).

Laparoscopic heminephrectomy was done in 17 consecutive patients with 19 affected units having ectopic ureter ($n=8$) or ureterocele ($n=7$), of which three had lower pole VUR. Follow-up was a mean of 57 months (8–115), during which time lower pole VUR resolved in 3/4 units. The only infections involved the stump and occurred in three patients (18 %) leading to removal. One patient had loss of function to the remaining lower pole. Two of seven with ureteroceles had persistent, but smaller, ureteroceles that were asymptomatic (Denes et al. 2007).

Lower Tract Surgery for Ureterocele

Ureterocele excision or unroofing with reimplantation, sometimes following prior puncture, resulted in new or persistent VUR in 12 %, reported by two series.

Postoperative fUTI was reported in 0–10 %. Complications from retained upper pole segments did not occur.

Fifty-seven patients, 94 % female, at mean age approximately 28 months, underwent ureterocele surgery at three institutions by four surgeons based on their preference. Thirty-nine (68 %) had prior puncture, and operations comprised ureterocele excision or unroofing and ureteral reimplantation. During mean follow-up of 55 months (6–234), new VUR occurred in seven (12 %) and fUTI in six (11 %), of which two had reflux. Outcomes for the new VUR were not described (Lewis et al. 2008).

A review was done in 16 children, 15 females, with duplex ureteroceles and nonfunctioning upper poles who had lower tract reconstruction without upper pole excision at two institutions. Thirteen had prior puncture, and all had ureterocele excision, bladder neck reconstruction, and reimplantation. Follow-up was a mean of 62 months (33–127). VUR was found in 2 (12.5 %), 1 observed and the other not further described, and there were no fUTIs. The retained nonfunctioning upper pole moiety did not cause hypertension or other recognized complication (Gran et al. 2005).

Another review included 31 children, 28 females, mean age 30 months (19 days–10 years) with duplex ectopic ureters. Twelve with functioning upper poles (visualization in IVP) had ureteral reimplantation of the ectopic ureter, while 18 with non-visualization had upper pole heminephrectomy; one kidney had no function. During follow-up a mean of 66 months (6 months–20 years), one patient in each treatment group had recurrent UTI (not otherwise described). None had incontinence, and none with reimplantation had further surgery (El Ghoneimi et al. 1996).

Simultaneous Upper and Lower Tract Reconstruction for Ureterocele

One study reported secondary surgery after "complete" reconstruction in 6 % of patients.

Retrospective review was done in 18 patients with 20 ureteroceles who all had VUR and underwent upper heminephrectomy ($n=11$) or upper pole ureteral tailoring ($n=9$) and ureterocele excision, bladder neck reconstruction, and cross-trigonal reimplantation. Duration of follow-up was not stated (mean 33 months for all patients in the series); new contralateral VUR occurred in 1, and two patients had postoperative complications, including bilateral obstruction after bilateral reimplantation and one requiring intermittent catheterization. There was no mention of postoperative UTI; 1 (6 %) patient had reoperation (not further described) (Gomes et al. 2002).

Ureteroureterostomy

Two series using different inclusion criteria reported secondary surgery in <10 % of children after ureteroureterstomy (UU).

Of 142 children undergoing surgery for duplex ureters, 39 (17 %), 86 % females, underwent 41 UUs. There were five with ectopic ureter and four with ureterocele who only had UU. Nine others with ectopic ureters with lower pole reflux had UU and reimplantation, as did another 12 with prior ureterocele puncture. The remaining patients had lower pole reflux without ectopic ureter or ureterocele. Mean follow-up was 12 months (3–34). Two cases of new contralateral VUR were corrected with endoscopic injection, as was one of two cases with ipsilateral persistent VUR, comprising secondary interventions in 8 %. There was no mention of postoperative UTI and "all showed improvement of dilation" on ultrasound (Chacko et al. 2007).

Another review included 23 consecutive children, (74 %) female, and 26 duplex systems with ectopic ureter ($n=18$) or ureterocele ($n=8$) and no lower pole reflux, who represented 37 % of patients with these conditions operated during a 4-year study period. Median patient age was 10 months (2–56), and two of seven patients with ureteroceles had prior puncture with resultant upper pole reflux. Mean follow-up was 26 months (2–48). Preoperative upper pole hydronephrosis occurred in 22 ureters and was SFU grades 3 and 4 in 13 (50 %); postoperative ultrasound at 12 weeks showed resolution ($n=17$) or reduction to grade 2 or less in all ureters. One patient had fUTI and was found to have new grade 1 ipsilateral VUR treated with endoscopic injection, for secondary surgery rate of 4 % (Prieto et al. 2009).

Renal Function

Our review found only two studies mentioning renal functional outcomes. One stated that 8 % of patients had a decrease >10 % in renographic differential renal function after heminephrectomy.

From a retrospective review of 101 patients with heminephrectomy renal function, data were available in 60, of which 42 had upper pole (ureterocele in 20) and 18 lower pole excision. Mean age at operation was 44 months, and follow-up was a mean of 25 months (3–64). Preoperative and postoperative MAG-3 or DMSA scans were obtained (date of postoperative study not stated). Mean preoperative differential function was 40 % (22–61 %), and 33 % (13–60 %) postoperatively (statistical analysis not reported). Five (8 %) had a decrease >10 %—one who had recurrent postoperative UTI and without known reason in others (Gundeti et al. 2005).

The retrospective study by Gran et al. (2005) described above, in which bladder but not renal level surgery was done, reported that no patient had loss of renal function by nuclear renography, but timing of studies and resultant data were not stated or shown.

Histology of Nonfunctioning Renal Segments

Histology of resected upper pole segments was reported in two studies to most often demonstrate inflammatory changes or dysplasia.

Retrospective review of the upper pole was done in 50 consecutive heminephrectomy specimens related to ureterocele ($n=30$) or ectopic ureter. Twenty-five demonstrated nonspecific inflammatory findings in the interstitial tissues, chronic inflammatory changes with collecting system involvement in 15, microabscesses in 3, xanthogranulomatous pyelonephritis in 2, and dysplasia (parenchymal disorganization with cysts, primitive ducts, cartilage) in 30 with nephroblastomatosis in 1. Only one was interpreted as normal. There were no apparent differences in patients with antenatal versus postnatal diagnosis, but age at surgery and presurgical morbidities, including fUTI, were not described. The implication of these findings, however, was that there was little expectation that earlier diagnosis and treatment would significantly improve upper pole findings (Abel et al. 1997).

The 16 upper pole specimens with ectopic ureters removed for non-visualization on IVP by El Ghoneimi et al. (1996) as described above demonstrated "lesions of chronic pyelonephritis" in 13 and "focal lesions of dysplasia" in 4.

The practice of routinely removing upper poles based on such histologic findings was challenged by a review article that addressed association of renal dysplasia to UTI, hypertension, and tumor potential and concluded that occurrence of these is so rare that it does not support extirpation (Husmann 1998).

Continence

One study reported no postoperative incontinence after surgery for ectopic ureter.

Of the 28 females with duplex ectopic ureters reported by El Ghoneimi et al. (1996) above, the upper pole ureter entered the bladder neck in six, posterior urethra in 5, vagina in seven, vestibule in six, and was unclear in 4. Preoperative incontinence occurred in 13 (46 %), corrected in all cases by either upper pole reimplantation or heminephrectomy.

Of 31 duplex systems with ectopic ureters in 30 females and one male reported by Plaire et al. (Plaire et al. 1997) above, the orifice of the ectopic ureter was identified in 19 (58 %), at the bladder neck or urethra in 15, and vagina or vestibule in 4. The authors did not mention postoperative incontinence.

Bladder Dysfunction

There are no reliable data to determine if children with ureteroceles and ectopic ureters have increased bladder dysfunction compared to normal children.

A retrospective series analyzed 34 children, 79 % females, after ureterocele management. Eighteen (53 %) had extravesical ureteroceles. Median age at surgery was 10 months (3–101) and involved heminephrectomy for ten, ureterocele excision and reimplantation in six, both upper and lower tract surgery in 15, and no incision or no treatment in 3. Of these, 32 had bladder function assessment at median 5 years of age (1–12). Infrequent voiding <4×/daily was diagnosed in 19 (59 %). Another three (9 %) had incontinence, none with prior bladder surgery, including one with a persistent ureterocele. Two (6 %) used CIC because of "high" PVR. UD was done in 27 children, with 55 % having measured capacity >150 % predicted for age and 11 % detrusor instability; all had normal compliance and mean PVR was 12 cc. Uroflow pattern was stated to be normal in all cases. The authors considered only eight (25 %) to have normal bladder function defined as normal capacity and PVR <5 cc, but they did not correlate factors they considered abnormal to clinical symptoms or complications, such as UTI (Abrahamsson et al. 1998).

The four-surgeon series with ureterocele excision and reimplantation by Lewis et al. (2008) described above reported voiding dysfunction (infrequent voiding, holding maneuvers, urgency) postoperatively in 11 (20 %). One other child had incontinence, possibly due to bladder neck dysfunction.

Symptomatic Stumps

Three retrospective series report removal of the remnant "stump" after partial upper pole ureterectomy in from 7 to 18 %, mostly due to UTI.

None reported postoperative UTI occurrence after stump excision.

Stump removal was done in 4 (7 %) of 55 patients with duplex ureters with ureterocele, ectopia, and/or VUR who underwent upper pole heminephrectomy as described by Ade-Ajayi et al. (2001) above. All had recurrent UTI (not described), but follow-up after removal and UTI occurrence, if any, in other patients with stumps was not stated.

Of the 32 patients described by Plaire et al. (1997) with duplex ectopic ureters who all had upper tract surgery (heminephrectomy in 23 and reconstruction in eight), 4 (12 %) had secondary surgery to remove the remnant stump, 1 during a reimplantation for persistent lower pole reflux, 1 for pain during voiding, and two for fUTI.

Laparoscopic heminephrectomy was done in 17 consecutive patients with 19 affected units having ectopic ureter ($n=8$) or ureterocele ($n=7$). Follow-up was a mean of 57 months (8–115), during which time infections involved the stump in three patients (18 %) and were removed (Denes et al. 2007).

References

Abel C, Lendon M, Gough DC. Histology of the upper pole in complete urinary duplication–does it affect surgical management? Br J Urol. 1997;80(4):663–5.

Abrahamsson K, Hansson E, Sillen U, Hermansson G, Hjalmas K. Bladder dysfunction: an integral part of the ectopic ureterocele complex. J Urol. 1998;160(4):1468–70.

Ade-Ajayi N, Wilcox DT, Duffy PG, Ransley PG. Upper pole heminephrectomy: is complete ureterectomy necessary? BJU Int. 2001;88(1):77–9.

Besson R, Ngoc BT, Laboure S, Debeugny P. Incidence of urinary tract infection in neonates with antenatally diagnosed ureteroceles. Eur J Pediatr Surg. 2000;10(2):111–3.

Byun E, Merguerian PA. A meta-analysis of surgical practice patterns in the endoscopic management of ureteroceles. J Urol. 2006;176(4 Pt 2):1871–7. discussion 7.

Chacko JK, Koyle MA, Mingin GC, Furness 3rd PD. Ipsilateral ureteroureterostomy in the surgical management of the severely dilated ureter in ureteral duplication. J Urol. 2007;178(4 Pt 2):1689–92.

Chertin B, de Caluwe D, Puri P. Is primary endoscopic puncture of ureterocele a long-term effective procedure? J Pediatr Surg. 2003;38(1):116–9. discussion 116–9.

Denes FT, Danilovic A, Srougi M. Outcome of laparoscopic upper-pole nephrectomy in children with duplex systems. J Endourol. 2007;21(2):162–8.

Direnna T, Leonard MP. Watchful waiting for prenatally detected ureteroceles. J Urol. 2006;175(4):1493–5. discussion 5.

el Ghoneimi A, Miranda J, Truong T, Monfort G. Ectopic ureter with complete ureteric duplication: conservative surgical management. J Pediatr Surg. 1996;31(4):467–72.

Gomes J, Mendes M, Castro R, Reis A. Current role of simplified upper tract approach in the surgical treatment of ectopic ureteroceles: a single centre's experience. Eur Urol. 2002;41(3):323–7.

Gran CD, Kropp BP, Cheng EY, Kropp KA. Primary lower urinary tract reconstruction for nonfunctioning renal moieties associated with obstructing ureteroceles. J Urol. 2005;173(1):198–201.

Gundeti MS, Ransley PG, Duffy PG, Cuckow PM, Wilcox DT. Renal outcome following heminephrectomy for duplex kidney. J Urol. 2005;173(5):1743–4.

Hagg MJ, Mourachov PV, Snyder HM, Canning DA, Kennedy WA, Zderic SA, et al. The modern endoscopic approach to ureterocele. J Urol. 2000;163(3):940–3.

Han MY, Gibbons MD, Belman AB, Pohl HG, Majd M, Rushton HG. Indications for nonoperative management of ureteroceles. J Urol. 2005;174(4 Pt 2):1652–5. discussion 5–6.

Husmann DA. Renal dysplasia: the risks and consequences of leaving dysplastic tissue in situ. Urology. 1998;52(4):533–6.

Husmann D, Strand B, Ewalt D, Clement M, Kramer S, Allen T. Management of ectopic ureterocele associated with renal duplication: a comparison of partial nephrectomy and endoscopic decompression. J Urol. 1999;162(4):1406–9.

Husmann DA, Strand WR, Ewalt DH, Kramer SA. Is endoscopic decompression of the neonatal extravesical upper pole ureterocele necessary for prevention of urinary tract infections or bladder neck obstruction? J Urol. 2002;167(3):1440–2.

Lewis JM, Cheng EY, Campbell JB, Kropp BP, Liu DB, Kropp K, et al. Complete excision or marsupialization of ureteroceles: does choice of surgical approach affect outcome? J Urol. 2008;180 Suppl 4Suppl 4:1819–22. discussion 22–3.

Plaire JC, Pope JC, Kropp BP, Adams MC, Keating MA, Rink RC, et al. Management of ectopic ureters: experience with the upper tract approach. J Urol. 1997;158(3 Pt 2):1245–7.

Prieto J, Ziada A, Baker L, Snodgrass W. Ureteroureterostomy via inguinal incision for ectopic ureters and ureteroceles without ipsilateral lower pole reflux. J Urol. 2009;181(4):1844–8. discussion 8–50.

Shankar KR, Vishwanath N, Rickwood AM. Outcome of patients with prenatally detected duplex system ureterocele; natural history of those managed expectantly. J Urol. 2001;165(4):1226–8.

14 Non-refluxing Megaureter

Patricio C. Gargollo and Warren T. Snodgrass

The primary goal in diagnosing and treating non-refluxing megaureters is to prevent ipsilateral renal function loss.

Secondary goals are to minimize associated comorbidities, including febrile UTI (fUTI) and pain.

A summary of evidence for these aims is presented:

Loss of ipsilateral renal function during observation was reported in ≤10 % of megaureters.

Recurrent obstruction occurs in <10 % after surgical repair.

Reported UTIs were generally not characterized as febrile versus nonfebrile:

- **Although most patients were males, no study reported circumcision status.**
- **All reviews of observation patients reported antibiotic prophylaxis in most or all patients during the first year of life.**
- **UTI incidence during observation varied from 6 to 71 %.**
- **No study randomized patients to prophylaxis or no treatment; no study related UTI occurrence to circumcision status, initial presentation with UTI or not, extent of hydronephrosis (HN), or renography drainage patterns.**
- **The review reporting the highest occurrence of UTI during observation, with 57 % of patients initially diagnosed following UTI, reported that prophylaxis reduced infections.**
- **Surgical series did not systematically report UTI occurrence postoperatively.**

One review found abdominal and/or flank pain as the presenting complaint in 16 % of diagnosed megaureters in children at a mean age of 6 years. Pain did not recur after surgery, or in those selected for observation.

Observation

Spontaneous resolution of non-refluxing megaureters was reported in between 34 and 72 % at a mean time ranging from 1.5 to 4 years in four retrospective studies.

Generally, initial distal ureteral diameter <1 cm predicted greater likelihood for resolution. Two studies reported that no ureter with initial diameter >15 mm resolved spontaneously.

One study reported 9 % of observed megaureters had renal functional loss from a mean 45–33 %, all within 6 months.

All reported antibiotic prophylaxis in some or all patients, especially in the first year of life. Reported UTI (not characterized as febrile vs. nonfebrile) widely ranged from 6 to 71 %.

None reported pain or other symptoms.

Surgical rates for various indications, including UTI, decreased function, increased HN, and solitary kidney, were 16–23 %.

P.C. Gargollo, M.D. • W.T. Snodgrass, M.D. (✉)
Department of Pediatric Urology, University of Texas Southwestern Medical Center and Children's Medical Center Dallas, 1935 Medical District Drive, MS F4.04, Dallas, TX 75235, USA
e-mail: warren.snodgrass@childrens.com

W.T. Snodgrass (ed.), *Pediatric Urology: Evidence for Optimal Patient Management*,
DOI 10.1007/978-1-4614-6910-0_14, © Springer Science+Business Media New York 2013

A retrospective study included 60 neonates, 80 % males, diagnosed with 72 non-refluxing megaureters defined as dilation of the distal ureter >6 mm by initial US and negative VCUG. Cases were detected by prenatal US (80 %) or by neonatal US done for other reasons. These patients received antibiotic prophylaxis for 12 months, and follow-up renal US at 3-month intervals for 1 year and then every 6 months. DTPA renography was done two times the first year and then annually. Resolution was defined as a distal ureter <6 mm. Surgical indications were "symptomatic" UTI despite prophylaxis, decrease renal function to <40 % or >10 % initial value, and solitary kidney. Mean follow-up for conservatively managed patients was 5 years (6 months–15 years):

- Mean presenting HN grade was 4±1 (based on possible five grades modified from SFU scale); mean initial ureteral diameter was 13±5 mm (6–22).
- Initial renogram diuretic drainage (reported as T 75, time for 75 % clearance) was <5 min in 58 %, 5–10 min in 28 %, and >10 min in 14 %.
- Resolution occurred in 38 ureters (53 %) at mean time 2 years (6 months–8 years).
- Megaureter persisted in 18 (25 %), including 10 not changed from initial assessment and 8 with decreased ureteral diameter still >6 mm.
- Surgery was done in 16 (22 %) at mean age 17 months (6–48); specific indications were not stated.

Time to resolution significantly increased with increasing initial HN grade; initial mean ureteral diameter of 9.5±2 mm in the group that resolved was significantly less than the 15.6±4.5 mm in the persisting group and the 16.7±3 mm in the surgical group. No case with diameter >15 mm resolved. Surgery was not done for any ureter with T75 <5 min, and for 30 % and 80 % of those with 5–10 and >10 min. No observed patient had renal function loss as defined (Arena et al. 2012).

Retrospective analysis was also done in 53 patients (66 % males) with prenatal US abnormalities found postnatally to have 67 dilated ureters due to presumed UVJO. Mean cross-sectional diameter of the ureter adjacent to the bladder on the first US was 8±4 mm. All had VCUG excluding VUR or PUV, and DTPA renography at age 1 month. All were prescribed antibiotic prophylaxis with trimethoprim for the first year of life. Mean follow-up was 3 years:

- Twenty three (34 %) megaureters resolved at a mean 1.6 years.
- Eleven (16 %) had surgical correction for UTI in 3, poor function (10 %) or solitary kidney in 2, and for decreased renal function in 6 followed ≤12 months, with initial mean function 45 % (39–56 %) decreasing to mean 33 % (26–39 %). Renal function was regained in half.
- Of 53 ureters with diameter <1 cm, 23 (43 %) resolved; of 14 ureters with diameter >1 cm, 0 resolved.
- Of 52 ureters with T1/2 ≤10 min, 22 (42 %) resolved; of 15 with T1/2 >10 min, 1 (7 %) resolved (Liu et al. 1994).

Another retrospective review identified 54 newborns, 67 % males, with abnormal prenatal US found to have 69 non-refluxing megaureter between 1993 and 1998. Antibiotic prophylaxis was given during the first year of life. Median follow-up was 26 months (2–72):

- Thirty nine patients (72 %) resolved.
- Ten patients (19 %) had surgical repair at mean age 10 months (4–25) for increasing HN in 3, "obstructive appearance on IVP" in 2, decreased renal function (31–22 %) in 1, high-grade HN in 2, solitary kidney in 1, and acute renal failure in 1.
- Median distal ureteral diameter on first US was 0.8 cm in those that resolved versus 1.1 cm in those with surgery, $p=0.04$ (McLellan et al. 2002).

A fourth retrospective study described outcomes in 49 children, 71 % males, with 56 non-refluxing megaureters. Of these, 20 were diagnosed prenatally while the others presented at a mean of 10 months (all but 1 with UTI). There were 35 (71 %) males. HN was SFU grade 1 in 10, grade 2 in 39, grade 3 in 5, and grade 4 in 1. Mean follow-up was 47 months (12–78):

- Fifty percent of megaureters resolved during observation; including all with ureteral diameter <8.5 mm versus 0 with >15 mm.
- Resolution was not predicted by initial HN grade or renogram washout.

- Thirteen (23 %) had surgery, four as initial therapy and nine for "later deterioration" (not defined).
- Six (11 %) had renal function <40 % at last follow-up, all with impaired function on initial scan (data not shown).
- Thirty-five (71 %) patients had UTI, with 36 % having more than two episodes (subjects were German, and males likely were not circumcised).
- Antibiotic prophylaxis reduced UTI incidence by 55 % (7 UTIs/199 patient months with vs. 19 UTIs/244 patient months without prophylaxis, or 0.4 vs. 0.9 UTIs/year, $p<0.05$). Prophylaxis seemed most beneficial in the first 6 months of life. Neither UTI occurrence nor prophylaxis use was described in those detected prenatally versus the 57 % who were diagnosed after UTI (Gimpel et al. 2010).

Dietl's Crisis

One review found that 16 % of diagnosed megaureters presented with pain.

A review was done of all patients diagnosed with megaureter from 1993 to 2009, from which 103 with primary megaureter (including patients with refluxing megaureter) were identified. Of these, 17 children (16 %) with 20 megaureters presented with acute pain at median age of 77 months (40–208). The authors then focused on the 10 who specifically had ipsilateral flank pain. Renography in eight showed function >40 % in all cases and variable drainage patterns: five with T1/2 >20 min, one "indeterminate," and two with "no obstruction." Cystography demonstrated no VUR. Repair was done in six patients with resolution or improvement in HN (not described) who then had follow-up a median of 54 months (33–99) without recurrent pain. Four children (two diagnosed with obstructed and two with non-obstructed megaureters) were initially observed for a median of 9 months (6–28), with one lost to follow-up, one demonstrating increasing HN (not described) leading to surgery, and two with stable or decreased HN and no pain continuing observation (Anderson et al. 2012).

Surgery

Three studies reported minimally invasive techniques, including double-J stenting alone, balloon dilation with stenting, and endoureterotomy, successfully resolved or decreased HN in from 50 to 70 % of ureters with mean follow-up of 3 years. None reported systematic posttreatment cystography.

In retrospective studies of ureteral plication, folding, or excisional tapering with reimplantation, all report reduction in HN with risk <10 % for postoperative obstruction.

Occurrence of postoperative UTI, if any, was not routinely stated, and those reported were not characterized as febrile or not.

Double-J Stenting

Stenting ≥6 months was reported successful in nearly 50 % of ureters in one study.

A retrospective review was done for 31 nonrefluxing megaureters that had double-J stent (3–4.7 Fr) placed as curative therapy without surgery. Median age at stent placement was 37 months (2 months–15 years); indications were progressive HN on serial US (not further described) in 20, decrease in renal function to <40 % in 7, and pyonephrosis or other symptoms in 4. Degree of HN and distal ureteral diameter were not reported. Duration of stenting was ≥6 months. Median follow-up subsequently was 39 months (24–110):

- Complications during stenting occurred in six (19 %)—two with UTIs and four with gross hematuria treated with tranexamic acid.
- Fifteen (48 %) units resolved HN.
- Fifteen had recurrent HN. Seven were treated with repeated stenting, of which five were successful.
- Eleven (35 %) had reimplant.

Stenting was accomplished in 36/38 attempts (95 %), with one resulting in perforation and reimplantation. Duration of time for recurrent HN to develop after initial stenting was not stated (Carroll et al. 2010).

Balloon Dilation

Balloon dilation with 8 weeks stenting for distal narrowed ureteral segments <2 cm, or combined with ureterotomy for segments 2–3 cm, was reported successful in 71 %.

Balloon dilation ± laser endoureterotomy was done in 17 non-refluxing megaureters at mean age 7 years (3–12). Retrograde pyelography defined the length of the distal narrowed segment, with those <2 cm undergoing balloon dilation ($n = 12$, 71 %), those 2–3 cm having dilation plus laser ureterotomy at 12 O'clock ($n = 5$), and those >3 cm reimplanted. All endoscopic cases were stented using two 4.7-Fr pigtail stents for 8 weeks. There were no perioperative or stent complications. Preoperative extent of HN and distal ureteral diameters were not reported; postoperatively, 12 (71 %) had "significant improvement" on US (not defined). Five had magnetic resonance urography when HN persisted, and were considered non-obstructed. Posttreatment cystography was not done. Follow-up was a mean of 3 years (2–6) (Christman et al. 2012).

Endoureterotomy

One study found endoureterotomy to be successful in 71 % of cases with distal narrowed segment <1.5 cm.

Fifty two non-refluxing megaureters with a distal narrowed segment <1.5 cm had endoureterotomy at 6 O'clock extending through the ureteral wall to detrusor muscle and double-J stent for 1 week. Success was defined as resolution of HN (or "mild pelvis fullness ± minor lower-ureteral dilation") and stable or improved renal function. Mean follow-up was 39 months (14–62), with 37 (71 %) considered successful and 10 (19 %) improved. There was no VUR postoperatively, but also any mention of postoperative cystography in the follow-up protocol. A second endoureterotomy was done in 6, and was successful in 5 (apparently counted among the 47 resolved or improved cases), while the other had reimplantation. Five (10 %) ureters needed open surgery for inability to place a ureteral stent to perform the procedure ($n = 3$), postoperative obstruction ($n = 1$), or recurrent UTI ($n = 1$). Renal functional data were not reported, nor were distal ureteral diameters (Kajbafzadeh et al. 2007).

End Cutaneous Ureterostomy

One study of end cutaneous ureterostomy as initial therapy in non-refluxing megaureter did not report preoperative extent of ureteral dilation. At reimplantation, 31 % were tapered.

fUTI occurred in 40 %.

A retrospective review was done to identify patients who had end cutaneous ureterostomy, 15 with primary megaureter (refluxing vs. nonrefluxing not stated; 2 had duplicated systems with lower pole VUR and upper pole obstruction). Age at diversion was not stated for this cohort. During diversion, six (40 %) had fUTI with positive cultures from the ureterostomy (time interval after diversion to UTI or recurrent UTI was not stated). None showed increasing HN. At take down of the ureterostomy done in 13 cases, 4 (31 %) were tapered. Size of distal ureter before end cutaneous ureteroscopy was not stated (Kitchens et al. 2007).

Plication

Two studies reported no obstructive complications, and one noted 6 % VUR after plication and reimplantation.

Over 50 % of renal units still demonstrated HN, in one including those with SFU grades ≥2.

One reported return of renal function loss in 50 % of those affected, while the other stated that mean function was unchanged by surgery.

Renogram drainage was reported improved or normal after surgery, but data were not shown.

Eleven of 67 megaureters managed by Liu et al. (1994) described above had surgical correction for breakthrough UTI in 3 at mean age 9 months, for poor function (10 %) or solitary kidney in 2, and for decreased renal function in 6 at mean age 6 months, with initial mean function 45 % (39–56 %) decreasing to mean 33 %

(26–39 %). Repair included excision of the distal aperistaltic segment, Starr plication, and cross-trigonal reimplantation. Postoperative UTIs were not described; decreased renal function in eight was regained in four and stable in four. There was persistent HN in 55 % (not described), but improved renogram drainage (not described). The authors stated that there were no postoperative complications. Indirect nuclear cystography was done postoperatively to evaluate for VUR, but results were not stated.

Retrospective analysis was done in 17 non-refluxing megaureters operated by distal segment excision and cross-trigonal reimplantation with or without Starr plication. Indications were impaired renogram drainage (not defined) in 11, fUTI in 4, failure to thrive in 1, and increasing HN in 1 (not described). The postoperative assessments described below were done at 3 months:

- Preoperative HN was SFU grade 1 in 2, grade 2 in 7, grade 3 in 7, and grade 4 in 1. After surgery, HN was SFU grade 0–1 in 6, grade 2 in 9, and grade 3 in 2; there was a reduction in 13, and 4 were unchanged.
- Preoperative median ureteral diameter by US was 11 mm (6–24); postoperatively, the distal ureter was not detected in 14 and was "greatly reduced" in 3.
- Preoperative renal function was normal (median 50 %, range 43–54 %) in 15 kidneys and 40 % in two kidneys; postoperative function was not described except to state that there was no significant change in mean renal function.
- Preoperative renogram drainage was "impaired" in 11 (65 %), described as T1/2 >15 min in 7 or "retention of >30 % isotope" 30 min after furosamide in 8 (disparity between 11 impaired kidneys vs. these 15 with delayed drainage was not explained); postoperative renograms were all stated to be normal.
- Postoperative UTIs occurred in two patients; the infant with poor feeding improved.
- No ureter developed obstruction after surgery, and one (6 %) had VUR (assessment done by either direct or indirect cystography; numbers of each not stated) (Aksnes et al. 2002).

Ureteral Folding

One report stated that ureteral folding with reimplantation significantly reduced distal ureteral diameter, with only one (4 %) obstruction. Mean preoperative ureteral diameter was 19 mm.

Technical results of distal segment excision and Kalicinski ureteral folding with Leadbetter–Politano reimplantation were reported in 26 non-refluxing megaureters. All were stented with a 6- to 8-Fr catheter for 1 week. One (4 %) developed postoperative stenosis leading to reoperation. Preoperative distal ureteral diameter was a significantly greater mean 19 mm versus 5 mm postoperatively (Perdzynski and Kalicinski 1996).

Excisional Tapering

A study of excisional tapering did not report preoperative ureteral diameter. Resolved or reduced HN without VUR was achieved in 87 %.

A retrospective study considered 31 patients undergoing excisional tapering of the distally dilated ureter followed by intra- ($n=15$) or extravesical reimplantation ($n=16$) based on surgeon preference. Preoperative ureteral diameter was not stated. "Indwelling stents" were used for 4–6 weeks. Follow-up was mean 3.5 years (8 months–12 years). Surgical success was defined as resolved or improved HN and no VUR (time for these evaluations was not stated), achieved in 13 (87 %) and 15 (94 %), $p=0.6$. Changes in HN were not described, nor were problems classified as "failure" in three patients (Defoor et al. 2004).

References

Aksnes G, Imaji R, Dewan PA. Primary megaureter: results of surgical treatment. ANZ J Surg. 2002;72(12):877–80.

Anderson CB, Tanaka ST, Pope JC, Adams MC, Brock 3rd JW, Thomas JC. Acute pain crisis as a presentation of primary megaureter in children. J Pediatr Urol. 2012;8(3):254–7.

Arena S, Magno C, Montalto AS, Russo T, Mami C, Baldari S, et al. Long-term follow-up of neonatally diagnosed primary megaureter: rate and predictors of spontaneous resolution. Scand J Urol Nephrol. 2012;46(3):201–7.

Carroll D, Chandran H, Joshi A, McCarthy LS, Parashar K. Endoscopic placement of double-J ureteric stents in children as a treatment for primary obstructive megaureter. Urol Ann. 2010;2(3):114–8.

Christman MS, Kasturi S, Lambert SM, Kovell RC, Casale P. Endoscopic management and the role of double stenting for primary obstructive megaureters. J Urol. 2012;187(3):1018–22.

DeFoor W, Minevich E, Reddy P, Polsky E, McGregor A, Wacksman J, et al. Results of tapered ureteral reimplantation for primary megaureter: extravesical versus intravesical approach. J Urol. 2004;172(4 Pt 2):1640–3. discussion 3.

Gimpel C, Masioniene L, Djakovic N, Schenk JP, Haberkorn U, Tonshoff B, et al. Complications and long-term outcome of primary obstructive megaureter in childhood. Pediatr Nephrol. 2010;25(9):1679–86.

Kajbafzadeh AM, Payabvash S, Salmasi AH, Arshadi H, Hashemi SM, Arabian S, et al. Endoureterotomy for treatment of primary obstructive megaureter in children. J Endourol. 2007;21(7):743–9.

Kitchens DM, DeFoor W, Minevich E, Reddy P, Polsky E, McGregor A, et al. End cutaneous ureterostomy for the management of severe hydronephrosis. J Urol. 2007;177(4):1501–4.

Liu HY, Dhillon HK, Yeung CK, Diamond DA, Duffy PG, Ransley PG. Clinical outcome and management of prenatally diagnosed primary megaureters. J Urol. 1994;152(2 Pt 2):614–7.

McLellan DL, Retik AB, Bauer SB, Diamond DA, Atala A, Mandell J, et al. Rate and predictors of spontaneous resolution of prenatally diagnosed primary nonrefluxing megaureter. J Urol. 2002;168(5):2177–80. discussion 80.

Perdzynski W, Kalicinski ZH. Long-term results after megaureter folding in children. J Pediatr Surg. 1996;31(9):1211–7.

15 Posterior Urethral Valves and Ureterovesical Junction Obstruction

Warren T. Snodgrass

Primary aims in the diagnosis and management of posterior urethral valves (PUV):

1. **To prevent acquired renal damage.**
2. **To improve bladder function.**

A secondary aim is to facilitate achievement of urinary continence.

Summary of evidence for these goals:

Case series report end-stage renal disease (ESRD) in from 3 to 42 % of patients during mean follow-up ranging from 4 to 12 years:

- **No prenatal finding (oligohydramnios, anamnios, renal hyperechogenicity, loss of corticomedullary differentiation) or fetal urine test accurately predicts postnatal renal function.**
- **Prenatal bladder drainage improves survival but not renal function.**
- **Neither prenatal versus postnatal diagnosis nor age at postnatal diagnosis predicts likelihood for ESRD.**
- **There are conflicting results from retrospective analyses regarding potential risk for CRF/ESRD by vesicoureteral reflux (VUR), recurrent febrile UTI (fUTI), bladder dysfunction, and/or pop-off mechanisms.**

Factors predicting poor renal functional outcomes are nadir creatinine >1 mg/dL and abnormal initial postnatal renal ultrasound with hyperechogenicity, volume loss, and/or loss of corticomedullary differentiation.

There are no reports of longitudinal objective analysis of bladder function after valve ablation:

- **One study compared UD in infants after ablation to control males with UTI, reporting no difference in median maximum voiding pressures.**
- **Three retrospective studies found increased bladder capacity and decreased end filling pressures in bladders after valve ablation versus urinary diversion, but did not account for selection bias.**
- **Continence is reported by age 5 in approximately 20–60 %.**
- **There are few data regarding indications and outcomes for medical bladder therapy in valve patients using anticholinergics, alpha-blockers, and/or CIC.**

One matched cohort study using validated questionnaires reported adult men mean age 37 years with prior valves had 2× greater LUTS than controls.

Prenatal Diagnosis

Despite advances in ultrasound technology, one retrospective study reported high sensitivity to diagnose PUV but low specificity to distinguish valves from bilateral VUR and PBS in male fetuses with bilateral HN. The best indicators were increased bladder thickness and dilation, whereas the keyhole sign was not diagnostic.

W.T. Snodgrass, M.D. (✉)
Department of Pediatric Urology, University of Texas Southwestern Medical Center and Children's Medical Center Dallas, 1935 Medical District Drive, MS F4.04, Dallas, TX 75235, USA
e-mail: warren.snodgrass@childrens.com

W.T. Snodgrass (ed.), *Pediatric Urology: Evidence for Optimal Patient Management*,
DOI 10.1007/978-1-4614-6910-0_15, © Springer Science+Business Media New York 2013

Table 15.1 Prevalence of prenatal ultrasound signs in those fetuses that were postnatally diagnosed with posterior urethral valves (PUV Group, $n=31$) and those that were diagnosed with other pathologies (non-PUV group, $n=23$)[a]

Sign	PUV group (n [%])	Non-PUV group (n [%])	P^{b}
Keyhole sign	16 (51.6)	8 (34.8)	0.27
Bladder dilatation	30 (96.8)	11 (47.8)	<0.0001[c]
Thickened bladder wall	29 (93.5)	9 (39.1)	<0.0001[c]
Oligohydramnios	19 (61.3)	7 (30.4)	0.024[c]
Dilated and thick-walled bladder	28 (90.3)	9 (39.1)	0.0001[c]
Dilated and thick-walled bladder with the keyhole sign	14 (45.2)	6 (26.1)	0.18

[a]Reproduced from Bernardes LS, Aksnes G, Saada J, Masse V, Elie C, Dumez Y, et al. Keyhole sign: how specific is it for the diagnosis of posterior urethral valves? Ultrasound Obstet Gynecol. 2009;34(4):419–23, with permission from John Wiley and Sons

[b]For difference between PUV-diagnosed and non-PUV diagnosed groups

[c]Statistically significant

A second retrospective series found prenatal ultrasound to have low sensitivity to detect PUV antenatally.

A retrospective study reviewed prenatal findings in 54 males with bilateral HN between 2000 and 2006 to determine ability to diagnose PUV versus bilateral VUR and PBS. Median gestational age at first diagnosis of HN was similar in those with PUV versus other etiologies (25 weeks [19–36] vs. 23 weeks [12–33]). Forty eight (89 %) had more than one prenatal ultrasound, with a mean of five (1–7). PUV was suspected prenatally in 42, confirmed postnatally in 29 (69 %); PUV was not suspected prenatally in 12, but found postnatally in 2 (17 %). Overall sensitivity and specificity of prenatal evaluation were 94 % (95 % CI 87–99 %) and 43 % (95 % CI 30–57 %). The keyhole sign was found in 52 % of those with PUV versus 35 % without PUV, $p=0.27$. Combinations of ultrasonographic findings are summarized in Table 15.1.

These findings indicate prenatal diagnosis continues to have poor specificity (Bernardes et al. 2009).

Another retrospective review evaluated 34 boys with PUV diagnosed between 1992 and 2004, reporting16 (47 %) had normal prenatal ultrasound. PUV was diagnosed in the other 18 at <24 weeks in 12 and >24 weeks in 6, whereas 6 of 16 not detected had an ultrasound at >24 weeks (Harvie et al. 2009).

Prenatal Assessment of Renal Function

There currently is no prenatal test able to accurately predict postnatal renal function.

A systematic literature review found that no fetal urine test is sufficiently accurate in predicting poor postnatal renal function to be clinically useful.

Three retrospective studies found neither oligohydramnios/anamnios nor abnormal fetal renal appearance (hyperechogenicity, loss of corticomedullary differentiation) correlated with postnatal renal function.

Fetal Urine Analysis

A systematic review of publications concerning accuracy of prenatal urine chemistries to predict poor postnatal renal function in fetuses with congenital bladder outlet obstruction included 23 articles involving 572 women. The two most accurate tests were calcium >95th percentile for gestation (LR+6.65 [0.23–190.96]; LR−0.19 [0.05–0.74]) and sodium >95th percentile for gestation (LR+4.46 [1.71–11.6]; LR−0.39 [0.17–0.88]). Beta (2)-microglobulin was less accurate (LR+2.92 [1.28–6.69]; LR−0.53 [0.24–1.17]). Since fetal urine anlaytes vary through gestation, becoming more hypotonic, results using the 95th percentile were more accurate than absolute thresholds. Nevertheless, the authors conclude that there currently is no accurate urinary analyte to predict poor postnatal renal function (Morris et al. 2007).

Fetal Ultrasound

A retrospective analysis was performed in 31 fetuses with proven PUV. Pregnancy was terminated at a median gestational age of 30 weeks (21–36) in six for oligohydramnios plus adverse biochemical markers. Shunting was not attempted. Of the other 25 delivered, 4 previously had urinary ascites (three undergoing prenatal shunt and the fourth delivered at 33 weeks). All patients underwent valve resection. Outcomes for these 25 with median follow-up of 40 months (12–79) included 1 death at day 16 from renal failure, and 4 (17 %) others with renal impairment (abnormal serum creatinine) at last assessment. Prenatal oligohydramnios/anamnios and timing of its onset did not predict postnatal renal function. Similarly, prenatal renal ultrasonographic features (hyperechogenicity, lack of corticomedullary differentiation) did not predict postnatal serum creatinine. Creatinine was normal in three of the four with prenatal ascites. It was also normal in 10 of 13 with oligohydramnios, including 4 with anamnios. Ten of 11 with bilateral hyperechogenicity had a normal creatinine, as did 7 of 8 with bilateral hyperechogenicity, loss of corticomedullary differentiation, and oligohydramnios (Bernardes et al. 2011).

A retrospective review of 30 patients with PUV diagnosed in utero with postnatal valve ablation and follow-up a mean of 4 years (1–8) reported 6 (20 %) had CRF (serum creatinine >2 SD for age)/ESRD. No prenatal factor predicted poor renal outcomes: diagnosis at gestational age <24 weeks (OR 0.15 [95 % CI 0.88–2.26]), oligohydramnios (OR 0.81 [95 % CI 0.11–5.63]), or hyperechogenic renal cortex (OR 0.25 [95 % CI 0.62–10.14]) (El-Ghoneimi et al. 1999).

Another retrospective review included all liveborn males with PUV and at least one documented prenatal sonogram. There was no mention of prenatal intervention. Valve ablation or vesicostomy with subsequent valve ablation was done postnatally shortly after birth or at diagnosis. There were 34 patients, 18 (53 %) with prenatal diagnosis and 16 with a normal antenatal evaluation. Of those with prenatal detection, no ultrasound parameter (oligohydramnios, HN, renal echogenicity) predicted renal functional outcomes (Harvie et al. 2009).

Prenatal Intervention Versus Observation

One systematic review of published interventions found prenatal bladder drainage improved postnatal survival but not renal function. Results from a RCT of prenatal shunting are pending.

To date no published RCT compares prenatal shunting versus observation in fetuses diagnosed with bladder outlet obstruction. The multicenter PLUTO (Percutaneous Shunting in Lower Tract Obstruction) trial was initiated with the primary objective to determine if prenatal shunting improves postnatal mortality and renal function (Morris and Kilby 2009). Recruitment has closed, but results are pending.

Systematic review of published antenatal intervention for bladder outlet obstruction identified 20 articles with 369 fetuses, of which a total of 261 had antenatal intervention. Most were percutaneous vesico-amniotic shunts, but 9 were open fetal surgeries and 26 were fetal cystoscopies with 14 valve ablations. Prenatal bladder drainage improved perinatal survival (likely due to fewer deaths from pulmonary complications) versus no treatment (OR 3.86 [95 % CI 2.00–7.45]), primarily in a subgroup with predicted poor prognosis on the basis of fetal urinalysis (OR 12.85 [95 % CI 1.25–153.03]). However, improvement in postnatal renal function was not found (OR 0.50 [95 % CI 0.13–1.90]) Complications included shunt dislodgement or occlusion in 34 % with vesico-amniotic shunting, two premature rupture of membranes, four cases of chorioamnionitis, three hernias, and one bladder rupture from shunting, and three patient deaths (Morris et al. 2010).

Prognosis Based on Prenatal Versus Postnatal Diagnosis

The likelihood that boys with PUV will develop CRF/ESRD does not vary by prenatal versus postnatal diagnosis.

Analysis was performed in 46 boys diagnosed with PUV between 1983 and 1997, with mean follow-up 12.5 years (5.5–20) using a prospective protocol. Antenatal diagnosis was made in 23/40 (57.5 %) at median gestational age 28 weeks (16–38). In the other 23, the diagnosis was made postnatally at median 31 days of age (1 day–1 year) for uremia/acidosis, UTI, respiratory symptoms, and/or weak urinary stream. Treatment was nearly identical in both cohorts, comprising valve ablation in 23 (50 %) or vesicostomy or supravesical diversion in 23 (50 %). CRF (GFR≤59 mL/m/1.73 m^2) developed in 6 (13 %) and ESRD in 8 (17 %), with no difference in antenatal versus postnatal detection (Ylinen et al. 2004).

A retrospective review of 34 boys with PUV compared prenatal versus postnatal diagnosis for risk of CRF (serum creatinine >2 SD for age)/ ESRD. Sixteen of 34 had normal prenatal ultrasound with postnatal diagnosis made at a median 3.5 months (2 day–5 year). Follow-up after valve ablation was a mean of 8 years. There was no difference in poor outcomes based on antenatal versus postnatal diagnosis (5/13 vs. 2/14, $p=0.4$) (Harvie et al. 2009).

Another retrospective review compared 30 boys with prenatally detected PUV and 10 with postnatal diagnosis at mean of 21 days (1–60). At mean follow-up of 4 years, 2/30 (7 %) and 1/10 (10 %) had ESRD. If another five with prenatal diagnosis leading to termination were included, poor outcomes remained similar (El-Ghoneimi et al. 1999).

Prognosis Based on Postnatal Parameters

Several reports analyzed factors potentially correlating with CRF/ESRD. All are retrospective, many involve few patients, the diagnosis of CRF varies (<90 mL/min/1.73 m^2 vs. <60–64 mL/min/m^2), and definitions of factors were not always stated.

Factors not predicting poor renal functional outcomes include age at diagnosis and VURD.

Factors correlating with poor renal functional outcomes are nadir creatinine >1 mg/dL and abnormal initial renal ultrasound (hyperechogenicity, loss of volume, loss of corticomedullary differentiation).

Abnormal bladder function is also associated with poor renal function, but usefulness of this observation is limited by lack of a consistent definition for diagnosis.

There are mixed findings concerning the relationships between urinomas, VUR, and UTI and CRF/ESRD. Although results of analyses of VUR and CRF/ESRD varied, no study reviewed found VUR grade to predict renal outcomes.

Age at Diagnosis

A retrospective review of 227 males with PUV undergoing primary valve ablation analyzed factors leading to ESRD. Mean age at diagnosis was 30 months (10 days–16 years), with only 2 diagnosed prenatally and 107 (47 %) during infancy. Mean follow-up was 7 years (0.5–16), during which time ESRD occurred in 27 (12 %), and was not influenced by presentation before versus after infancy (Ansari et al. 2010).

A similar retrospective analysis of 120 males undergoing primary valve ablation between 1987 and 2004 considered factors potentially associated with ESRD. Age at diagnosis was a mean of 2 years (1 day–15 years), presenting with urinary retention, UTI, stranguria/dysuria, and incontinence. With follow-up a median of 3.6 years, ESRD occurred in 18 (15 %). Age at presentation did not correlate with renal function (although statistical means to evaluate age, i.e., <1–2 years vs. >2 years mentioned in discussion, or as a continuous variable, were not described) (Sarhan et al. 2011).

Another retrospective evaluation also found age at presentation not predictive of renal functional outcomes. This study included 52 males with PUV divided into two groups, those diagnosed and treated before ($n = 39$, mean age 30 days at surgery) versus after 1 year of age ($n = 13$, mean age 3.8 years at surgery). Those with late diagnosis presented with UTI, voiding dysfunction, or failure to thrive. Follow-up was a mean of 7 years after valve ablation, but specific times for the two groups were not stated. ESRD did not vary significantly between the two groups (8 % vs. 0 %, $p = 0.55$) (Kibar et al. 2011).

Nadir Serum Creatinine

Retrospective analysis was performed in 227 males with PUV undergoing valve ablation between 1992 and 2008, at mean age 30 months (10 days–16 years) and mean follow-up 7 years (0.5–16). ESRD developed in 27 (12 %). Multivariable logistic regression analysis found nadir serum creatinine >1 mg/dL correlated with renal failure (OR 23.79 [95 % CI 8.20–69.05]). Twenty two of 27 patients with ESRD had nadir creatinine >1 mg/dL, although a creatinine >1 mg/dL was also found in 18/200 without renal failure (Ansari et al. 2010).

A retrospective analysis of renal functional outcomes evaluated presenting and nadir serum creatinine in a series of 120 males with primary valve ablation. Mean age at treatment was 2 years (1 day–15 years), with follow-up a mean 4.4 years. CRF was defined as GFR (determined by Schwartz formula) ≤59 mL/min/1.73 m^2. Patients with CRF ($n = 44$) were compared to those with normal or less severe renal insufficiency ($n = 76$). Mean initial serum creatinine (1.7 mg/dL vs. 0.8 mg/dL), mean nadir serum creatinine (1 mg/dL vs. 0.55 mg/dL) and mean initial calculated GFR (34 mL/min vs. 117 mL/min) were all significantly different between the two groups. Nevertheless, 24 % of patients with a nadir creatinine <1 mg/dL still developed CRF, while 16 % with nadir creatinine >1 mg/dL did not (Sarhan et al. 2010).

Retrospective analysis was done in 42 males, median age 0.97 months (interquartile range 0.03–58.49) with PUV treated between 1983 and 2009 that segregated patients into 23 with normal renal function versus 19 with GFR (using Schwartz formula) <90 mL/min/1.73 m^2 throughout mean follow-up of 5.2 years. Serum creatinine levels at age 1 year were available in 19/23 and 14/19 patients in the two groups, with median calculated GFR 112 mL/min/1.73 m^2 (IQR 96.0–134.0) in those with preserved normal renal function versus 24.5 mL/min/1.73 m^2 (IQR 14.0–62.3) in those with renal insufficiency, $p < 0.001$ (Pohl et al. 2012).

Renal Ultrasound Parameters

Retrospective analysis reported by Pohl et al. (2012) mentioned above evaluated renal ultrasound parameters from the first postnatal study in 42 PUV patients diagnosed at median age <3 months and compared them to functional outcomes of normal calculated GFR versus CRF (<90 mL/min/1.73 m^2). Total renal volume less than the third percentile was significantly more common in those with CRF (OR 17.42 [95 % CI 3.28–92.61]), with 79 % of those with CRF having hypoplastic kidneys. Similarly, hyperechogenicity greater than the liver or spleen (OR 21.33 [95 % CI 2.37–192.03]) and loss of corticomedullary differentiation (OR 28 [95 % CI 3.11–252.48]) correlated with CRF.

The retrospective review by Sarhan et al. (2011) referenced above including 120 males with PUV diagnosed at mean age 2 years (1 day–15 years) with follow-up a median 3.6 years also considered first renal ultrasound appearance versus calculated GFR. However, in this study, CRF was defined as ≤59 mL/min/1.73 m^2. Univariable analysis found significant differences in hyperechogenicity occurring in 12/76 (16 %) with normal GFR versus 16/44 (36 %) with CRF, $p = 0.014$.

VUR

VUR was not predictive for CRF (<90 mL/min/1.73 m^2) in the retrospective analysis reported by Pohl et al. (2012) mentioned earlier. VUR was initially diagnosed in 21/40 (52.5 %)

(no information was available in 2), which was unilateral in 12 and bilateral in 9 patients for a total of 30 renal units. VUR was grades 1–2 in 9 and 3–5 in 21 renal units. No difference in VUR was noted in patients with normal versus reduced renal function (OR 2.89 [95 % CI 0.79–10.57]).

Similarly, the retrospective analysis by Sarhan et al. (2011) discussed above that defined CRF as calculated GFR ≤59 mL/min/1.73 m^2 found that VUR was not a predictive factor on univariable analysis that compared no, unilateral, and bilateral VUR but did not report grade differences, if any.

Another retrospective review identified 142 patients with PUV treated between 1975 and 2005, of which 119 had sufficient data for analysis at mean follow-up of 7 years (3–24). Fifteen (13 %) progressed to ESRD. Although VUR grades III–V occurred in 93 % with ESRD versus 48 % in patients without ESRD, multivariable logistic regression analysis found differences were not significant (OR 2.0 [95 % CI 0.2–24]) (DeFoor et al. 2008).

In contrast, one retrospective analysis did find bilateral VUR a risk factor for ESRD in multivariable logistic regression. There were 116 males with PUV presenting at mean age of 13 months (0–120) who underwent primary valve ablation, followed by diversion in 32 (28 %) by Sober ureterostomies (31) or vesicostomy (1) for "severe VUR and HN" (22) or poor renal function (9). Subsequent follow-up was a mean of 10 years (18 months–22 years), during which time 49 (42 %) developed ESRD. VUR was found in a total of 52/116 (45 %) patients, including 18/49 (37 %) with ESRD, unilateral in 10 and bilateral in 8. Bilateral VUR, found in 16 % of those with ESRD, was reported a significant risk factor in multivariable logistic regression, but the OR was not stated. However, neither high-grade VUR (3–5) nor unilateral VUR was found to be a risk factor (Ghanem et al. 2004).

The retrospective analysis by Ylinen et al. (2004) of 46 boys reported VUR initially in 32 (70 %), unilateral in 17 and bilateral in 15 (grades not stated). Both unilateral and bilateral VUR increased risk for CRF (<60 mL/min/1.73 m^2)/ESRD versus no VUR. Among patients with VUR, there was no difference in renal outcomes for grades 1–2 versus 3–5.

UTI

Recurrent fUTI was another risk factor for ESRD considered by DeFoor et al. (2008), occurring in 58/119 (49 %) patients despite antibiotic prophylaxis for VUR, bladder dysfunction requiring CIC, and/or "severe" HN. These infections were equally likely in patients with preserved renal function versus those with ESRD.

The analysis by Ansari et al. (2010) discussed above also reported that recurrent fUTI (not further defined) did not correlate with progression to ESRD in 227 males presenting at mean age of 30 months. Seventy seven (34 %) had fUTI during mean follow-up of 7 years, with no difference in those with versus without ESRD.

One study that specifically defined fUTI similarly found it was not a significant risk factor for renal function > than or <90 mL/min/1.73 m^2 calculated GFR, occurring in a total of 33/42 (79 %) patients (OR 3.72 [95 % CI 0.67–20.63]). However, >3 fUTIs (occurring in 50 %) did correlate with reduced renal function (OR 6.40 [95 % CI 1.65–24.77]) (Pohl et al. 2012).

However, Ylinen et al. (2004) reported that UTIs occurred in 30/46 (65 %) boys with PUV, with a mean of 1.9 episodes of fUTI in 22 of them, and that these patients were more likely to have CRF (<64 mL/min/1.73 m^2)/ESRD than those without UTI.

Bladder Dysfunction "Valve Bladder"

Ansari et al. (2010) defined bladder dysfunction for their retrospective multivariable analysis as the presence of one or more factors: end filling pressure >40 cm H_2O, post-void residual urine >30 % of the maximum cystometric bladder capacity, myogenic failure, and/or need for CIC. By these criteria, 21/27 (78 %) with ESRD had bladder dysfunction versus 38/200 (19 %) patients without ESRD (OR 5.67 [95 % CI 1.90–16.93]).

A retrospective analysis included urodynamic findings in 116 boys with PUV presenting at mean age 13 months (0–120) and then undergoing primary valve ablation, with 31 also having Sober ureterostomies and 1 a vesicostomy. A total of 52 (45 %) developed ESRD. Age and number of UDs (assuming some had more than one study) were not stated. Studies were done transurethrally with a 7-Fr catheter at a filling rate of 5–10 cc/min. Expected bladder capacity was determined by formula (age + 2) × 30 cc; "loss" of bladder compliance was not defined, although used as a factor in logistic regression. Eighty percent of all patients had abnormal bladder parameters. Univariable analysis found bladder compliance and/or detrusor overactivity to be significant predictive factors for ESRD, specific results of multivariable analysis for these factors were not stated (Ghanem et al. 2004).

Bladder dysfunction leading to CIC was found on retrospective chart review in 37/119 (31 %) patients with PUV, generally due to low capacity and filling pressures >40 cm H_2O in younger patients or myogenic failure with retention in older patients ("low capacity, younger, older, retention" were not defined). These patients were found on multivariable logistic regression to have increased risk for ESRD (OR 8.9 [95 % CI 1.1–73]) (DeFoor et al. 2008).

In contrast, Sarhan et al. (2011) reported that bladder dysfunction occurring in 35 % of toilet-trained boys did not correlate with ESRD. However, definition of "bladder dysfunction," means to diagnose it, and time to diagnosis after valve ablation that was done at mean age 2 years, were not stated.

Ylinen et al. (2004) simply defined bladder function as total urinary continence (day and night) and compared achieving this threshold at age <5 years versus >5 years. By this definition, bladder function did not correlate with CRF/ESRD (OR 0.45 [95 % CI 0.13–1.65]).

VURD/Urinary Extravasation

The analysis by Ylinen (2004) of 46 PUV boys included VURD, defined as unilateral VUR into a nonfunctioning kidney, which was found in nine patients, with three developing ESRD. Urinary extravasation was noted in four patients, one progressing subsequently to ESRD. Neither "pop-off" mechanism was found protective of renal function.

"Pop-off" mechanisms, including VURD, large bladder diverticulum, urinoma, and/or ascites, were considered a single factor in the retrospective analysis of 120 PUV cases by Sarhan et al. (2011). Presence of these did not predict future renal function.

Another retrospective study involved 73 consecutive patients with PUV presenting at mean age of 1.6 years (0–11). Of these 35 had VUR, with VURD (unilateral VUR with renal dysplasia) in 21. Follow-up was a mean of 5.6 years (1–17). Logistic regression analysis was not done, but chi square analysis found no differences in patients with versus without VUR, or in those with VURD versus others having VUR without VURD (Hassan et al. 2003).

A retrospective review divided 89 consecutive patients with PUV diagnosed as neonates and treated between 1989 and 2009 into the 9 (10 %) with urinomas versus those without to determine impact, if any, on renal function. These urinomas were bilateral in one and unilateral in the remainder, ranging in size from 4×3×4 to 9×9 cm. Median initial nadir creatinine after valve ablation or vesicostomy was significantly lower in those with urinomas (0.35 mg/dL [0.2–0.5] vs. 0.5 mg/dL [0.2–6.5], $p < 0.01$). Ipsilateral renal function was not reported. Initial management of the urinomas was conservative, although four underwent percutaneous drainage due to respiratory or feeding impairment; neither the time of drainage nor the time for resolution of those observed was stated (Wells et al. 2010).

Diagnosis by VCUG

Our review found no report on the sensitivity and specificity of VCUG in diagnosis of PUV. Two studies agreed that the catheter in the urethra during voiding imaging does not impair diagnosis of PUV.

Three radiologists reviewed preoperative VCUGs in 48 patients with cystoscopically confirmed PUV to determine if the urethral catheter used in the test impacted visualization of the valve. Studies were done leaving the catheter in the urethra in 28, without in 17, and both in 3. Valves were diagnosed in 25/28 (89 %) with the catheter versus 15/17 (88 %) without (Ditchfield et al. 1995).

In another study, 123 males had VCUG using a 6- or 8-Fr catheter at median age 2.6 months during investigations of prenatal HN or UTI. For inclusion, four voiding phase images were required, two with and two without the catheter; only 80 studies met this criteria. Of these, three showed PUV, seen in views with and without the catheter (Chaumoitre et al. 2004).

Initial Management

No RCT compares outcomes for treatment in newborns by primary valve ablation versus diversion by vesicostomy or supravesical diversion.

Our review found only one study comparing primary valve ablation versus vesicostomy for newborn management of PUV, with selection determined by whether or not the urethra admitted a 9-Fr resectoscope. Preoperative mean serum creatinine and mean serum creatinine at 1 year were reported as similar in the two groups.

Another review of patients <1 year at surgery found no difference in renal insufficiency or ESRD based on initial valve ablation versus supravesical diversion, although reasons for different interventions were not stated.

Within the limitations of retrospective chart reviews and the potential for selection bias in deciding valve ablation versus diversion, our review found no report indicating diversion superior to ablation.

Valve ablation can be done by a variety of methods, including fulguration, laser, or cold knife incision. Our review found few descriptions of technique and outcomes.

"Residual valves" have been reported by several authors, described by one as leaflets that could be engaged with a cold knife hook but not defined by others. Two studies using objective urethral ratios to diagnose persistent posterior urethral dilation reported residual valves in those with ratios above the medians of controls (1.73, 2.6) during follow-up VCUG 6–12 weeks later. Re-ablation resulted in normalization of ratios.

Urethral strictures occurring in up to 50 % of newborns and infants when 10-Fr or larger resectoscopes were used prompted vesicostomy or ablation using either hooked electrodes without direct visualization or bugbee electrodes introduced through smaller cystoscopes. Today 9-Fr resectoscopes potentially allow more primary ablations under direct vision in newborns with less concern for urethral trauma. Our review found only one contemporary study reporting inability to use a 9-Fr resectoscope in newborns, occurring in 47 %, and none concerning stricture presence or absence after ablation.

Ablation Technique

Thirteen neonates at mean age 9 days underwent transurethral YAG laser valve ablation at maximum power of 25 W via an 8-Fr cystoscope. Vaporization began centrally and moved peripherally, leaving a small rim circumferentially. VCUG was repeated at 4 weeks, with subsequent follow-up to a mean of 2.3 years (6 month–5 years). No strictures occurred, and no delayed repeat ablations were reported. Four infants who had ureteral reimplantation, apparently within 6 months of ablation, also had cystoscopy stated to demonstrate no residual valves (Biewald and Schier 1992).

Adequacy of Valve Ablation

The retrospective report from Sarhan et al. (2011) with 120 PUV patients treated at mean age 2 years stated that all underwent primary valve ablation, done in 65 (54 %) with a cold knife versus fulguration using a hot loop or bugbee hook electrode (43 [36 %] and 12 [10 %]). Repeat VCUG was obtained 1–3 months later, with "adequate valve ablation" in 85 %. The remaining 18 (15 %)

underwent a second ablation. Specific findings to determine adequate ablation on VCUG were not defined, nor were findings at residual fulguration described or correlated with initial surgical methods.

Retrospective analysis was done in 31 consecutive patients with post-ablation cystoscopy during a 2-year period from 2006 to 2008. Ablation was done using an 11-FR cold knife ($n=21$) or 3-Fr point electrocautery ($n=9$) and was unknown in one. Further details (location and number of incisions) were not stated. Follow-up cystoscopy and VCUG were done in all at median 5 months (3–12). VCUG reported resolution in 10, improvement in 8, and persistence of posterior urethral dilation in 12 (39 %). Cystoscopy found valves sufficient for further ablation in 16 (52 %). Cold knife ablation was done in all but one, and these incisions were described: at 5, 7, 12 O'clock ($n=5$); at 5, 7 O'clock ($n=8$); at 7 or 12 O'clock only in one each. Potential clinical relevance for these valve remnants was assumed by ability to engage them with the hook of the cold knife. Based on secondary ablation, the positive/negative predictive value of visualized valves plus persistent posterior urethral dilation on VCUG was 83 %/75 %, but either valve or posterior urethral dilation alone was only 40 %/50 %. (Smeulders et al. 2011).

In another retrospective analysis, 20 patients underwent valve ablation at median age 1.5 months (1–12) and then had urethral ratios (transverse midpoint diameter of posterior urethra/transverse diameter at widest point of bulbar urethra during voiding without catheter) determined by repeat VCUG 6–8 weeks later. Ablation was performed using an 11-Fr resectoscope with Collins knife and cutting diathermy current or a 9-Fr cystoscope with 2.4-Fr electrode, with location and number of incisions not stated. Controls were similarly aged boys undergoing VCUG "for suspected urinary tract pathology." Median urethral ratio in 13 patients with available studies before valve ablation was 8.6 (4–14.7) versus post-ablation median in 20 patients of 3.4 (1.9–15) and controls of 2.6 (1.3–5.5). Repeat cystoscopy was selective, in five patients with persistent dilation a mean of 8 (5–15.5), who all had secondary ablation and resultant decrease in urethral ratio to 3.1 (2.9–6.4) (Bani Hani et al. 2006).

VCUG and repeat cystoscopy was done in 30 patients 8–12 weeks after valve ablation at a median age of 13 months (1 day–11 years). Ablation was performed using either a 7- or 10-Fr cystoscope with bugbee electrode, but otherwise technical details (location and number of fulgurations) were not described. There were 30 controls for urethral ratio undergoing VCUG for "suspected urinary tract pathology." Mean urethral ratio in controls was 1.73 ± 0.57, versus pre-ablation mean in patients of 4.94 ± 2.97, $p < 0.001$ (21/30 had ratios >2.3). Mean post-ablation ratio was 2.13 ± 1.19, which was not different from controls. However, two patients had persistently abnormal post-ablation ratios (6.5) and both had residual valves not seen in others (Gupta et al. 2010).

Urethral Stricture After Ablation

A review of 28 patients with transurethral valve ablation noted that strictures, diagnosed by VCUG, all occurred in newborns and infants. Ablation was done using a loop electrode via a 10-Fr ($n=2$) or 12-Fr ($n=12$) resectoscope, and strictures developed in 7/14 (50 %), located in the membranous ($n=2$), bulbar ($n=4$) or anterior ($n=1$) urethra (Myers and Walker 1981).

Urethral stricture at the site of prior ablation occurred in 3/82 (4 %) patients in one retrospective series in which all newborns and infants underwent vesicostomy with subsequent closure and valve ablation at age 9–12 months. Fulguration was done using a 9-Fr resectoscope with a loop electrode applied at 5, 7, and 12 O'clock. VCUG was done 6 months after ablation. Of the three strictures, one occurred following urethral trauma with a false passage and "profuse bleeding" done elsewhere, with re-fulguration subsequently done for residual valves. The other two had preliminary diversion. Means of diagnosis, time after ablation to stricture, and any associated symptoms were not stated, nor were treatment and results for the strictures described (Lal et al. 1998). Considering the subgroup of patients

<12 months old at presentation (comprising those with diversion before ablation) strictures occurred in 2/38 (5 %).

TUR Valves Versus Urinary Diversion

A review of 45 newborns with PUV managed between 1997 and 2002 found that 24 underwent primary valve ablation, while 21 had vesicostomy because the urethra would not admit a 9-Fr scope. Mean preoperative serum creatinine was similar in the two groups (1.6 ± 1.5 mg/dL vs. 1.7 ± 1.5). Nine were lost to follow-up, and six died before 12 months (four valve ablation, two vesicostomy). Apparently, diverted patients still had vesicostomy at 12 months. Mean postoperative serum creatinine at 1 year was 0.7 ± 0.2 mg/dL in 12 patients after ablation versus 0.9 ± 0.7 mg/dL in 9 with vesicostomy, which was said to be similar by chi square analysis (Narasimhan et al. 2004).

Another review included 46 patients, 23 prenatally detected and 23 diagnosed within 1 year of life. In each group approximately 50 % underwent primary valve ablation or supravesical diversion, but decision making was not described. During a mean observation period of approximately 12 years, six (13 %) developed renal insufficiency (<59 mL/min/1.73 m^2) and eight (17 %) ESRD, with no differences in outcomes based on initial surgical management (Ylinen et al. 2004).

A retrospective review included 100 consecutive patients with PUV born before 1985 and reported in 1996. Forty-two presented at less than 1 month of age, and 56 at less than 1 year (mean, median, range not reported). Initial management included valve ablation (74), vesicostomy (13), or supravesical diversion (9); after valve ablation, three also had supravesical diversion without further improvement in serum creatinine, and four others had vesicostomies, with one then having decreased creatinine. Median follow-up was 11 years, but follow-up for each group was not stated. Data were presented as Kaplan Meier curves, showing no statistical differences in risk for ESRD based on initial therapy (Smith et al. 1996). Selection of patients for primary valve ablation versus urinary diversion was not described, nor was analysis presented to demonstrate if patient groups had similar initial renal function.

Another retrospective review included 67 patients treated between 1985 and 2000, 38 undergoing primary valve ablation, 25 vesicostomy for a small urethra, and 4 ureterostomy for "gross pyuria and sepsis with dilated and tortuous ureters, or failure of serum creatinine to diminish with catheter drainage." Patients undergoing vesicostomy were significantly younger at a mean of 16.3 ± 29.1 months versus 37.2 ± 36.1 and 40.5 ± 17.9 months for valve ablation or ureterostomy. Initial renal function for each of the three groups was not stated or compared, nor was timing for post-surgical analysis of renal function described—the authors only stating that improvement in serum creatinine levels was not significantly different in diverted patients versus those with valve ablation (Puri et al. 2002).

Bladder Function

Although bladder dysfunction is a potential risk factor for ESRD in boys with PUV, we found no published systematic protocol to diagnose and manage patients. While functional characteristics of the bladder may evolve over time after valve ablation, our review found no studies describing longitudinal UD evaluations.

Two studies reported bladder capacity and compliance better after primary valve ablation versus diversion by vesicostomy or supravesical diversion, although selection bias for diversion could account for this observation.

One study with UD performed in infants within 2 weeks of valve ablation found no difference in median maximum detrusor pressures during voiding compared to age-matched controls evaluated after UTI.

Bladder dysfunction is also suspected from urinary incontinence in boys after the usual age of toilet training, reported in 42–80 %, but few reviews described ages at which continence was achieved, and none was found that used objective assessments to define normal versus altered

bladder function. Potential contributing factors, such as detrusor overactivity, poor compliance, and/or polyuria, have not been systematically assessed when continence is delayed.

Few studies report medical therapy with anticholinergics, alpha-blockers, and/or CIC in patients after valve ablation. Indications, age at initiation of therapy, duration of treatment, and results have not been systematically reported.

One study found imipramine abolished detrusor overactivity in nearly 90 % and improved compliance in 43 % of patients treated, with symptomatic improvement reported in 59 %.

Two studies reported alpha-blocker therapy using terazosin for PVR >10 % predicted bladder capacity reduced post-void residuals from a mean of approximately 15 cc to a mean of 2 cc.

One matched cohort study of adult men using a validated questionnaire found symptoms of voiding dysfunction reported by 32 % of former valve patients, who also had significantly greater urge and/or stress incontinence compared to age-matched controls.

Urodynamics

A retrospective study created two groups: 11 patients treated from 1970 to 1983 who underwent supravesical diversion versus 8 undergoing primary valve ablation from 1980 to 1983. Indications for diversion were small urethra, "severe urinary tract infections and failure to stabilize renal function or improve a poor clinical condition despite bladder drainage via a urethral catheter and medical treatment." Mean patient age at surgery was 10.2±8.1 months (diversion) versus 11.8±11.2 months (valve ablation), and mean duration of diversion was 57±39 months. All had "rapid fill" UD testing at mean ages of 13.6±2.2 years (diversion) versus 11±4.1 years. Mean maximum bladder capacity adjusted for age by the formula age+2×30 was significantly greater in those ablated (1.37±0.19 %) versus diverted (0.9±0.3 %), and end filling pressure at this capacity was significantly less in ablated (8±2.6 cm H_2O) versus diverted (19.3±4 cm H_2O) bladders (Podesta et al. 2002).

The retrospective analysis of 67 patients treated initially by primary valve ablation ($n=38$) versus vesicostomy ($n=25$) or supravesical diversion ($n=4$) mentioned above (Puri et al. 2002) included UD testing in all patients. Studies were performed using an 8-Fr transurethral catheter at a filling rate of 10 % expected bladder capacity for age. A significant difference was found in maximum bladder capacity between ablated versus vesicostomy patients (mean % 96±33 vs. 62±28). Compliance of <10, 10–20, and >20 cc/cm H_2O was also significantly better in ablated versus vesicostomy patients. Age at which UD was performed, time interval from valve treatment, and number of UDs performed per patient were not described.

UD was obtained in 116 patients who underwent valve ablation at mean age 14 months (6 days–164 months), followed by supravesical diversion in 32 (28 %) for "severe VUR and HN" in 22 and "poor renal function" in 9 for an unreported duration. Time after ablation for UD testing, the number of tests obtained per patient or, if more than one study was done, which was selected for analysis, were not stated. Filling was done via a 7-Fr transurethral catheter at 5–10 mL/min. Abnormal bladder parameters were found in 93 (80 %). Cystometric capacity was greater than expected by formula for age in 34 (29 %) and less in 33. Compliance loss was reported for 30 (26 %) and detrusor overactivity in 44 (38 %). Patch EMG electrodes indicated impaired pelvic floor relaxation in 31 (27 %), while retention >10 % voided volume was noted in 47 (41 %). Although 80 % of patients were considered to have abnormal bladder function, when the authors categorized them further, 86 (74 %) had normal compliance (61 without and 25 with detrusor overactivity), while 30 (26 %) had decreased compliance (13 without and 17 with detrusor overactivity). Definitions of increases/decreases in capacity, decreased compliance, or abnormal pelvic EMG were not stated. Differences, if any, between those with ablation versus ablation plus diversion were not discussed. Multivariable regression analysis found only bilateral VUR, and not bladder dysfunction, to independently predict ESRD (Ghanem et al. 2004).

Another retrospective analysis identified 25 males evaluated from 1994 to 2007 at a median age of 0.5 month (0–10.2). UD was performed in six boys 2–6 days before valve ablation, and in the other 19 at median 2 days (0–15) after ablation. Detrusor pressures were monitored using 4-Fr catheters, presumably transurethrally, with infusion done at 2–5 cc/min using a second 4-Fr tube placed suprapubically in 8. A control group of males without PUV was created from infants having UD after UTI at median age 3.3 months (1.5–9.6). Median maximum detrusor pressure during voiding was similar in PUV patients (112 cm H_2O, 40–331) and controls (91 cm H_2O, 48–191, $p=0.39$). Repeat UD was obtained at 12 months after valve ablation in 17 patients, finding a significant increase in median bladder capacity and decrease in median maximal voiding pressures to 100 cm H_2O, 60–193, $p=0.01$ (Taskinen et al. 2009).

Urinary Continence

Continence was assessed in 100 boys with PUV, excluding an unspecified number who died or had ESRD before age 5 years. Total continence (dry day and night) occurred in 19 % of boys by age 5, 46 % by age 10, and in 99 % by age 20, with no significant differences based on initial therapy by valve ablation versus urinary diversion (Smith et al. 1996). Additional therapies (anticholinergics, CIC), if any, were not described.

In another study of 46 patients diagnosed either prenatally or within the first year of life and then undergoing either valve ablation or supravesical diversion, total urinary continence was achieved in 17 (37 %) by age 5 years, and in 22/27 (81 %) with follow-up to 10 years. Differences, if any, based on initial surgery were not described (Ylinen et al. 2004).

In another retrospective series, 63/65 cases of PUV diagnosed prenatally underwent primary valve ablation. During follow-up a median of 6.8 years, 55 patients were toilet-trained, of which 32 (58 %) were dry at mean age 3 years. Of the remaining 23, 7 were dry using anticholinergics ± alpha-blockers, 3 were dry on CIC, 3 had nocturnal enuresis (presumably dry during the day), and 10 were wet day and night (Sarhan et al. 2008).

Of 70 boys presenting at mean age 7.5 years (2–14), 33 (47 %) had diurnal incontinence. Following valve ablation, incontinence resolved in 24 at an unspecified interval and persisted in 9 (27 %). In four of nine, symptoms were controlled with medication (desmopressin, anticholinergics), but use in others was not stated. Incontinence resolved in six of nine patients during a mean of 11 months (4–18) and persisted in two receiving medical therapy; one was lost to follow-up (Schober et al. 2004).

Bother from bladder dysfunction can extend into adulthood. A study from Finland identified 106 patients with PUV treated after 1953, and received a response from 68 (64 %) to a validated LTUS questionnaire. These data were compared to age-matched controls at a 4:1 ratio (272 controls: 68 PUV patients) at median age of 37.5 years (18–57). Of PUV patients, 32 % reported at least one moderate or severe symptom, versus 16 % of controls ($p=0.002$). Overall, patients had 2× increase in LTUS (hesitancy, weak stream, incomplete emptying, straining) over controls. Urge incontinence was reported by 15 % PUV patients versus 5 % of controls ($p=0.014$), while stress incontinence occurred in 12 % versus 3 % ($p=0.005$) (Tikkinen et al. 2011).

Medical Bladder Therapy (Anticholinergics, Alpha-Blockers, CIC)

A longitudinal study involved 30 PUV patients, all ≥5 years of age (5–20, mean or median not stated), who had UD testing and were treated with imipramine. Indications for investigation of these patients versus others of similar age, if any, were not described. Although all were considered toilet-trained, 27/30 had symptomatic voiding dysfunction described as diurnal incontinence in 22 and only nocturnal enuresis in 5. UD used an 8-Fr transurethral catheter with filling rates at 10 % expected capacity for age by formula, and needle electrodes for sphincter

EMG. All were considered to have abnormal UD, with detrusor overactivity in 18 (60 %) and compliance <10 mL/cm H_2O in 21 (70 %). Imipramine was used at 1.5–2 mg/kg/24 h in a single or divided doses. "Significant" symptomatic improvement occurred in 16/27 (59 %). Repeat UD was reported at 1 and 2 years. Detrusor overactivity resolved on medication in 16/18 (89 %), while compliance improved in 9/21 (43 %) (Puri et al. 2005).

As mentioned above, of 23 toilet-trained boys with prenatally diagnosed PUV and primary valve ablation, 7 (30 %) were dry using anticholinergics ± alpha-blockers, 3 were dry on CIC, 3 had nocturnal enuresis (presumably dry during the day), and 10 were wet day and night. Specific indications for these therapies were not described (Sarhan et al. 2008).

Another retrospective analysis of 119 patients undergoing valve ablation reported 37 (31 %) were started on CIC for "hostile bladder dynamics" (DeFoor et al. 2008). The authors generally described these patients in two categories: "younger" ones who had low capacity and high-end fill pressures that also received anticholinergics, and "older" ones with myogenic failure and retention who did not need anticholinergics. The number of older versus younger patients, age at initiation of medical therapy, and response to treatment were not described.

Forty two patients were diagnosed with post-void residual volumes by ultrasound >10 % of expected bladder capacity for age 1 week after valve ablation. Age ranged from neonates to >5 years, with 69 % less than 1 year. Terazosin, 0.02–0.4 mg/kg, was given daily, with 25 % increases in dose every 2 weeks until residual volumes were <10 % capacity. After 6 months of successful therapy, medication was weaned. Mean pretreatment residual volume was 16 cc (34 % expected capacity) versus mean residual 2 cc (1.5 % expected capacity) on therapy. Symptomatic hypotension occurred in one, and another two boys did not respond. Four had therapy successfully ended after 14 months, while others apparently continued medication at mean follow-up 17 months (2 months–6 years) (Abraham et al. 2009).

In another retrospective series of 65 consecutive patients undergoing valve ablation at median age 1.5 months (1 day–13 years), post-void residuals were measured by ultrasound during outpatient follow-up, with those having PVR >10 % expected bladder capacity started on terazosin 0.04–0.4 mg/kg/day. Patient age, interval after ablation before alpha-blocker treatment, duration of therapy, and number of patients treated were not stated. Mean PVR pretreatment was 15 and 2.5 cc with terazosin (Sudarsanan et al. 2009).

Radiologic Changes After Valve Ablation

Posterior urethral dilation decreases within 12 weeks, with persistent dilation suggesting inadequate valve ablation (reviewed above).

VUR occurs in approximately 50 % of patients with PUV and is reported to resolve in 25 % to 80 % of renal units, often within a year of valve ablation. Resolution is more likely and occurs more rapidly in grades 1–3 versus 4–5 VUR.

Two studies reported decreased HN in 70 % of renal units within 6–12 months of valve ablation.

Posterior Urethral Dilation

Thirty patients underwent repeat VCUG 12 weeks following valve ablation, with urethral ratio (transverse midpoint posterior urethral diameter/transverse widest anterior urethral diameter) measured and compared to controls without PUV undergoing VUCG after UTI. Median age of patients at ablation was 13 months (1 day–11 years) and 12 months (2 days–16 years) in controls. Mean pre-ablation urethral ratio was 4.94 ± 2.97, mean post-ablation was 2.13 ± 1.19 ($p<0.001$), and was 1.73 ± 0.58 in controls ($p<0.001$ vs. pre-ablation and $p=0.1$ vs. post-ablation). Two patients with persistent dilation (ratios 5,6) after ablation were both found to have residual valves (Gupta et al. 2010).

VUR

A prospective observational study included 20 patients undergoing valve ablation at median

15 months (12 days–5.5 years), of which 12 had VUR into19 renal units (grade 1 in 2, grade 3 in 4, grade 4 in 6, and grade 5 in 7). Follow-up VUCG was obtained at 3 and 6 months. By 6 months VUR had resolved in 15 (79 %) renal units, leaving one case each with grade 1–4 and no grade 5 (Priti et al. 2004).

A retrospective review concerned VUR in 127 patients and 200 renal units treated from 1953 to 2003. Data were available for 141 refluxing ureters after valve ablation. Resolution occurred at median 1.28 years (0.04-15.16) in 88 (62 %) renal units, while another 24 (17 %) were removed for poor function, and 29 (21 %) were reimplanted. Resolution was significantly faster for unilateral VUR (median 0.7 vs. 1.36 years), and for grades 1–3 (median 0.68 years) versus grades 4 and 5 (median 1.47 years), and was not influenced by ipsilateral renal function (<10 %, found in 22/73 with scintigraphy). Likelihood for specific grades to resolve was not stated (Heikkila et al. 2009).

Of 73 consecutive patients with PUV, 35 (48 %) had VUR, unilateral in 18. There was mean follow-up of 5.6 years (1–17) in this retrospective analysis, during which resolution occurred in 11/44 (25 %) units at a mean of 12 months. There was no difference in unilateral versus bilateral reflux resolution, nor in resolution according to ipsilateral function <20 % versus greater, but grades 1–3 were more likely than grades 4–5 to resolve (6/9 [67 %] versus 5/35 [14 %], $p=0.0038$) (Hassan et al. 2003).

Another retrospective series included 65 consecutive boys with PUV treated from 2001 to 2007 with primary valve ablation at median age 1.5 months (1 day–13 years). VUR occurred in 26 (40 %), unilateral in 18. During median follow-up of 24 months (6–75), 11/32 (34 %) ureters resolved (grades not stated). (Sudarsanan et al. 2009).

Hydronephrosis

The prospective study by Priti et al. (2004) also reported renal ultrasonography findings at ablation and repeated 3 and 6 months following ablation, reported as grades 0–3. All initially had HN, which was bilateral in 90 %. During follow-up HN resolved in one patient, but diminished significantly in the remainder; of 17 renal units with moderate to severe dilation, 5 (29 %) had persistent moderate to severe HN at 6 months after ablation.

Fifty consecutive patients, mean, median age 2 years (1–12), undergoing valve ablation during a 3-year period from 2004 to 2007 had follow-up a mean of 30 months and minimum of 1 year. Pre-ablation HN was described as 0 in 8 (16 %), grade 1 in 10 (20 %), grade 2 in 12 (24 %), grade 3 in 14 (28 %), and grade 4 in 6 (12 %) (grading system not defined). At 1 year after ablation, 31 (62 %) had grade 0, 4 (8 %) had grade 3, and none had grade 4 HN (Gupta et al. 2009).

Ureteral Reimplantation or Endoscopic Injection

As discussed above, VUR often resolves within a year of valve ablation, and it is unclear if VUR represents a modifiable factor for renal function.

One study found less postoperative VUR after excisional tapering with versus without psoas hitch reimplantation.

VUR was present in 38/54 (70 %) boys in a retrospective study. Spontaneous resolution occurred in 9/38 (24 %) after ablation, and nephrectomy was done in 7 patients for nonfunction. Twenty patients had surgical reflux resolution, by reimplant in 5 and by injection with polytetrafluoroethylene in 15 patients and 24 ureters (grade 4 in 6, grade 5 in 18). Indications for intervention were not described. Age at injection was a mean of 2.2 years (8 months–6 years), and all but one (with UTI) had injection ≥12 months after valve ablation. A single injection resolved VUR in 17/24 (71 %) ureters, and with up to three injections all were reported successful. The number and results of any subsequent VCUGs, if done, were not discussed (Puri and Kumar 1996).

A retrospective review of 106 boys with PUV found 20 patients undergoing ureteral surgery, by reimplantation in 25 renal units and transureteroureterostomy in 7 renal units. Of these, 5 patients and 12 ureters had VUR, while the remaining 15 patients and 20 ureters had UVJ obstruction (discussed below). Mean interval from valve ablation to reimplant was 1.8 years (6 months–4.5 years) for the entire group, and grade of VUR was not clearly stated, but was grade 4 or 5 "in most." Excisional tapering to 10–12-Fr was done in all 25 reimplanted ureters, with a psoas hitch in 18 and not in the other 7, whose technique was not further described. Four out of five refluxing patients had persistent VUR; grades were not stated. Of the entire group undergoing surgery for either obstruction or VUR, psoas hitch reimplantation had significantly less postoperative VUR than did repairs without hitch (2/18 ureters with hitch vs. 7/7 ureters without hitch, $p<0.004$) (El-Sherbiny et al. 2002).

Ureterovesical Junction Obstruction

Impaired ureteral drainage across the ureterovesical junction generally has been attributed to valve bladder and/or intrinsic ureteral dysfunction rather than UVJ obstruction. Our review found only one article specifically reporting UVJ obstruction in 12 % of PUV patients.

El-Sherbiny et al. (2002) diagnosed UVJ obstruction in13/106 (12 %) boys and 20 renal units following valve ablation at a mean of 1.8 years (6 months–4.5 years). All had bilateral "grade 3 or 4" HN (grading scale not defined). Diuretic renography demonstrated T1/2 >20 min in 7 patients and 11 renal units, while Whitaker test found renal pressures >22 cm H_2O over bladder pressures in 6 patients and 9 renal units with supravesical diversion before repair.

Nephrectomy to Reduce Urine Output

One study reported that unilateral nephrectomy reduced polyuria by 40 % before renal transplant.

A retrospective study evaluated consecutive patients undergoing unilateral or bilateral native nephrectomy from a total of 126 consecutive pediatric kidney transplants. These nephrectomies were done a median of 1.9 months (0–41) before transplant. The indication was polyuria, defined as sustained urine output >2.5 cc/kg/h, in 22 children, of which 10 had congenital urinary tract anomalies that were not further described. Of these 22 children, 15 had unilateral surgery (sometimes the first of staged removal) and median urine output decreased from 3.9 cc/kg/h to 2.4 cc/kg/h, a change of −40 % from 2.1 to 1.4 L per day (Ghane Sharbaf et al. 2012).

Renal Transplantation

Several cohort studies indicate that graft survival is similar in patients with renal failure due to PUV versus those with medical renal disease.

A retrospective cohort study compared graft survival after living unrelated donor transplantation in 15 PUV patients, mean age 12.5 ± 2.8 years, to 45 matched controls of similar age also receiving living unrelated grafts and all managed with a similar immunosuppressive protocol. Preoperative urologic assessment included VCUG, cystoscopy, and UD; of these 15 patients, 4 took anticholinergics, 2 used CIC, and 9 had prior ileocystoplasty. There were no differences in acute or chronic rejection episodes between patients and controls, and mean graft survival was 7 years in patients and 6.2 in controls, $p=0.9$ (Otukesh et al. 2008).

Another retrospective study compared renal graft outcomes in 18 PUV patients transplanted at mean age 9.1 years (1–18) 1:1 with a selected control group with medical renal disease of similar age, donor type, and immunosuppressive therapies. No pre-transplant UD or bladder reconstruction was done in any patient, but no mention was made of other medical therapies for bladder management, if any, and the authors admitted there were neither UD data nor voiding histories for any PUV patients before or during 10 years of post-transplant follow-up. Nevertheless, 10-year graft survival was not significantly different between patients and controls, 54 % versus 41 % $p=0.35$ (Indudhara et al. 1998).

A third retrospective matched cohort study compared cadaveric transplantation in 19 PUV patients at mean age of 10 years (1.3–17) to 62 controls with glomerulonephropathies and 42 controls with renal dysplasia—neither control group including patients with known bladder dysfunction. There were no differences in PUV patients versus controls for graft survival at 1, 5, or 10 years. In this series, all PUV patients underwent pre-transplant UD, which diagnosed "severe" bladder dysfunction in 8 (42 %) described as detrusor overactivity, poor compliance, reduced bladder capacity, and bladder sphincter "incoordination" (none specifically defined). Pre-transplant augmentation was performed in five of these. All transplant reimplantations were antirefluxing done into the native bladder. No patient had pre-transplant bilateral nephrectomies, but eight had unilateral nephrectomy before or during the transplant, and six had unilateral nephrectomy afterwards, resulting in three with bilateral removal of native kidneys. Another patient had bilateral nephrectomy after transplant, so that altogether 4/19 (21 %) received bilateral nephrectomies. Indications for nephrectomy were not clearly stated (Mendizabal et al. 2006).

References

Abraham MK, Nasir AR, Sudarsanan B, Puzhankara R, Kedari PM, Unnithan GR, et al. Role of alpha adrenergic blocker in the management of posterior urethral valves. Pediatr Surg Int. 2009;25(12):1113–5.

Ansari MS, Gulia A, Srivastava A, Kapoor R. Risk factors for progression to end-stage renal disease in children with posterior urethral valves. J Pediatr Urol. 2010;6(3):261–4.

Bani Hani O, Prelog K, Smith GH. A method to assess posterior urethral valve ablation. J Urol. 2006;176(1): 303–5.

Bernardes LS, Aksnes G, Saada J, Masse V, Elie C, Dumez Y, et al. Keyhole sign: how specific is it for the diagnosis of posterior urethral valves? Ultrasound Obstet Gynecol. 2009;34(4):419–23.

Bernardes LS, Salomon R, Aksnes G, Lortat-Jacob S, Benachi A. Ultrasound evaluation of prognosis in fetuses with posterior urethral valves. J Pediatr Surg. 2011;46(7):1412–8.

Biewald W, Schier F. Laser treatment of posterior urethral valves in neonates. Br J Urol. 1992;69(4):425–7.

Chaumoitre K, Merrot T, Petit P, Sayegh-Martin Y, Alessandrini P, Panuel M. Voiding cystourethrography in boys. Does the presence of the catheter during voiding alter the evaluation of the urethra? J Urol. 2004;171(3):1280–1.

DeFoor W, Clark C, Jackson E, Reddy P, Minevich E, Sheldon C. Risk factors for end stage renal disease in children with posterior urethral valves. J Urol. 2008;180(4 Suppl):1705–8. discussion 8.

Ditchfield MR, Grattan-Smith JD, de Campo JF, Hutson JM. Voiding cystourethrography in boys: does the presence of the catheter obscure the diagnosis of posterior urethral valves? AJR Am J Roentgenol. 1995;164(5):1233–5.

El-Ghoneimi A, Desgrippes A, Luton D, Macher MA, Guibourdenche J, Garel C, et al. Outcome of posterior urethral valves: to what extent is it improved by prenatal diagnosis? J Urol. 1999;162(3 Pt 1):849–53.

El-Sherbiny MT, Hafez AT, Ghoneim MA, Greenfield SP. Ureteroneocystostomy in children with posterior urethral valves: indications and outcome. J Urol. 2002;168(4 Pt 2):1836–9. discussion 9–40.

Ghane Sharbaf F, Bitzan M, Szymanski KM, Bell LE, Gupta I, Tchervenkov J, et al. Native nephrectomy prior to pediatric kidney transplantation: biological and clinical aspects. Pediatr Nephrol. 2012;27(7): 1179–88.

Ghanem MA, Wolffenbuttel KP, De Vylder A, Nijman RJ. Long-term bladder dysfunction and renal function in boys with posterior urethral valves based on urodynamic findings. J Urol. 2004;171(6 Pt 1):2409–12.

Gupta SD, Khatun AA, Islam AI, Shameem IA. Outcome of endoscopic fulguration of posterior urethral valves in children. Mymensingh Med J. 2009;18(2):239–44.

Gupta RK, Shah HS, Jadhav V, Gupta A, Prakash A, Sanghvi B, et al. Urethral ratio on voiding cystourethrogram: a comparative method to assess success of posterior urethral valve ablation. J Pediatr Urol. 2010;6(1):32–6.

Harvie S, McLeod L, Acott P, Walsh E, Abdolell M, Macken MB. Abnormal antenatal sonogram: an indicator of disease severity in children with posterior urethral valves. Can Assoc Radiol J. 2009;60(4): 185–9.

Hassan JM, Pope JC, Brock 3rd JW, Adams MC. Vesicoureteral reflux in patients with posterior urethral valves. J Urol. 2003;170(4 Pt 2):1677–80. discussion 80.

Heikkila J, Rintala R, Taskinen S. Vesicoureteral reflux in conjunction with posterior urethral valves. J Urol. 2009;182(4):1555–60.

Indudhara R, Joseph DB, Perez LM, Diethelm AG. Renal transplantation in children with posterior urethral valves revisited: a 10-year followup. J Urol. 1998;160(3 Pt 2):1201–3. discussion 16.

Kibar Y, Ashley RA, Roth CC, Frimberger D, Kropp BP. Timing of posterior urethral valve diagnosis and its impact on clinical outcome. J Pediatr Urol. 2011;7(5):538–42.

Lal R, Bhatnagar V, Mitra DK. Upper-tract changes after treatment of posterior urethral valves. Pediatr Surg Int. 1998;13(5–6):396–9.

Mendizabal S, Zamora I, Serrano A, Sanahuja MJ, Roman E, Dominguez C, et al. Renal transplantation in children with posterior urethral valves. Pediatr Nephrol. 2006;21(4):566–71.

Morris RK, Kilby MD. An overview of the literature on congenital lower urinary tract obstruction and introduction to the PLUTO trial: percutaneous shunting in lower urinary tract obstruction. Aust N Z J Obstet Gynaecol. 2009;49(1):6–10.

Morris RK, Quinlan-Jones E, Kilby MD, Khan KS. Systematic review of accuracy of fetal urine analysis to predict poor postnatal renal function in cases of congenital urinary tract obstruction. Prenat Diagn. 2007;27(10):900–11.

Morris RK, Malin GL, Khan KS, Kilby MD. Systematic review of the effectiveness of antenatal intervention for the treatment of congenital lower urinary tract obstruction. BJOG. 2010;117(4):382–90.

Myers DA, Walker 3rd RD. Prevention of urethral strictures in the management of posterior urethral valves. J Urol. 1981;126(5):655–7.

Narasimhan KL, Kaur B, Chowdhary SK, Bhalla AK. Does mode of treatment affect the outcome of neonatal posterior urethral valves? J Urol. 2004;171(6 Pt 1): 2423–6.

Otukesh H, Basiri A, Simfroosh N, Hoseini R, Fereshtehnejad SM, Chalian M. Kidney transplantation in children with posterior urethral valves. Pediatr Transplant. 2008;12(5):516–9.

Podesta M, Ruarte AC, Gargiulo C, Medel R, Castera R, Herrera M, et al. Bladder function associated with posterior urethral valves after primary valve ablation or proximal urinary diversion in children and adolescents. J Urol. 2002;168(4 Pt 2):1830–5. discussion 5.

Pohl M, Mentzel HJ, Vogt S, Walther M, Ronnefarth G, John U. Risk factors for renal insufficiency in children with urethral valves. Pediatr Nephrol. 2012;27(3): 443–50.

Priti K, Rao KL, Menon P, Singh N, Mittal BR, Bhattacharya A, et al. Posterior urethral valves: incidence and progress of vesicoureteric reflux after primary fulguration. Pediatr Surg Int. 2004;20(2):136–9.

Puri P, Kumar R. Endoscopic correction of vesicoureteral reflux secondary to posterior urethral valves. J Urol. 1996;156(2 Pt 2):680–2.

Puri A, Grover VP, Agarwala S, Mitra DK, Bhatnagar V. Initial surgical treatment as a determinant of bladder dysfunction in posterior urethral valves. Pediatr Surg Int. 2002;18(5–6):438–43.

Puri A, Bhatnagar V, Grover VP, Agarwala S, Mitra DK. Urodynamics-based evidence for the beneficial effect of imipramine on valve bladders in children. Eur J Pediatr Surg. 2005;15(5):347–53.

Sarhan O, Zaccaria I, Macher MA, Muller F, Vuillard E, Delezoide AL, et al. Long-term outcome of prenatally detected posterior urethral valves: single center study of 65 cases managed by primary valve ablation. J Urol. 2008;179(1):307–12. discussion 12–3.

Sarhan O, El-Dahshan K, Sarhan M. Prognostic value of serum creatinine levels in children with posterior urethral valves treated by primary valve ablation. J Pediatr Urol. 2010;6(1):11–4.

Sarhan OM, El-Ghoneimi AA, Helmy TE, Dawaba MS, Ghali AM, Ibrahiem el HI. Posterior urethral valves: multivariate analysis of factors affecting the final renal outcome. J Urol. 2011;185(6 Suppl):2491–5.

Schober JM, Dulabon LM, Woodhouse CR. Outcome of valve ablation in late-presenting posterior urethral valves. BJU Int. 2004;94(4):616–9.

Smeulders N, Makin E, Desai D, Duffy PG, Healy C, Cuckow PM, et al. The predictive value of a repeat micturating cystourethrogram for remnant leaflets after primary endoscopic ablation of posterior urethral valves. J Pediatr Urol. 2011;7(2):203–8.

Smith GH, Canning DA, Schulman SL, Snyder 3rd HM, Duckett JW. The long-term outcome of posterior urethral valves treated with primary valve ablation and observation. J Urol. 1996;155(5):1730–4.

Sudarsanan B, Nasir AA, Puzhankara R, Kedari PM, Unnithan GR, Damisetti KR. Posterior urethral valves: a single center experience over 7 years. Pediatr Surg Int. 2009;25(3):283–7.

Taskinen S, Heikkila J, Rintala R. Posterior urethral valves: primary voiding pressures and kidney function in infants. J Urol. 2009;182(2):699–702. discussion –3.

Tikkinen KA, Heikkila J, Rintala RJ, Tammela TL, Taskinen S. Lower urinary tract symptoms in adults treated for posterior urethral valves in childhood: matched cohort study. J Urol. 2011;186(2):660–6.

Wells JM, Mukerji S, Chandran H, Parashar K, McCarthy L. Urinomas protect renal function in posterior urethral valves–a population based study. J Pediatr Surg. 2010;45(2):407–10.

Ylinen E, Ala-Houhala M, Wikstrom S. Prognostic factors of posterior urethral valves and the role of antenatal detection. Pediatr Nephrol. 2004;19(8): 874–9.

Neurogenic Bladder

16

Warren T. Snodgrass, Micah A. Jacobs, and Patricio C. Gargollo

Primary reasons to diagnose and manage neurogenic bladder:

1. **Prevent acquired renal injury.**
2. **Prevent acquired loss of bladder compliance.**

Secondary aims:

1. **Achieve urinary (and bowel) continence.**
2. **Improve self-care and/or facilitate management by other caregivers.**

Summary of evidence for these goals:

Renal scar has been diagnosed by DMSA in 25–32 % of patients with spina bifida in retrospective series. No longitudinal data relates UD findings or management of neurogenic bladder to renal scarring.

Although UD findings are the cornerstone for therapeutic decision-making, technical aspects of the test (catheter size, filling rates, temperature of infused fluids, seated versus supine positioning, number of cycles) are not standardized, and no study reports inter- and intra-observer agreement in their interpretation for neurogenic bladder.

One prospective study showed 20 % of newborns had end filling pressures >40 cm H_2O, with medical management (CIC plus AC) decreasing pressures to <40 cm H_2O in all. Of newborns with initial UD end filling pressures <40 cm H_2O, 10 % had loss of compliance at median age 9 months, with reduction again to <40 cm H_2O with CIC plusAC.

No prospective study reports impact of detrusor leak-point pressure (DLPP) on future bladder compliance.

No prospective series reports overall rates of spontaneous voiding, urinary continence with medical management, or evidence of sphincter incompetency leading to surgery in a cohort of consecutive children with spina bifida.

Optimal medical management (frequency of CIC, overnight catheter drainage, AC regimens and doses) for detrusor overactivity or decreased compliance before augmentation is not standardized.

Many retrospective, and a few prospective, series report outcomes from bladder neck surgery ± augmentation, with dryness in 50–90 %. Generally, LMS, AUS, and bladder neck closure more reliably achieve dryness than slings or bladder neck injections.

One-third or fewer of patients undergoing bladder outlet surgery without augmentation will manifest decreased compliance on postoperative UD. Most respond to medical therapy.

Health-related quality-of-life surveys found no differences reported by patients before versus after surgery for incontinence, but reported improved independence and self-esteem following ACE.

ACE procedures can improve self-esteem and independence with bowel care.

W.T. Snodgrass, M.D. (✉) • M.A. Jacobs, M.D., M.P.H.
P.C. Gargollo, M.D.
Department of Pediatric Urology,
University of Texas Southwestern Medical
Center and Children's Medical Center Dallas,
1935 Medical District Drive, MS F4.04,
Dallas, TX 75235, USA
e-mail: warren.snodgrass@childrens.com

W.T. Snodgrass (ed.), *Pediatric Urology: Evidence for Optimal Patient Management*,
DOI 10.1007/978-1-4614-6910-0_16, © Springer Science+Business Media New York 2013

Few series comparing ACE to retrograde enemas report no additional benefit of ACE to achieve fecal continence.

LACE uses less irrigation volume and requires less toilet time than ACE.

Complications after ACE occur in 15 % to more than 50 % in published series, most commonly stoma stenosis or leakage. Pain with irrigation is also reported in some series with phosphate, saline, or tap water enemas.

Series reporting >5-year follow-up indicate that 10–45 % of patients no longer use the ACE.

Definition

There is no consensus definition for "neurogenic bladder" in children, which generally refers to bladder dysfunction diagnosed by a combination of symptoms, imaging, and/or UD findings in patients with neurologic conditions.

Prevalence of Neurogenic Bladder with Spinal Cord Anomalies

Myelodysplasia

UDs appear normal in 25–33 % of newborns with spina bifida. Spontaneous continence rates in these, and in newborns observed despite abnormal UDs, have not been reported.

Three studies with UD assessments in consecutive newborns with myelomeningocele reported abnormal findings in ≥75 % (Sidi et al. 1986; Sillen et al. 1996; Granberg et al. 2011).

A retrospective analysis of 502 children with myelomeningocele referred to a multi-specialty center reported that neurogenic bladder occurred in 275/283 (97 %) patients evaluated at median age 12 years (2 months to 42 years) (Torre et al. 2011).

Lipomeningocele

Two studies reported neurogenic bladder in approximately one-third of patients with spinal cord lipoma.

UD in 29 consecutive patients with lipomyelomeningocele evaluated at a mean age 1.9 years (1 month to 13 years) were considered abnormal in 11 (38 %) (Dushi et al. 2011).

A retrospective analysis of 502 children with spinal dysraphism referred to a multi-specialty center at median age 12 years reported neurogenic bladder occurred in 33/98 (34 %) with spinal lipoma. Neurogenic bladder was diagnosed in significantly more with lipomyelomeningocele (18/31, 58 %) versus lipomyeloschisis and phylum lipomas (33/98, 34 %) (Torre et al. 2011).

Sacral Agenesis/Caudal Regression

Fifty to seventy-five percent of children referred with sacral agenesis have a neurogenic bladder, with one study reporting the likelihood increasing with increasing extent of the sacral deformity.

A retrospective analysis of 502 children with spinal dysraphism referred to a multi-specialty center at median age 12 years reported neurogenic bladder occurred in 54/90 (60 %) with caudal regression syndrome (Torre et al. 2011).

Another retrospective analysis reported that 11/15 (73 %) children with sacral agenesis had a neurogenic bladder confirmed by UD at mean age 40 months (for the entire series of 28 patients that included others with anorectal malformations). Those with normal bladder function were described as having minor sacral defects in only parts of S4 and S5 pedicles versus those with neurogenic bladders having total S5 and partial S4 absence (Boemers et al. 1994).

A 20-year retrospective review of all patients evaluated in a neurourology clinic with sacral agenesis found 22 cases initially evaluated at median 10.5 (2–24) years of age. UD was performed in each, and all were abnormal, with detrusor overactivity in 19 (86 %) and DSD in 14 (64 %) (Wilmshurst et al. 1999).

Primary Tethered Cord

Primary tethered cord is diagnosed during evaluation for orthopedic deformities or cutaneous

lesions (generally in patients before toilet training) and for urinary incontinence in older children. Retrospective series report abnormal UD in 20–87 % of patients with orthopedic and/or cutaneous lesions, mostly detrusor overactivity.

A retrospective review analyzed all cases of tethered cord releases during a 7-year period to identify infants and children <3 years of age with a primary tethered cord. Underlying diagnoses included spinal cord lipoma, fatty filum, and diastematomyelia presenting due to cutaneous manifestations or musculoskeletal disorders. UD was obtained in 66/79 patients before neurosurgery done at mean age 10 months, and was considered abnormal in 30 (45 %), with varying findings of overactivity, "hypotonia," DSD, poor compliance, and high voiding pressures. The authors did not consider isolated uninhibited contractions abnormal (Macejko et al. 2007).

Another retrospective review of cases undergoing tethered cord release identified 48 nonsyndromic children that were subdivided into three groups based on clinical presentation:

- Group 1—orthopedic deformities/scoliosis: 19 patients, mean age 8 years (8 months to 14 years); 4 had daytime urinary incontinence; UD showed detrusor overactivity in 3 (16 %).
- Group 2—cutaneous lesions: 16 patients, mean age 1 year (1 month to 11 years), with only 1 patient beyond the age of toilet training; UD diagnosed detrusor overactivity in 4 (25 %), while the remainder were considered normal.
- Group 3—diurnal incontinence: 13 patients, mean age 9 years (4.5–14). Preoperative UD indicated detrusor overactivity in 11 and areflexia in 2 (DLPP not stated) (Nogueira et al. 2004).

A third retrospective review considered 24 patients diagnosed with a tethered cord, presenting at median age 6 years (1 month to 12 years). Nineteen (79 %) had cutaneous lesions, 15 (62 %) had orthopedic deformities/scoliosis, and 7 (of 14 toilet trained) had incontinence. Preoperative UD was abnormal in 21 (87.5 %): 17 with detrusor overactivity and 4 with decreased compliance (Guerra et al. 2006).

MRI spinal cord findings varied in these studies: Nogueira et al. stated that a conus positioned at the midpoint or below the second vertebra diagnosed tethered cord, but a thickened filum alone did not. In contrast, Guerra et al. and Macejko et al. reported a variety of lesions, including thickened filum, lipoma, syearinx, diastematomyelia, and spina bifida occulta.

Other Etiologies for Neurogenic Bladder

Cerebral Palsy

Three retrospective studies reported that the most common abnormal UD findings in children with cerebral palsy referred for urologic evaluation were detrusor overactivity in approximately 50 % and DSD in ≤10 %.

A retrospective report comprised 57 children with cerebral palsy referred from ages 2 to 20 years with voiding complaints, including incontinence in 49 (86 %), isolated urgency and frequency in 3, and retention in 1. UD was performed (with needle electrode EMG for external sphincter function). Findings included detrusor overactivity in 34 (60 %), DSD with retention in 3, reduced capacity in 2, and "hypertonia" in 2. The authors considered findings consistent with an upper motor neuron injury in 49 (86 %) patients, while 6 (11 %) had EMG evidence of an incomplete lower motor neuron injury (Decter et al. 1987).

Another retrospective review of 31 consecutive children with cerebral palsy at median age 10 years (4.5–17) reported 7 (23 %) were voiding and continent, 3 (10 %) used CIC plus AC, and the remainder wore diapers. UD demonstrated detrusor overactivity in 16 (52 %) (Richardson and Palmer 2009).

A third retrospective study included 36 children with cerebral palsy evaluated at mean age 8 years (4–18), of which 24 (67 %) had voiding symptoms. UD was abnormal in 21 (58 %), with detrusor overactivity in 17 (47 %) and DSD in 4 (11 %) (diagnosed using patch EMG electrodes) (Karaman et al. 2005).

Anorectal Malformations

Prevalence of neurogenic bladder in children with anorectal malformation is 12–35 %, with

two studies reporting most, but not all, associated with spinal/sacral anomalies.

Ninety consecutive children, mean age 17 months (1–128), with anorectal malformations (29 % high, 51 % low) had a mean of two UD evaluations. Neurogenic bladder was diagnosed in 22 (24 %), all but 1 of which also had partial sacral agenesis. UD in 52 patients with a normal sacrum found uninhibited detrusor contractions in 5 that were considered possibly normal for patient age and so were not considered evidence of neurogenic bladder (Boemers et al. 1996).

Another study included 89 patients with anorectal malformation classified as low in 39 (44 %), high in 45 (51 %), and as cloaca in 5 (6 %). Sixty had UD at mean age 5 years, done in 54 because of spine abnormalities, with neurogenic bladder diagnosed in 31/89 (35 %) with detrusor overactivity in 21 and areflexia in 10. These occurred in both low (40 %) and high (51 %) malformations. Of the 31 patients, spinal/sacral anomalies were found in 28 (90 %) (Mosiello et al. 2003).

A German registry of patients with anorectal malformation was used to identify 267 individuals who then were visited at home by physicians using standardized forms to collect data. Thirty-two (12 %) had neurogenic bladder dysfunction (not defined) (Maerzheuser et al. 2011).

Urodynamics

Even though urodynamic assessment is a cornerstone in the diagnosis and treatment of neurogenic bladder, best practices in its performance and terminology to describe its results remain ill-defined.

Since technical factors described below potentially impact UD findings, caution is needed in clinical decision-making based on urodynamic assessment.

Furthermore, no study shows inter- and intra-observer agreement in UD interpretation in children with neurogenic bladder. Consequently, urologists analyzing the same patient might draw different conclusions regarding bladder function, and readers studying published reports cannot be certain the authors categorized patients as they would have.

Urodynamics: Technical Considerations

DLPP is potentially increased by larger transurethral catheters (7, 10 Fr versus 5 Fr) and faster infusion rates (25 cc/min versus 2.5 cc/min).

Uninhibited contractions are reported more likely seen with UD performed in the seated than supine position, in the first versus second cycle, and with room temperature versus body temperature infusions.

There are no published standards for technical aspects of the examinations.

One study performed UD in 23 children 5 weeks to 21 years of age with neurogenic bladder (20 myelomeningocele, 1 lipomeningocele, 1 spinal cord injury, and 1 sacral agenesis). Infusion was done by gravity at a rate of 15–22 cc/min. Studies were performed using first a 7-Fr and then 10-Fr triple-lumen catheter, and finally with two 5-Fr feeding tubes transurethrally. DLPP increased in 75 % of cases with larger catheter size. Extent of change was not described, except to state that in 8 (35 %) there was no leakage despite bladder distention when a 7- or 10-Fr catheter was used, and that in seven patients DLPP was <40 cm H_2O using 5-Fr and >40 cm H_2O using larger catheters. These differences occurred in patients up to age 14 years (Decter and Harpster 1992).

Although transurethral catheters can create partial obstruction, no study has compared suprapubic to transurethral pressure measurements in children.

Infusion rates may also impact DLPP. One study compared filling at approximately 25 cc/min to 2.5 cc/min via a 7-Fr catheter in 38 children ranging in age from 16 days to 18 years (mean 3 years) with myelodysplasia. In 26 cases there was no variation in detrusor pressure based on infusion rate, while in the other 12 (32 %) there was a significant increase of >15 cm H_2O with more rapid than slower infusion. In 14 (37 %) DLPP exceeded 40 cm H_2O with rapid infusion but not with slower inflow (Joseph 1992).

A prospective randomized trial compared both room temperature versus body temperature (heated) saline infusion in 58 children mean age 9 years (for larger cohort of 101 patients) with spinal dysraphism and reported room temperature studies had significantly greater (16 %) bladder capacity, pressure during filling, and uninhibited detrusor contractions (Chin-Peuckert et al. 2004).

A nonrandomized study sequentially allocated patients to undergo urodynamic evaluation supine versus sitting. The study population was not defined, except for mean age 10 years with spinal dysraphism in 19/48 patients. No differences were noted for bladder capacity or DLPP, but detrusor overactivity (60 % versus 53 %) and observed incontinent episodes (42 % versus 35 %) were significantly more common in patients sitting (Lorenzo et al. 2007).

Concordance of findings in two consecutive studies performed during one session was reported in a retrospective study of 66 children a mean age of 7.4 years with varying diagnoses, including spinal dysraphism in 43 (65 %), but also non-neurogenic conditions (posterior urethral valves, voiding dysfunction). These patients were selected from a larger cohort of 112 children to include those who underwent two trials during a single session using the same inflow rate and patient position. Why these patients had two tests while others did not was not stated. Maximum bladder capacity, end filling pressure, and DLPP were not significantly different between the two studies, although detrusor overactivity was more often observed during the first than second trial (Chin-Peuckert et al. 2003).

Bladder Capacity

One study reported capacity in myelodysplastic children to age 9 years is 25 % less than predicted using the common age-based formula [capacity cc = (age + 2) × 30].

UD results from patients studied between 1983 and 1994 were reviewed to determine if age-based formulas [capacity cc = (age + 2) × 30] accurately predict bladder capacity in children with myelomeningocele. Filling was done at a rate of 3–5 % of expected capacity per minute using a 6- or 7-Fr dual-channel urethral catheter in 506 children at mean age 5 years. Patients received no anticholinergic or sympathomimetic medications, and prior bladder surgery and VUR were exclusions. Capacity was defined as the volume when there was leakage or voiding, or discomfort, or infusion spontaneously stopped. Capacity was found to be related to age through 9 years, and approximately 25 % less in patients with myelodysplasia versus neurologically normal children (Palmer et al. 1997).

ICCS Recommendations

Based on expert opinion, the ICCS recommends UD be performed using "as small a catheter as possible" at a rate in cc/min calculated from body weight (kg)/4, or 5–10 % expected bladder capacity for age (Neveus et al. 2006).

Leak Point Pressure >40 cm H_2O

DLPP >40 cm H_2O has been widely accepted as an indicator of bladder pressure posing a high risk for development of hydronephrosis, VUR, and loss of detrusor compliance, based on a single retrospective study.

Technical factors in UD studies discussed above potentially impact DLPP and so could result in an error in diagnosis of high risk.

In addition, storage time at pressure >40 cm H_2O before leakage occurs varies between patients, potentially creating different exposures to high pressures even in children with identical DLPP.

DLPP is defined as the lowest detrusor pressure at which urine leakage occurs in the absence of either a detrusor contraction or increased abdominal pressure (Abrams et al. ICS 2002).

A retrospective analysis was reported in 42 patients with myelodysplasia followed a mean of 7 years (3–15), without further description of age, number of UD, or other inclusion/exclusion criteria. UD findings were compared to IVP and

VCUG. UD was done using a transurethral triple-lumen catheter (size not stated), or two 8-Fr catheters, with "slow filling" (infusion rate not stated). In five patients, a Foley balloon was used to occlude the bladder neck because of leakage at low bladder volume. Seven of 42 (17 %) were described as having "a reflex detrusor response" to filling that was considered normal in 4 and DSD in 3. The other 35 had areflexia, with 30 having decreased compliance and 5 having no increase in pressure during filling. Of the entire cohort, intravesical pressure at urine leakage was less than 40 cm H_2O in 20, none of whom had VUR and 2 had ureteral dilation. DLPP was greater than 40 cm H_2O in 22, with VUR in 15 (68 %) and ureteral dilation in 18 (81 %), $p<0.001$. Actual DLPP were not provided, and the number of patients with DLPP >40 cm H_2O having neither VUR nor dilation was not stated (McGuire et al. 1981).

DMSA-Based Acquired Renal Damage

One endpoint in patient management is avoidance of acquired renal damage, but our review found only one study describing DMSA results in newborns, and two retrospective studies reporting DMSA findings in children, with myelomeningocele.

No longitudinal study analyzes risk factors for renal scarring in patients with neurogenic bladder.

Baseline DMSA

DMSA scintigraphy in newborns with myelodysplasia has only been reported in one prospective observational study, finding 8 % to have abnormalities considered congenital.

One prospective study obtained DMSA as a baseline evaluation in 38 consecutive newborns at approximately age 6 weeks. Of these, 35 (92 %) were normal, while 1 showed a focal cortical defect and another 2 had differential function <45 % (1 with ipsilateral grade 5 VUR)—all considered by clinical history to represent congenital abnormalities (Granberg et al. 2011).

Risk Factors for Renal Scar

Three retrospective studies reported that DMSA scintigraphy found renal scar in 15–32 % of myelodysplastic patients.

VUR and febrile UTI were significant risk factors, but two studies reported urodynamic parameters (DLPP, compliance) were not.

No longitudinal study reports initial and follow-up DMSA to determine baseline findings and risk for subsequent acquired renal damage.

A retrospective analysis included DMSA and UD obtained in 113 sequential patients from 2005 to 2007, from which a study cohort of 64 patients over 10 years of age (mean 16, 10–23) was selected. All had a history of CIC. Function <40 % or focal scar were considered abnormal, and were found in 16 (25 %). Risk factors for abnormal DMSA included VUR (OR 2.06 [95 % CI 1.43–2.97]) and febrile UTI (OR 9.53 [95 % CI 2.674–34.34]) but not DLPP (44 ± 20 versus 46 ± 28 cm H_2O) or detrusor compliance (8.8 ± 5.9 versus 12 ± 11) (Shiroyanagi et al. 2009).

Another retrospective study also obtained UD and DMSA scintigraphy in all referred children and adolescents for incontinence and/or recurrent UTI from 1996 to 2004. Renal scar was defined as focal cortical defects, while children with "shrunken kidney or renal atrophy and diffuse scarring" were excluded as possibly having congenital nephropathy. In patients with mean age 7 ± 4 years, renal scarring was found in 30/95 (32 %) with neurogenic bladder due to myelodysplasia (79 %), sacral agenesis (6 %) and spinal cord tumors, myelitis, etc. (14.6 %). At presentation, 40 % were on AC and 33 % used CIC, the authors commenting that treatments were started "late in life." Univariable analysis found febrile UTI and VUR as risk factors for renal scar, but not neurogenic versus non-neurogenic incontinence (evaluated in another 15 children). Multivariable analysis reported only VUR correlated with scarring, OR 8.12 (95 % CI 2.92–23.14). Of the entire cohort of 120 patients, mean pressure at maximum bladder capacity was 25 ± 23 cm H_2O, with 14 having pressures >40 cm H_2O. No urodynamic parameter, including end pressure at capacity, decreased compliance with end pressure >40 cm H_2O, detrusor overactivity, or DSD, predicted renal scarring (Leonardo et al. 2007).

A third retrospective study reviewed DMSA and VCUG results in 180 children with myelomeningocele evaluated between 1970 and 1988, with DMSA introduced in 1983 but then obtained in all patients. Mean age at DMSA evaluation was not stated. UD was done selectively in an unspecified number of patients, with neither results nor treatments for neurogenic bladder described. VUR was found in 72 (40 %) patients, and renal scar (focal cortical defects) in 28 (15.5 %) patients. Of these 28 patients with scar, 21 (75 %) had VUR grades 2–5 (Cohen et al. 1990).

Newborn Assessment

Initial Imaging and Urodynamics

Three prospective studies reported that 21–32 % of newborns had UD that was considered normal. In these three studies, detrusor pressures >40 cm H_2O were found in 15–25 % of newborns.

Initial US and VCUG were described in two of these studies, with 21 % of newborns reported to have hydronephrosis (8 %) and/or VUR (15 %).

Three prospective, consecutive patient series describe newborn imaging (Table 16.1).

Thirty newborns with myelodysplasia underwent renal ultrasound and VCUG between 1981 and 1984. Reported imaging results combined HN, VUR, and bladder trabeculation (without definition) and stated that 11/30 (36 %) had abnormal findings. Grades of HN and VUR were not stated (Sidi et al. 1986).

Thirty-four consecutive newborns with myelodysplasia underwent imaging, with 7 (21 %) having HN (n=2, 6 %) or VUR (n=5, 15 %), without describing grades (Sillen et al. 1996).

Imaging in 71 consecutive patients <6 months of age reported 14 (20 %) to have HN (n=6, 8 %) or VUR (n=11, 15 %). HN was bilateral in five of six, and was SFU grade 2 (n=3), 3 (n=2), and 4 (n=1). VUR was bilateral in four, and grade 1 (n=2), 2 (n=4), 3 (n=1), 4 (n=1), and 5 (n=3) (Granberg et al. 2011).

UD in these three series are summarized in Table 16.2. Differences in methodologies and terminologies limit direct comparisons of results between these.

UD studies by Sidi et al. (1986) used a 7-Fr transurethral double-lumen catheter infusing CO_2 at 10–15 cc/min, and a monopolar 27-gauge needle electrode in the external urethral or anal sphincter in 30 consecutive newborns. Nine of 30 (30 %) were considered to have normal, coordinated detrusor and sphincter activity. Three of 30 (10 %) had DSD, 3 (10 %) had no detrusor contraction with no pressure rise from baseline, and 15 (50 %) had no detrusor contraction associated with rising pressures, of which 6 (20 %) exceeded 40 cm H_2O. No patient was diagnosed with detrusor overactivity.

Sillen et al. (1996) reported that 34 consecutive infants underwent UD at 1 month of age using a 6-Fr transurethral catheter with inflow between 1.6 and 8 cc/min and patch EMG electrodes. Areflexia was defined as including contractions <20 cm H_2O, and poor compliance as pressures >20 cm H_2O. Patch EMG tracings obtained were unsatisfactory to diagnosis DSD. Eleven of 34 (32 %) studies were considered normal, 8 (23 %) had areflexia, and 15 (44 %) had detrusor overactivity. Pressures >20 cm H_2O was only seen in those with detrusor overactivity, occurring in 14/15, of which 8 exceeded 40 cm H_2O.

The prospective observational study by Granberg et al. (2011) evaluated 71 consecutive newborns and infants <6 months of age, using a 5-Fr transurethral urodynamic catheter, inflow at 10 cc/min and patch EMG electrodes. No attempt was made to diagnose DSD. Sixteen of 71 (23 %) were considered normal. Eleven (15 %) had no detrusor contraction and all had end filling pressures <25 cm H_2O. The remaining 45 (63 %) had detrusor overactivity with filling pressures (baseline from which contractions occurred) <25 cm H_2O in 15, between 25 and 40 cm H_2O in 17 and >40 cm H_2O in 11.

Table 16.1 Upper tract imaging in newborns with spina bifida

Authors	No. patients	Age at imaging	Total abnormal	Hydronephrosis (SFU grades)	VUR (grades)
Sidi et al. (1986)	30	<1 month	11 (36 %)[a]	NS	NS
Sillen et al. (1996)	34	1 month	7 (21 %)	2 (6 %) (NS)	5 (15 %) (NS)
Granberg et al. (2011)	71	<6 months	14 (20 %)	6 (8 %) SFU 2:3 3:2 4:1	11 (15 %) G 1:2 2:4 3:1 4:1 5:3

NS not stated
[a]Included hydronephrosis, VUR, and/or bladder trabeculation

Table 16.2 UD findings in consecutive newborns with myelomeningocele

	"Normal" (%)	DSD (%)	No contraction (%)	Overactivity (%)
Sidi et al. (1986) $n=30$	30	10[a]	60	0
Sillen et al. (1996) $n=32$	32	0[b]	23	44
Granberg et al. (2011) $n=71$	23	0[b]	31	46

[a]Used needle electrodes
[b]Used patch electrodes; findings considered inconclusive for DSD

Changes in Imaging and Urodynamics

One retrospective study reported 50 % of newborns considered to have a normal UD voided spontaneously after age 3. Another 33 % developed abnormal UD patterns, all considered due to tethered cord.

Two prospective studies reported 5 and 15 % of newborns considered by UD to be low risk (normal findings, or pressures <40 cm H_2O) developed pressures 40 cm H_2O and/or new hydronephrosis or VUR within 2 years.

A retrospective review found 25 newborns considered to have normal UD from among 204 studied between 1979 and 1998. Follow-up included imaging and annual UD. Eight of 25 (32 %) had adverse urodynamic changes, six without clinical symptoms, UTI in one, and urge incontinence in the other. All eight were diagnosed with tethered cord and underwent release that was restored initial UD patterns in two. None developed hydronephrosis or VUR. Twelve children were over age 3 years who retained a normal UD study without prior deterioration, and all were described as voiding "voluntarily with complete, or nearly complete, continence and bowel elimination" (Tarcan et al. 2001).

The 30 newborns reported by Sidi et al. described above were divided into two groups based on initial UD-based risk assessment and followed a mean of 18 months (4–42) with periodic imaging (Fig. 16.1):

- Nine were considered at high risk, including three with DSD and six with no contractions and end pressures >40 cm H_2O. Of these, five with abnormal radiologic findings underwent therapy (CIC plus anticholinergics or vesicostomy), while four with initial normal radiology were observed. At a mean of 13 months (6–22), all four had radiologic changes (not defined) leading to CIC plus anticholinergics.
- Twenty-one newborns with normal urodynamic tests or no detrusor contraction with end pressures <40 cm H_2O were considered low risk. Initially, six had abnormal radiology, and all were observed with only antibiotic

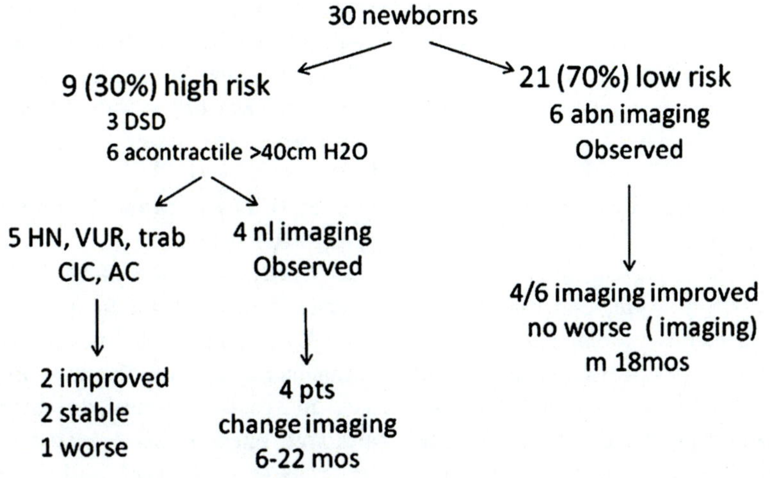

Fig. 16.1 UD-based selective therapy. Created with data from Sidi et al. (1986)

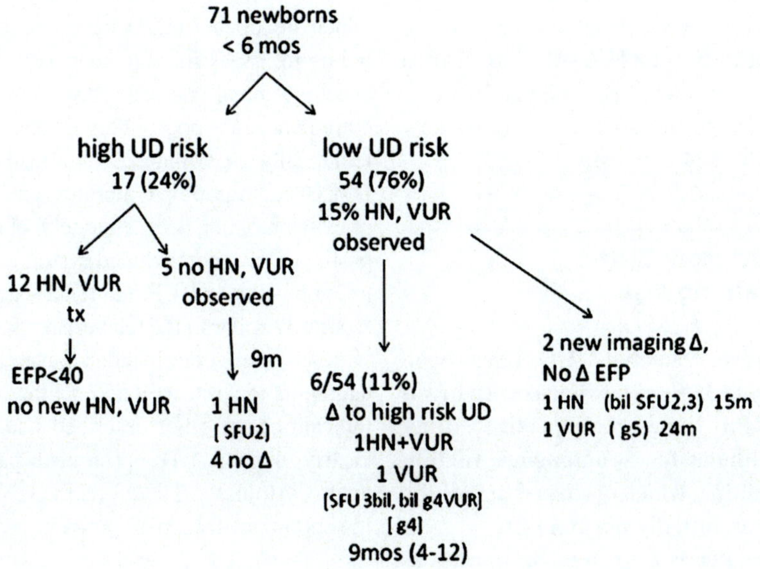

Fig. 16.2 UD-based selective therapy. Created with data from Granberg et al. (2011)

prophylaxis, with four becoming normal in one to more than 2 years, one remaining stable, and one progressing VUR from grade I to IV, with repeat UD showing decreased compliance, resulting in treatment by reimplantation, CIC, and anticholinergics. The remaining 15 with normal imaging had no adverse changes on subsequent imaging.

During follow-up in both groups, adverse changes were initially diagnosed on the basis of imaging that prompted repeat UD, which otherwise were not done in stable or improved patients. Adverse changes specifically in those thought to be at low risk occurred in only 1/21 (5 %).

The prospective trial described by Granberg et al. (2011) followed a similar protocol for 71 newborns (Fig. 16.2): therapy for those with high-risk UD and abnormal imaging versus observation in those with low-risk UD regardless of imaging results:

- Seventeen (24 %) considered high risk had detrusor overactivity with end filling pressures >40 cm H_2O, of which 12 started CIC and anticholinergics, while 5 with normal imaging were observed. Of the five that were observed, one developed new SFU grade 2 hydronephrosis, while four others remained stable a mean of 9 months later.
- Fifty-four (76 %) were considered low risk with normal UD, or having either no detrusor contraction or detrusor overactivity with end filling pressures <40 cm H_2O, observed with renal US every 6 months and repeated UD at 12 and 36 months. Of these, 6 (11 %) converted to DLPP over 40 cm H_2O at mean of 9 months later (4–12), with new bilateral SFU 3 HN and bilateral VUR grade 4 in one, and new unilateral VUR grade 4 in another. Two others who did not have conversion on UD to increased DLPP >40 cm H_2O still had a change in imaging, one having new bilateral SFU 2 and 3 HN at 15 months and the other new grade 5 VUR at 24 months.

Management from Birth to Toilet-Training Age

As noted above, "normal" UD have been reported in up to 33 % of newborns with myelodysplasia. Only one retrospective study reported likelihood for spontaneous voiding after toilet training, which occurred in half the children with an initially normal UD.

Twenty-five percent or less of newborns with myelodysplasia have UD findings of bladder pressures >40 cm H_2O. Up to 15 % of those thought to be low risk and observed convert to high risk within 2 years.

Therefore, ≥60 % of newborns and infants are not at high risk for renal damage or loss of bladder compliance in the first 3 years of life, based on UD findings of detrusor pressures <40 cm H_2O.

Three newborn assessment and management options have been proposed:

- **Initial evaluation and follow-up with imaging**
- **Universal CIC and anticholinergics**
- **Selective UD-based assessment and treatment**

All have a limited evidence basis for the goals of avoiding acquired renal damage or adverse changes in bladder compliance.

CIC in newborns and infants, started in those with HN and/or VUR with end filling pressures >40 cm H_2O was associated with greater fUTI rates than was observed in one prospective study.

A Cochrane review of RCTs found no difference in rate or time for onset of symptomatic UTI based on sterile versus clean catheterization, single versus multiple catheter use, or coated versus uncoated catheters, although participants reported coated catheters were easier to insert and remove.

Available data for each of three management options are summarized below, but most reports are retrospective, with long study periods during which treatments might have changed, and endpoints to assess management, specifically avoidance of renal damage and loss of bladder compliance, are poorly defined and were not systematically determined. As already mentioned, DMSA scintigraphy to monitor renal function and scarring has not been routinely obtained. Some protocols have not included cystography, yet a correlation between VUR and renal scarring has been reported similar to the relationship seen in patients without neurogenic bladder. Several reports note augmentation rates related to therapy, although indications were not described and there are no clearly defined UD or clinical parameters for enterocystoplasty. Therefore, the level of evidence to support any treatment protocol is poor.

Imaging-Based Observation

A retrospective review of new patients with myelomeningocele evaluated between 1975 and 2000 identified 184 patients, 83 of which were ≤6 months of age and comprised the study group. Initial assessment was renal US and physical examination to detect urinary retention. Eighteen (22 %) patients were defined as high risk because of HN ($n=6$ [7 %]) or retention ($n=12$ [14 %]). Sixteen of 18 high-risk patients had various interventions (CIC, AC, vesicostomy). Twenty-nine of 65 (45 %) initial low-risk patients were later considered high-risk at mean age of 3 years (2 months to 12 years), on the basis of f UTI ($n = 13$), new HN ($n = 5$), finding of VUR during assessment for continence ($n = 5$) or urinary retention ($n = 5$). However, some of these patients had been started on CIC, presumably for continence, as 4/13 with f UTI were being catheterized. Based on new HN alone, 5/65 (8 %) initially observed had adverse upper tract changes. Renal deterioration defined as failure of renal growth or renal scar on ultrasound was noted in 2/83 patients, but DMSA imaging was not routinely obtained. The number of children with UD testing was not stated, and since VCUG was not systematically done the prevalence of VUR was not reported (Hopps and Kropp 2003).

Universal CIC and Anticholinergics

A retrospective review reported patients treated on a protocol from 1988 to 2001 that placed all newborns on CIC, AC, and antibiotic prophylaxis (frequency of CIC and type/dosing of medications not stated). Renal US and serum creatinine were obtained at initial assessment, with baseline UD performed at approximately 3 months of age, and then annually (technique only described as "standard 5 channel"). DMSA was obtained for suspected renal abnormality on US (number obtained not stated). There were 144 total patients, of which 35 (24 %) had spina bifida occulta. Follow-up was a mean of 81.6 months (5.4–162.2). Initial renal US was normal in 271/288 (94 %) renal units, and showed "mild" or "gross" dilation in 5 and 4. During follow-up, repeat renal ultrasonography remained normal in 262 (91 %) renal units, while (new) mild and gross dilation were found in 7 and 1, and 10 were thought to have new renal scarring confirmed with DMSA in 6 (4 %). Continence outcomes were reported for 82 children >6 years of age. Twenty-two were voiding, indicating universal CIC was discontinued at some point, 34 (41 %) had undergone augmentation, and presumably the other 26 continued on CIC and AC (Dik et al. 2006). There was no comparison group without treatment, and the number of patients not compliant with therapy was not stated.

Urodynamic-Based Selective Therapy

The prospective observational study by Sidi et al. (1986) described earlier divided newborns with myelodysplasia into high- versus low-risk categories based on UD (see Fig. 16.1). The endpoint in this evaluation was imaging deterioration, but the authors did not separately describe VUR versus HN. There were no data regarding acquired renal functional loss or scarring, and no follow-up UD data after the initial newborn assessment.

The prospective trial described above by Granberg et al. (2011) followed a similar UD-based risk assessment for 71 consecutive newborns (see Fig. 16.2). Imaging and UD changes from initial high- and low-risk designations are described earlier. Baseline DMSA data were available in 38, also reported above, but follow-up DMSA results were pending.

Two retrospective studies reported early therapy reduced later need for augmentation specifically in patients considered at high risk on UD.

In the first, a chart review identified and compared two patient groups thought to have high risk for renal damage based on initial UD, those with CIC and AC begun at <1 year of age versus those presenting later with similar therapy starting after age 4 years. High risk was defined as "positive perineal patch EMG activity and narrowing of membranous urethra on VCUG (presumably representing DSD), detrusor contractions to >30 cm H_2O, and/or poor compliance at volumes less than expected capacity." Treatment was CIC every 3 h plus oxybutynin 0.1 mg/kg 3× daily.

The 46 beginning treatment at age <1 year were considered comparable to the 52 with initiation of therapy at age >47 months, with HN in 14 (30 %) versus 13 (27 %), bladder trabeculation in 10 (22 %) versus 12 (23 %), VUR in 9 (20 %) versus 12 (23 %), and "high pressure on cystometry" in 45 (98 %) versus 47 (90 %):

- There was no difference in response to medical therapy determined by changes in renal US ("improvement" in 8/14 [57 %] versus 6/13 [47 %]; persistence in 6 [43 %] versus 7 [54 %]).
- There was no difference in persistent VUR (2/9 [22 %] versus 5/12 [42 %]).

- Continence, defined as no pads, was similarly achieved in 18/ 46 (39 %) versus 20/54 (38 %).
- The only significant difference was in rate of enterocystoplasty, 5/45 (11 %) versus 14/52 (27 %) $p<0.05$, which was performed for "recurrent symptomatic UTI, worsening HN, or nontolerance to therapy"—none of which was found to be different between groups.

Mean age was significantly greater during follow-up in the late presenting group (143 versus 85 months) (Wu et al. 1997). Since initial and subsequent assessments were similar for all parameters between the two groups, the difference in augmentation rate may only have indicated follow-up to an older age in those presenting after age 4 years versus those beginning therapy as infants.

The second also retrospectively identified and assessed two cohorts, but these were all infants less than 1 year of age considered to be at high risk for bladder deterioration based on initial UD showing DSD and/or high filling pressures (>30 cm H_2O at 75 % predicted capacity) or high voiding pressures (>80 cm H_2O in males and >65 cm H_2O in females). Forty-seven infants observed after testing between 1978 and 1984 did not begin medical therapy until a mean of 4 years (1–14) were compared to 18 similar patients after 1985 who had CIC and AC (oxybutynin 0.2 mg/kg given 2–4x daily) instituted at less than 1 year of age. Deterioration was defined as incontinence and/or HN ± VUR. During follow-up, 6/47 (13 %) versus 3/18 (17 %) had incontinence; 5/47 (11 %) had HN and/or VUR versus 0/18; and augmentation was eventually done in 11/47 (23 %) versus 3/18 (15 %), $p=0.74$ (Kaefer et al. 1999).

Consequently, neither retrospective study demonstrated a difference in objective outcome variables based on early versus delayed medical therapy in patients considered to have high-risk UD.

Febrile UTI

Febrile UTI occurred in 25 % of newborns and infants in one prospective observational study, 9/17 (53 %) considered high risk on initial UD (end filling pressures >40 cm H_2O plus HN and/or VUR) versus 9/54 (17 %) with low-risk UD. These fUTIs were more likely in children on CIC, 10/18 (56 %) CIC versus 8/53 (15 %) being observed, $p=0.001$ (Granberg et al. 2011).

Development of symptomatic UTI (positive urine culture and symptoms) was the primary endpoint of a Cochrane review of RCTs comparing catheterization techniques (three trials of sterile versus clean, six trials for single versus multiple use, one comparing standard lubricant to antibiotic gel) and catheter types (four trials of coated versus uncoated, two comparing coated versus multiuse uncoated catheters) in both adults and children. No trials were found comparing self versus caregiver catheterization or comparing catheter cleaning techniques. A total of 565 participants were enrolled, with 74 % completing. Key findings included:

Sterile Versus Clean CIC

- No difference in symptomatic UTI.
- No difference in time to onset of symptomatic UTI, with mean times ranging from 1 to 4 weeks in the three studies.

Single-Use (Sterile) Versus Multiple-Use (Clean)

- No difference in symptomatic UTI.
- No difference in time to onset of symptomatic UTI.

Coated Versus Uncoated Catheters

- One of four trials reported marginally significant fewer UTIs with coated catheters; three studies found no difference.
- Two trials reported participants scored coated catheters better for insertion, extraction, and comfort (Moore et al. 2007).

Medical Management

Few management studies describe AC dose or interval, clinical or UD efficacy, or discontinuation due to side effects.

Initial therapy in infants and children is oxybutynin 0.2 mg/kg/dose given 2–4× daily, with one study reporting reduction in end filling pressures to <40 cm H_2O in all infants treated.

One trial reported patients intolerant or having insufficient response to oxybutynin XL had dose adjustment to a tolerable level plus either tolterodine LA or solifenacin for two-drug AC therapy. Incontinent episodes decreased and mean bladder capacity increased, with no patient having side effects to discontinue treatment.

Systematic review of intravesical oxybutynin reported therapy decreased end filling pressures a pooled mean of −16 cm H_2O. Intravesical and oral therapy can also be combined.

Systematic review of botox injection in children with neurogenic bladder reported therapy decreased incontinent episodes and detrusor end filling pressures, with effects sustained to ≤6 months.

Oral Anticholinergics

One report described treatment in newborns using oral oxybutynin 0.2 mg/kg/dose given 2–4× daily, with conversion to intravesical oxybutynin (regimen not described) for side effects. The number of infants treated 2× versus 4× daily, the number changed to intravesical AC, and the impact of treatment on UD parameters were not described (Kaefer et al. 1999).

The prospective series by Granberg et al. (2011) reported medical management in 71 newborns and infants. AC was started in those with both end filling pressures >40 cm H_2O and HN and/or VUR using oxybutynin 0.2 mg/kg given 2–4× daily. Twelve met criteria for therapy after their initial UD and radiologic assessment and another eight initially observed began medical therapy for increased end filling pressure to >40 cm H_2O (two with new unilateral or bilateral grade 4 VUR) or adverse imaging changes without increased pressures (new unilateral grade 5 VUR, new bilateral HN grades 2, 3). Subsequent UD and imaging demonstrated pressures <40 cm H_2O and resolution or decrease in HN in two with resolution or decrease grade VUR in two. Side effects were not described.

Another series of 502 patients with neurogenic bladder treated at median age 12 years (2 months to 42 years) prescribed oxybutynin 0.3 mg/kg/day in two or three divided doses that was increased to a maximum of 0.5 mg/kg/day. Neither response nor side effects were described (Torre et al. 2011).

Twenty-six consecutive patients, mean age 8 years (3–17), had bladder neck sling without augmentation and were managed with oral oxybutynin 0.2 mg/kg given 3–4× daily, or extended-release 2× daily. Intravesical oxybutynin 5 or 10 mg given 2× daily for children and teens was added to those with side effects or insufficient UD improvement. Eight patients with postoperative increased detrusor pressures and/or uninhibited contractions had increased AC therapy, comprising an increase from 3 to 4× daily in five and addition of intravesical instillation in three. One patient did not comply, and another resumed prior dosing due to side effects, with subsequent UD showing no change, while the other six had decreased end filling pressures to <40 cm H_2O (Snodgrass et al. 2010).

Double Oral Anticholinergic Therapy

A prospective open label protocol added a second oral anticholinergic when a first single agent failed. The study included 19 children, mean age 13.5±3 years, with neurogenic bladder initially treated with oxybutynin XL (maximum 30 mg). Non-responders and those with intolerable side effects had the oxybutynin reduced to the greatest dose tolerated and then tolterodine LA (4 mg) or solifenacin (5–10 mg) was added. Mean number of incontinence episodes daily diminished from 4.5±2.1 to 0.09±0.5, and mean UD bladder capacity increased from 210±98 to 428±159 mL. Side effects included dry mouth, blurred vision, constipation, and headache in 10/19 (53 %), although the authors stated no patient discontinued therapy during median duration 18 months (3–42) (Bolduc et al. 2009).

Intravesical Anticholinergics

A systematic review found eight studies (two prospective and six retrospective) concerning intravesical oxybutynin in children with neurogenic bladder. These encompassed 297 children who started therapy, of which 66 (27 %) discontinued it due to side effects in 28 (9 %) or other causes, including the inconvenience of crushing pills to create the solution. Mean change in bladder compliance was only reported in two studies, both +7 cc/cm H_2O, while pooled mean change in pressure at capacity was −16.4 cm H_2O (95 % CI −22.8 to −10). Dosing is not standardized, with the eight studies reviewed using a maximum of 0.2 mg/kg/day or 20 mg/day (Guerra et al. 2008).

Botox Injections

One systematic literature review identified six studies concerning botox injection in children with neurogenic detrusor overactivity; all were small open-label trials involving fewer than 26 patients with follow-up 12–26 weeks (1–52 weeks). Together these trials enrolled a total of 108 patients at mean age 9.8 years, with 93 % having myelodysplasia. Dose injected varied from 5 to12 U/kg, maximum 300 U, injected throughout the dome and base sparing the trigone. All reported decreased incontinence, with >65 % patients dry. Maximum detrusor pressures also decreased in all studies, while mean bladder compliance increased. However, not all these observations in all studies were statistically significant. Improvement was noted generally within 2 weeks of injection, lasting from 2 weeks to 6 months. Neuromuscular side effects were not reported. There are no data regarding possible injury to the detrusor musculature from repeated injections over time (Game et al. 2009).

Management for Continence

No longitudinal study has reported how many infants with myelodysplasia will be able to void voluntarily with continence versus achieve continence with medical therapy versus require surgery.

Therapy to achieve social continence begins around ages 3–4 years in children not already on medical therapy. CIC ± AC are used initially.

Patients with persistent incontinence due to sphincteric incompetency require outlet surgery to achieve continence.

Enterocystoplasty increases bladder capacity and compliance, but specific indications have not been defined.

One prospective analysis of health-related quality of life before and after surgical reconstructions for spina bifida in 31 children and adolescents reported no significant overall changes despite improved continence.

Medical Therapy

See above.

Surgery for Sphincteric Incompetency

Urine leakage in the absence of a detrusor contraction defines an incompetent urethral closure mechanism.

Surgical options to achieve continence include implantation of the artificial urinary sphincter, bladder neck revision and/or sling, and bladder neck closure.

The role of enterocystoplasty in these patients is ill-defined.

Definition of Sphincteric Incompetency

The ICCS (2002) defines an incompetent urethral closure mechanism as one allowing leakage of urine in the absence of a detrusor contraction.

Clinical reports of children undergoing bladder outlet surgery have further characterized sphincter incompetency in children with neurogenic bladder as having stress incontinence, or incontinence despite CIC and AC with areflexia, a smooth bladder contour,

and open bladder neck on cystography. Reported mean DLPP was ≤45 cm H_2O.

A retrospective series described 36 consecutive patients with neurogenic bladder, 2 with exstrophy/epispadias and 1 with cecoureterocele as having stress incontinence secondary to intrinsic sphincteric deficiency that was treated by bladder neck sling. Mean DLPP was ≤38 cm H_2O (range not stated) (Perez et al. 1996).

Another retrospective review concerned 16 patients with myelodysplasia and 2 with spinal cord injury with incontinence despite CIC, AC, and sympathomimetics. Twelve had SUI, and 15 demonstrated "reflex incontinence" (not stated if this was before or despite AC therapy) with UD findings of mean DLPP 23 ± 10 cm H_2O and mean stress leak point pressure 42 ± 19 cm H_2O. All had an "incompetent bladder outlet" on cystography (Austin et al. 2001).

Criteria for sling was defined in a retrospective review of 63 patients with neurogenic bladder as DLPP <45 cm H_2O, open bladder neck on cystography, and SUI (Castellan et al. 2005).

Sphincter incompetency was diagnosed in two additional retrospective series with 89 and 17 patients as DLPP ≤30 cm H_2O in patients incontinent despite CIC and AC (Chrzan et al. 2009; Salle et al. 1997).

A prospective series of 30 children with neurogenic incontinence reported bladder outlet procedures were done for SUI and/or leakage despite CIC and AC to achieve areflexia. There were four with SUI, and DLPP or end filling pressure (in those without UD leakage) ranged from 8 to 53 cm H_2O (mean 22). Cystography in 28 showed a smooth bladder; the bladder outlet was not described (Snodgrass et al. 2007).

Leadbetter/Mitchell Bladder Neck Revision Plus Sling

One prospective study found Leadbetter/Mitchell bladder neck revision plus sling (LMS) had better initial and long-term continence than did sling alone in both males and females undergoing bladder outlet surgery without augmentation.

LMS reduces the bladder outlet diameter by 50 % to improve coaptation by sling.

A prospective study compared initial and long-term continence in 37 consecutive patients with neurogenic bladder undergoing LMS to 34 prior consecutive patients undergoing sling alone. Of the entire series, 39/71 (55 %) were male, 44 (62 %) were ambulatory, and mean age was 8 years (3–18), with no differences between the two cohorts. Preoperative UD found mean bladder capacity of 85 % (28–200 %) predicted capacity by formula age +2 × 30, and mean DLPP 21 cm H_2O (3–50), also similar between the two groups. No prior or simultaneous augmentations were done, and all had a Mitrofanoff procedure. There were no differences in outcomes based on gender, age at surgery, or ambulatory versus wheelchair status. Initial continence (dry, no pads) determined at 6 months after surgery was significantly different: 29/37 (78 %) LMS versus 18/34 (53 %) sling, $p = 0.04$. Kaplan Meier curves initially showed dry sling patients to have recurrent incontinence during follow-up to nearly 100 months, leaving fewer than 25 % still dry, versus no loss of continence in LMS patients after 18 months, with 60 % still dry at maximum follow-up of 55 months. Postoperative compliance changes in these patients are discussed below (Granberg et al. 2011).

Sling

Reported dryness after slings ranges from 37 to 88 % of children, with similar results in males and females, and augmented versus non-augmented patients.

Prior or simultaneous augmentation has been done in less than 10–100 % of patients in reported series.

Persistent incontinence after sling was due to persistent sphincteric incompetency in all series reviewed below.

A prospective study performed tight 360° rectus fascial sling with Mitrofanoff and no prior or simultaneous augmentation in a consecutive series of 30 children (18 males) with neurogenic bladder at a mean age of 8.6 years (3–17), comprising all patients operated during the study period for neurogenic outlet insufficiency. With mean follow-up 22 months (6–60), 17/30 (57 %) were dry, with no differences in outcomes by gender, age, or ambulatory status. Postoperative UD found DLPP increased a mean of 12 cm H_2O (−5 to 42). Five (17 %) without improvement all had persistent outlet incompetency on postoperative UD (Snodgrass et al. 2007). Bladder response to outlet surgery without augmentation is discussed below.

Subsequent longer follow-up in these patients found new incontinence over time due to recurrent outlet insufficiency (sling failure), resulting in 25 % dryness at 100 months, as mentioned in the section above (Granberg et al. 2011).

Bladder outlet suspension versus 360° tight wrap using rectus fascia was reported in a retrospective review of 27 children with neurogenic incontinence. Nineteen (70 %) had simultaneous augmentation (indications not described). With follow-up ranging from a mean of 2–3.5 years, 10 (37 %) were dry, with no difference based on surgical technique or augmentation versus no augment. Fourteen that remained completely wet had persistent outlet incompetency, including four without augmentation (Barthold et al. 1999).

A retrospective study was done in 89 children (46 male) undergoing rectus fascial sling at mean age 10 years (2–14). During follow-up at a mean of 6 years (2–14), 42 (47 %) were dry. Detrusorraphy was done simultaneously in 59 (66 %) and augmentation in 11 (12 %) for capacity less than 80 % predicted for age and/or compliance with filling pressures >20 cm at 70 % predicted capacity. There were no differences in continence outcomes between those undergoing only sling versus sling with detrusorraphy or augmentation, or in males versus females (Chrzan et al. 2009).

Another retrospective study described 39 children (24 female) with mixed etiology incontinence (34 myelodysplasia) who underwent rectus fascial sling at mean age 9 years (4–17). Sling alone was performed in four, with all others having either prior or simultaneous augmentation (criteria for augmentation not stated). Twenty-three of 39 (59 %) were dry after surgery with mean follow-up of 17 months (8–31). Results did not vary by gender. Nine wet patients were all stated to have no change in postoperative DLPP, implying continued sphincteric incompetency (Perez et al. 1996).

A retrospective series reported outcomes of slings and augmentation in 58 children (15 males) with neurogenic bladder operated at a median age of 11.4 years (4–40) and followed postoperatively for a mean of 4 years (1–10). "Complete passive continence" was achieved in 51 (88 %) (the time point at which this observation was made was not stated, nor was loss of continence in those previously dry described). Postoperative UD performed in 28 patients found DLPP increased a mean of 9 cm H_2O (0–20). Persistent incontinence was due to persistent outlet incompetency in all cases (Castellan et al. 2005).

Artificial Urinary Sphincter

Artificial urinary sphincter (AUS) implantation achieves continence in approximately 60–90 % of patients.

A stated advantage to AUS is potential to empty without CIC, reported in 20–45 % after surgery.

Ten-year device survival varies from less than 10–80 %, with mechanical revisions needed in 25–50 % of patients.

Reported prior or simultaneous augmentation rates vary from a total of 5–43 %.

AMS 800 was implanted in 35 children with neurogenic bladder at mean age 14.4 years (11–18); the indication "sphincteric incompetence" was not defined. During follow-up a mean of 5.5 years (5 months to 11 years), dryness was achieved in 32 (91 %), with 28 (80 %) using CIC. The device was placed at the bladder neck with cuff pressure 61–70 cm H_2O. Implantation without augmentation was done for filling pressure <15 cm H_2O at 50 % of predicted bladder capacity for age (formula used not stated). Enterocystoplasty was done simultaneously in 13 (37 %). Nine mechanical failures occurred in seven (20 %) patients, and device removal for erosion in three (at 2–48 months). In total, 36 devices were implanted into these 35 children, with 32 functioning at the study's end (Lopez Pereira et al. 2006).

A retrospective study reported outcomes in 30 males with myelodysplasia undergoing AMS 800 device placement at the bladder neck. Indications were only defined as incontinence with mean DLPP 38 mmHg (0–70). Mean age at implantation was 12.6 years (9–19), and with mean follow-up 4.7 years, 19 (63 %) were dry, with 22 (73 %) using CIC. Prior or simultaneous augmentation was done in four (13 %) for "small capacity, low compliance or unstable bladders." Mean device survival was 4.7 years (3 months to 15 years), with only four (8 % of originally and subsequently implanted devices) functioning after 8 years. Thirty-two revisions in 17 patients were done for mechanical failure/malfunction (9), reservoir leak (13), erosion (5), infection (6) or too large a cuff (4) (Spiess et al. 2002).

A retrospective analysis of results at a postoperative mean of 12.5 years (5–22) in 79 patients (75 myelodysplasia, 5 bladder exstrophy) reported that 57 (72 %) were dry for 4 h and 36/63 (57 %) with an intact device used CIC. The indication for implantation was incontinence with no detrusor overactivity in bladders with "near normal" capacity and compliance. Simultaneous augmentation was done in four (5 %) patients to achieve these criteria. Age at surgery was a mean of 11.7 years (5–18). The study period included use of three different AUS models (AMS 742 [3], 792 [41], 800 [35]) but found no outcome differences among them. Varying cuff pressures were also used (61–70 [36], 71–80 [36], 81–90 [9]) with no outcome differences, but reasons for selecting these were not stated. A functioning device remained in 63/79 (80 %). Device failure required revisions in 18 (23 %) patients, and erosion in 16, including 4/5 with exstrophy, led to device removal at a mean of 5.6 years (1–11) (Hafez et al. 2002).

Another retrospective analysis included 134 patients, of which 107 had neurogenic bladder. Indications for AUS were not specifically described, except as an option to increase outlet resistance. Mean age at implantation was 10 years (3–39). Prior or simultaneous augmentation (indications not defined) was done in 38 and 19, for a total of 57 (43 %). Dryness for all patients was realized in 115 (86 %) with series follow-up at 7 years. One advantage attributed to AUS use was postoperative ability to empty without CIC, which was reported in 72 % of those with neurogenic bladders preoperatively and 33 % postoperatively. In contrast to Hafez et al., mechanical malfunction was reported more often with AMS 742/792 devices versus AMS 800 (38/59 [64 %] versus 33/109 [30 %], $p < 0.0001$; occurring every 7.6 versus 16 patient-years, $p = 0.0001$). Ten-year device survival was 62.5 % for AMS 800 (Herndon et al. 2003).

Salle Bladder Neck Repair

Two retrospective studies reviewed the Salle bladder neck procedure, including simultaneous augmentation in 50 and 76 %, reporting that 61 and 69 % of patients were dry.

Fistulas shortening the continence mechanism were reported in one study as occurring in 12 %.

Difficulty with urethral CIC occurred in 17 and 29 %.

The Salle repair creates a midline anterior bladder wall flap extending cephalad from the bladder neck, which is sewn to a mucosal strip on the floor of the bladder between the ureteral orifices to lengthen the sphincteric mechanism.

A retrospective report of 17 children (7 males) with mean age 9 years having mixed-etiology incontinence (13 neurogenic bladder) reported Salle repair with follow-up at a mean of 26 months (9–49) with 9/13 (69 %) dry. Thirteen of 17 (76 %) had simultaneous augmentation. The postoperative follow-up protocol was not described, nor was new HN or VUR mentioned. UD results and anticholinergic use were not discussed. Urethrovesical fistula shortening the continence mechanism occurred in two, and three patients had difficulties catheterizing though the repair (Salle et al. 1997).

Another retrospective review involved 18 children (11 males) with neurogenic incontinence despite CIC and "pharmacologic treatment" operated with Salle repair at median age 7 years (3–14), including simultaneous augmentation in 9 (50 %) and Mitrofanoff procedure in 4. At median follow-up of 2 years (7 months to 3 years), 11 (61 %) were dry, and 12 (67 %) needed anticholinergics. Four of 14 (29 %) performing transurethral CIC had difficulty (Jawaheer and Rangecroft 1999).

Bladder Neck Injection

Injection has been done as primary therapy or for persistent incontinence after sling or bladder neck revisions, with prior or simultaneous augmentation in 0–39 %.

Less than 33 % of reported patients became dry, regardless of gender, primary versus secondary treatment, injected volume, injection antegrade versus retrograde, or bladder augmentation or not.

Two studies found second injections successful in <10 % of patients undergoing therapy after failed sling.

A prospective trial injected Dx/HA in 27 children with neurogenic bladder (4 after failed sling). Augmentation was only described for other patients with exstrophy/epispadias. With follow-up a mean of 26 months (6–84), 8 (30 %) were dry. A maximum of three injection sessions were used, with mean volume per session of 4 cc (1.6–12). All injections were done transurethrally, in males at the bladder neck and the external sphincter, whereas in females Dx/HA was injected all along the urethra. A suprapubic catheter was used for continuous drainage for 5 days post-injection. The time at which continence was determined, the number of injections needed and duration of continence were not described. Male versus female outcomes were similar for the entire group, which included patients with exstrophy/epispadias (Lottmann et al. 2006).

A study using polydimethylsiloxane in 44 patients (19 males) with neurogenic bladder at mean age 13 years (7–17) reported 15 (34 %) became dry at median follow-up of 28 months (6–53). All were injected transurethrally at the bladder neck, with additional injections lateral and distal to the verumontanum in males. Mean injected volume was 3.5 cc per session and 5.7 cc per patient. One injection was done in 23, with two or more injections in the remainder, the authors noting that three to four injections were only successful in one of four patients. For 20 children, treatments were primary, while 24 had prior Young-Dees bladder neck repair or a suspension, and 17 (39 %) had prior augmentation. Postoperative CIC continued per urethra without suprapubic drainage. There was no significant difference in results based on gender, primary versus secondary therapy, or augmented versus non-augmented patients (Guys et al. 2001).

A retrospective evaluation was reported for 27 patients with persistent outlet incompetency after fascial sling without augmentation at median age 8.5 years who then underwent injection with either Dx/HA (3) or polydimethylsiloxane (24), performed transurethrally in 16, antegrade in 8 and both in 3. A single injection was done in 15, with two to three in the remainder, using 4–8 cc per injection (mean not stated). At mean follow-up of 8 years (2.4–14), 2 (7 %) were dry. Repeat injections were not effective (de Vocht et al. 2010).

Twenty-six consecutive children (16 males) with neurogenic bladder and persistent outlet incompetency after bladder neck sling ($n = 17$) or LMS ($n = 9$) underwent one to two Dx/HA injections done antegrade (8), transurethrally (1), or both (5). None were augmented. Six of 24 (23 %) with follow-up were dry (Fig. 16.3). Median age was 8.9 years (4.6–17.8). Mean injected volume was 2.2 cc (1.5–3). Of nine dry after one injection, five remained dry at mean 27 months (6–52); of 14 with a second injection, one remained dry at 39 months. Injected volume, injection method, initial bladder neck surgical technique, and patient gender did not correlate with outcomes (DaJusta et al. 2012, in press).

Bladder Neck Closure

Primary bladder neck closure was reported in two studies, achieving dryness in 77 and 88 %.

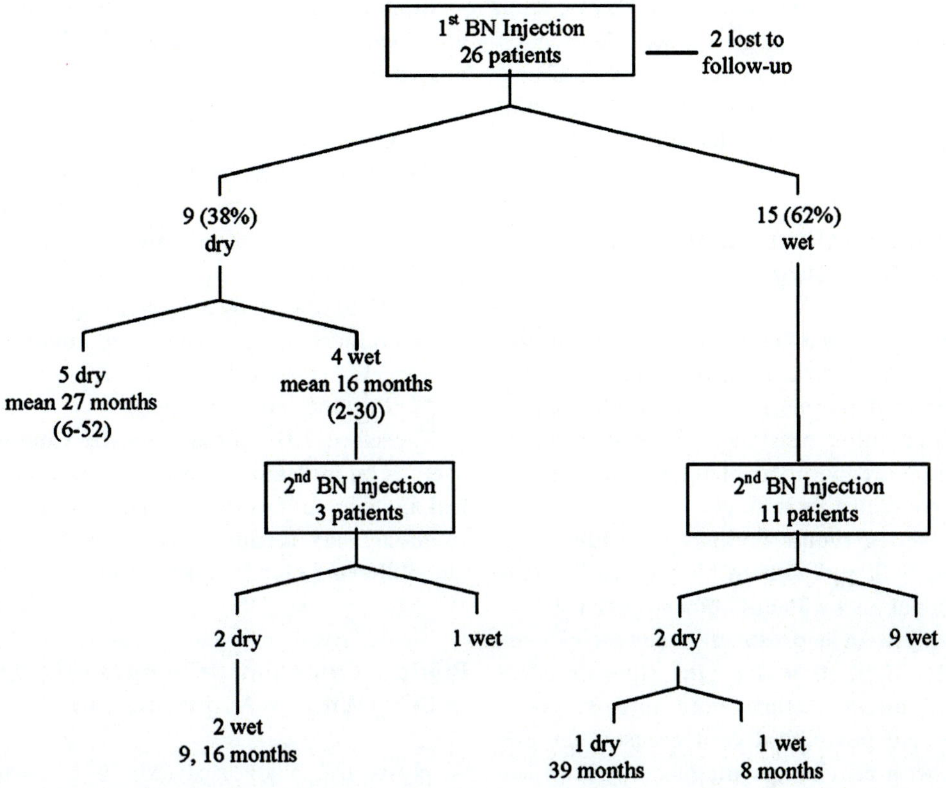

Fig. 16.3 Results of bladder neck injection for incontinence after sling

Closure after failed outlet surgery was reported in one study with 100 % dryness.

Prior or simultaneous augmentation was done in 9–81 %, with 9 % developing bladder perforation in one report.

Bladder neck re-canalization was described by two reports occurring in 2 and 23 %.

A retrospective review included 52 patients (23 male) with mixed-etiology incontinence (36 with myelodysplasia, 3 with sacral agenesis) undergoing bladder neck closure as primary surgery after failed medical therapy. Indications were persistent incontinence despite CIC and AC in non-ambulatory patients with BMI ≥ 30 and "low" DLPP (not defined). Mean age was 13.9 years (1.5–58). Simultaneous augmentation was done in 41 (81 %) apparently for "inadequate bladder capacity" (not defined). At mean follow-up 20 months (2–68), 44/50 (88 %) were dry with CIC every 3 h. Six (12 %) developed stomal stenosis requiring urgent intervention, while overall stomal complications developed in 17 (33 %), including stenosis in 12 and urinary leakage in 5. Re-canalization of the bladder neck was found in one (2 %). Bladder stones developed in 7/51 (14 %) and bladder perforation in 4/44 (9 %) (assuming all occurred following augmentation) (Bergman et al. 2006).

Twenty-one patients with myelodysplasia (15 males) underwent bladder neck closure as primary surgical therapy at mean age 8 years (3–16) and had mean follow-up at 20 years (15–23), reporting that 17 (80 %) were dry. Simultaneous augmentation was done in two (9 %). Re-canalization of the bladder neck occurred in 5 (23 %); stomal complications developed in 15 (68 %), including stenosis in 9 and leakage in 5 (Liard et al. 2001).

Another retrospective review included 17 children, mean age 13.5 years, with mixed-etiology incontinence (10 with myelodysplasia); prior outlet surgery had been done in 12 (71 %). Prior or simultaneous augmentation was done in 13 (76 %).With mean follow-up of 35 months, all patients were dry; difficulty with catheterization occurred in eight (47 %) (Hoebeke et al. 2000).

Bladder Compliance Changes After Bladder Neck Surgery

Decreased bladder compliance after the outlet procedures described above could indicate a change in detrusor dynamics in response to increased outlet resistance, or only represent the true preoperative bladder status previously concealed by leakage.

No series report findings in studies performed with and without bladder neck occlusion in patients with outlet incompetency.

Analysis of a prospective cohort of consecutive patients undergoing sling or LMS without augmentation found approximately 25 % had postoperative decreased compliance, with all changes diagnosed within the first postoperative year and successfully treated with increased AC and overnight continuous catheter drainage.

Need for secondary augmentation is unclear given that retrospective reports often do not state when adverse changes first occurred or what changes in medical management preceded augmentation:

- **Two retrospective series of sling without augmentation reported 0 and 5 % of patients.**
- **One report of AUS without augmentation having follow-up at 18–48 months stated that no delayed enterocystoplasties were done. Other series had secondary augmentation rates of 3, 32, and 44 %.**
- **One report of Dx/HA bladder neck injection noted that 19 % of patients manifested decreased compliance leading to augmentation.**

As there is no agreed indication for augmentation, selection bias is inevitable, both for those undergoing simultaneous enterocystoplasty during bladder outlet procedures and those thought to need subsequent augmentation.

Bladder capacity (and therefore compliance) can also *increase* after bladder outlet procedures:

- **One study with consecutive patients undergoing sling without augmentation reported increased bladder capacity ranging from 12 to 437 % (mean 90 %) over preoperative volume in 65 % of patients. This included 4/5 patients with preoperative capacity <50 % predicted by age-based formula.**
- **Mean increase in capacity and compliance was also reported in patients undergoing AUS without augmentation.**

Therefore, UD bladder capacity cannot be used as an indicator for enterocystoplasty, as leakage may underestimate true capacity and small-capacity bladders may increase in volume following bladder outlet procedures.

Bladder Compliance Changes After LMS or Sling Without Augmentation

A prospective study analyzed 26 consecutive patients undergoing 360° tight sling and having two postoperative UD within 18 months of operation, the first a mean of 7 months (3–12) and the last at a mean of 39 months (19–94). Preoperative bladder capacity at pressures <40 cm H_2O ranged from 70 to 500 cc, corresponding to 26–120 % predicted [based on formula of capacity = (age + 2) × 30], with 5 (19 %) having <50 % predicted volume. DLPP was <40 cm H_2O in 24 (92 %). Eight of 26 (31 %) patients had decreased compliance and/or uninhibited contractions on the first postoperative UD managed with an increase in anticholinergics. Volumes at last UD versus preoperative UD ranged from −45 to +437 %, and were decreased in 5, stable in 4, and increased in 17 (65 %). Increased volume ranged from 12 to 437 %, averaging 90 %, and occurred in 4/5 with preoperative capacity <50 % predicted by formula. All adverse findings were found on the initial postoperative UD, with no trend towards progressive compliance loss. No patient developed new HN, VUR, or bladder trabeculation (Snodgrass et al. 2010).

A subsequent publication from the same institution concerned a total of 71 patients (including the

26 described above) after sling versus LMS. Postoperative compliance changes leading to increased medical therapy occurred in 16/71 (23 %) that were all detected less than a year after surgery on initial UD and that responded to increased oral anticholinergics (oxybutynin 5 mg 4× daily± intravesical oxybutynin 5–10 mg 2× daily) and overnight catheter drainage. New HN grades 2–4 was found on postoperative imaging at any time during follow-up in 4/71 (6 %), and new VUR in 10/71 (14 %), grade 1 in 2, grade 2 in 6, grade 3 in 1, and grade 4 in 1 patient. Augmentation was done in three (4 %), one for loss of compliance and two others after second opinions for persistent incontinence or pubic pain. There were no differences in these outcomes between sling versus LMS, but initial and durable continence was significantly greater for LMS (Granberg et al. 2011).

The review by Chrzan et al. (2009) mentioned above included 89 patients undergoing sling, of which 11 had augmentation and 59 detrusorectomy for preoperative filling pressures >20 cm H_2O at <70 % predicted capacity (formula not stated). At mean follow-up at 6 years (2–14), 15/19 (79 %) who had sling alone were dry or improved (sporadic incontinence, no diapers). Apparently one (5 %) had subsequent augmentation, but indications and attempted medical therapies were not described. Postoperative UD and imaging findings also were not described.

Austin et al. (2001) also described the above reported sling in 18 patients with neurogenic incontinence, of which 12 (66 %) did not have augmentation, while 2 had prior and 4 simultaneous enterocystoplasty (indications not stated). At mean follow-up of 21 months (6–57), mean compliance (27±10 mL/cm H_2O) was unchanged in the 12 non-augmented children. Imaging changes, if any, were not reported.

Bladder Compliance Changes After AUS Without Augmentation

A retrospective series involved 44 children (35 with neurogenic bladder) with AUS and no augmentation, an unknown additional number with "severe detrusor instability and low compliance" excluded from study. During follow-up a minimum of 18 months, dryness was achieved in 28 (64 %). Eight (18 %) used CIC. Preoperative and postoperative UDs were compared with maximum follow-up of 48 months (mean and range not stated), finding mean capacity and compliance for the entire group studied increased. The actual numbers of patients with increases versus decreases was not stated. HN developed in 2 % and resolved with CIC; new VUR, if any, was not reported. No patient had augmentation (Churchill et al. 1987).

Of 35 patients with neurogenic incontinence undergoing AUS described by Lopez Pereira et al. (2006), 22 (63 %) with detrusor filling pressures <15 cm H_2O at 50 % of predicted capacity for age [capacity=(age +2)×30] did not have augmentation. During mean follow-up of 5.5 years (3 months to 11 years), 7 (32 %) underwent enterocystoplasty. All were using CIC. The decision for augmentation was reached a mean of 3 years postoperatively (1–6) based on poor compliance in patients only described as having incontinence (2) or VUR (5) without clinical symptoms. Postoperative medical therapy before augmentation and preoperative and postoperative UD findings were not described.

Similarly, Spiess et al. (2002) reported AUS without augmentation in 27 males with neurogenic continence and bladder capacity "corresponding to age," of which 12 (44 %) underwent postoperative augmentation for decreased compliance. Time for this occurrence and use of alternative treatments (CIC, AC) before proceeding to augmentation were not described.

In contrast, only 3 % of patients in the retrospective review by Hafez et al. (2002) had post-AUS augmentation. Of 79 patients (74 with neurogenic incontinence), the bladder preoperatively was described as having "near normal compliance and age-adjusted capacity" except for 4 with "poor compliance" who had simultaneous augmentation. With follow-up a mean of 12.5 years (5–22), postoperative detrusor overactivity developed in 13/75 (17 %) not augmented, which was managed by AC in 8, spinal cord detethering in 3, and enterocystoplasty in only 2 (3 %).

Bladder Compliance Changes After Bladder Neck Injection

Lottmann et al. (2006) described Deflux bladder neck injection without augmentation in 27 children with neurogenic bladder (four after failed sling). With follow-up a mean of 26 months (6–84), six (22 %) manifested diminished compliance following injection, with five undergoing augmentation (interval to change in bladder parameters, extent of pressure changes, upper tract changes, or changes in medical therapy used were not stated) (Lottmann et al. 2006).

Enterocystoplasty

Bladder augmentation using ileum or colon segments increases bladder capacity and compliance.

No randomized trial compares ileum versus colon regarding improvement in compliance versus complications.

Potential complications after enterocystoplasty include metabolic acidosis, B_{12} deficiency, bladder calculi, persistent decreased compliance, bladder rupture, and malignancy.

One prospective study reported that colon had greater complication rates than ileum, and one retrospective study found sigmoid augments more likely than other enterocystoplasties to rupture.

One study reported data obtained on a prospective protocol in 86 children undergoing augmentation for various reasons, including neurogenic bladder in 52 (60 %). Augmentation was done using ileum (32), colon (30), or stomach (18), and bladder replacement was done using colon (6) at mean age of 12.5 years (4–21) with follow-up a mean of 8.6 years (1–20). Fifty-six of 86 (65 %) had 105 complications that included 39 (10 %) bladder calculi, 5 (6 %) ruptures, 3 (3 %) inadequate bladder compliance, 3 (3 %) premalignant histological changes, and 4 (5 %) epididymoorchitis. Overall complications and bladder calculi were more frequent after colocystoplasty (Kispal et al. 2011).

A retrospective review identified 500 augmentations done at mean age 11.8 years for patients with conditions that included myelomeningocele ($n=272$, 54 %) or other causes of neurogenic bladder ($n=87$, 17 %), and bladder exstrophy ($n=42$, 8 %) or other nonneurogenic etiologies ($n=99$, 20 %). Augmentation used ileum (297, 59 %), sigmoid (85, 17 %), cecum/ileocecum (46, 9 %), ileo-sigmoid (8, 2 %), stomach (38, 8 %), stomach/bowel (7, 1 %), ureter (8, 2 %), and ureter/ileum (3, 0.6 %) With mean and median follow-up of 13 years, 169 (34 %) had complications specifically related to augmentation, resulting in 254 additional operations: 3 (0.6 %) malignancy with death, 43 (9 %) perforations with 1 death, 16 (3 %) bowel obstructions, 47 (9 %) repeat augmentation, 75 (15 %) bladder calculi. Multivariable analysis was not reported to determine potential contributions of underlying diagnosis, segment used for augmentation, Mitrofanoff channel, or bladder neck surgery to likelihood for complications (Metcalfe et al. 2006a).

Inadequate Bladder Compliance or Bowel Contractions

Systematic postoperative UD assessment has not been reported to determine rate or timing of changes in neobladder dynamics, including bowel segment contractions.

Phasic contractions were found in a retrospective review of postoperative UD in 13/29 (45 %) children 1 year after ileo- ($n=22$) or colo- ($n=7$) cystoplasty. Mean pressure was 35 ± 13 cm H_2O. Subsequent UD 10–14 years later found these contractions in 11 patients, new in 4 and resolved in 6, occurring in 6/22 (27 %) ileal versus 5/7 (71 %) colon augments, $p=0.07$. Medical therapy, if any, was not stated (Lopez Pereira et al. 2009).

In the report by Kispal et al. (2011) described above, 3/86 (3 %) bladders were found to have decreased capacity, compliance and/or "deteriorating renal morphology" 3–8 years after colocystoplasty (2) or gastrocystoplasty (1), leading to re-augmentation. Additional clinical information regarding symptoms, length of the original bowel segment, or therapy before re-augmentation was not described (Kispal et al. 2011).

Re-augmentation was done in 47/500 (9.4 %) patients reported by Metcalfe et al. (2006a) for decreased compliance with upper tract changes or incontinence at a mean time of 7.5 years (3 months to 23 years) postoperatively. This occurred less often after ileal augmentation than sigmoid (OR 0.22, 95 % CI 0.089–0.52), gastric (OR 0.23, 95 % CI 0.075–0.72), or cecal/ileocecal (OR 0.11, 95 % CI 0.044–0.28) augments (Metcalfe et al. 2006a).

Metabolic Acidosis

No metabolic acidosis was found in children with both preoperative and postoperative electrolytes and venous blood gases following enterocystoplasty.

Follow-up in the series reported by Lopez Pereira et al. (2009) included serum electrolytes and venous blood gases "at regular intervals." With mean postoperative assessment to 11 years, only 1/29 (3 %) had metabolic acidosis requiring alkali therapy, and this patient had metabolic acidosis before enterocystoplasty.

One study retrospectively analyzed preoperative and postoperative electrolytes and venous blood gases collected by protocol in 71 children with spina bifida after ileal or colonic augmentation, reporting no changes to suggest new metabolic acidosis or respiratory compensation during follow-up a mean of 46.8 months (1–138) (Adams et al. 2010).

B_{12} Vitamin Deficiency

Two retrospective studies report asymptomatic B_{12} deficiency, without megaloblastic anemia, found ≥7 years post-iliocystoplasty in 17 and 13 % of tested patients.

One short-term study found oral B_{12} replacement effective to restore normal levels within a mean of 4 months.

One study reported postoperative B_{12} levels in children after iliocystoplasty that used 15–20 cm of ileum taken 15 cm from the ileocecal valve, finding increased likelihood of subnormal values with greater duration of follow-up, especially after 7 years. The study population comprised 86 patients with B_{12} data from >300 ileal augments performed. Of these, only 25 patients had two levels obtained. In 29 patients tested ≥7 years postoperatively, 5 (17 %) had low values (defined as ≤200 pg/mL), without megaloblastic anemia in any case. Neurologic examinations were not done, and there were no control patients or testing for serum homocysteine or methylmalonic acid to determine if observed low B_{12} levels were clinically significant (Rosenbaum et al. 2008).

Another series of 105 children who had annual B_{12} levels a mean of 50 ± 30 months (2–183) after iliocystoplasty were retrospectively reviewed, finding two had decreased values (< 150 pg/mL) at more than 7 years after surgery. This occurred in 15 children (13 %) having follow-up ≥80 months. Neither had megaloblastic anemia; potential neurologic changes were not sought (Blackburn et al. 2010).

Oral B_{12} replacement (250 μg daily) was prescribed to 36 asymptomatic children with low (<200 pg/dL) or low normal (200–300 pg/dL) levels. With three monthly levels obtained, values increased to >300 pg/dL in all patients with mean follow-up of 4 months (Vanderbrink et al. 2010).

Bladder Calculi

Bladder stones develop in approximately 10–25 % of children after augmentation at a mean time of ≥4 years.

These calculi occur significantly more often after enterocystoplasty versus gastrocystoplasty, and during CIC via Mitrofanoff versus transurethrally.

Most are struvite or calcium apatite.

Recurrence after treatment is reported in approximately 33 %, with no difference in intact stone removal versus lithotripsy.

Two reports suggest neither daily nor weekly bladder irrigation reduced stone development. No RCT evaluates impact of irrigation on bladder stone formation or recurrence.

A retrospective review of 403 children using CIC created four cohorts: transurethral CIC, no augment (227); Mitrofanoff, no augment (18); transurethral CIC and augment (100); Mitrofanoff and augment (58). All augments used sigmoid or ileum. A total of 28 (7 %) developed stones, but mean follow-up intervals were not stated. There was no difference in prevalence among the four groups. Stones formed in augmented patients at a mean of 43 months (3–132), and in non-augmented children a mean of 103 months (36–204). Recurrence after treatment occurred in 9/28 (32 %) at a mean of 23 months. New calculi formed in 4/6 with lithotripsy versus 6/22 with intact removal, $p=0.15$. Analysis reported apatite (11), struvite (10), urate (2), and oxalate (2), with a foreign-body nidus, hair, or suture in 2 (Barroso et al. 2000).

Bladder stones occurred in 20/86 (23 %) augmented children, and recurred after treatment in ten followed after surgery on a protocol that included ultrasonography annually for 4 years and every other year thereafter. Underlying etiologies were mixed, with myelodysplasia (43) and exstrophy/epispadias (24) predominating. Mean time to the first episode was 4 years (5 months to 13 years). These developed significantly more often after colocystoplasty than after iliocystoplasty or gastrocystoplasty (29/30, 3/32, 1/18, $p=0.000$), and in those catheterizing via a Mitrofanoff versus transurethrally (18/56 versus 2/30, $p=0.007$). Irrigation was "strongly recommended" but its impact, if any, was not reported (Kispal et al. 2011).

One retrospective evaluation of 500 children after augmentation reported bladder calculi occurred in 75 (15 %), a mean of 5.6 years postoperatively. Recurrent stones developed in 28 (37 %). There were no differences in stone formation in ileal versus sigmoid augments, but both enterocystoplasties had a greater rate than did gastric augments, with no stones after stomach and one in a gastric/ileal composite. Mitrofanoff channel increased risk for stones (OR 2.2, 95 % CI 1.3–3.6). There was no difference in recurrence after cystolithotomy versus cystolithotripsy (OR 0.30, 95 % CI 0.06–1.5) (Metcalfe et al. 2006a).

Another retrospective study involved 105 patients (myelodysplasia in 41) after augmentation using ileum (37), colon (18), and stomach (50) with subsequent follow-up a minimum of 1 year and a median of 8.4 years (2–15) follow-up. Twelve (11 %) formed bladder calculi, 10/37 (27 %) with ileum, 1/18 (6 %) with colon, and 1/50 (2 %) with stomach, at a mean time of 5.2 years (1.4–14). Stones developed in 12/68 catheterizing per Mitrofanoff versus 0/37 per urethra, $p=0.007$. Stone analysis reported calcium apatite/struvite (7), ammonium acid urate (4), and calcium phosphate/oxalate (1). Recurrent calculi occurred in 4/12 (33 %) despite recommendations for "high volume" saline irrigation after the first episode (DeFoor et al. 2004).

Three patient cohorts followed a prospective management protocol. Thirty patients without augmentation underwent CIC alone, while another 30 patients with augmentation and "continent diversion" (presumably Mitrofanoff procedure) and 30 patients with augmentation alone all performed weekly bladder irrigations with sterile water (volume not stated). If urine demonstrated debris, irrigation was done more frequently during the week until clear. Etiologies of bladder dysfunction were diverse, but neurogenic bladder accounted for 38/60 (63 %) augmented children, while need for CIC in the medically treated group was not defined. Iliocystoplasty was done in 57, colocystoplasty in 2, and ureterocystoplasty in 1. All patients were followed >2 years, with mean of 4.7–5.7 years in the three cohorts. Stones occurred in no patient on CIC alone, versus five (17 %) of those augmented with Mitrofanoff and two (7 %) only augmented, $p=0.053$. The occurrence of stones in augmented patients at a similar rate as reported without systematic irrigation questioned efficacy of the weekly regimen to reduce stone risk (Brough et al. 2009).

Lopez Pereira et al. (2009) stated that all patients were instructed to irrigate their augmented bladder using saline once daily, using 50–100 cc rinsed three to four times. During follow-up a mean of 11 years (8–14.5) in 29 children with ileal (22) or sigmoid (7) enterocystoplasties, 3 (10 %) developed a stone.

Ventriculoperitoneal Shunt Infection or Dysfunction

Two retrospective studies report shunt complications after augmentation, occurring in 15 and 20 %.

A retrospective analysis included 20 children with myelodysplasia and VP shunts with no revision within 12 months of augmentation, and having at least 12 months follow-up after augmentation. Three-day mechanical and antibiotic bowel preparation had been done, and during surgery the shunt was packed in gauze away from the operative field. Postoperative parenteral antibiotics (not described) continued a mean of 9 days, and peritoneal drains were used for a mean of 16–18 days. VP shunt infection developed in 4 (20 %) and presented within 12 months with fever. Cultures grew *Staphylococcus epidermidis* or gram-negative organisms (Matthews et al. 1996).

Another retrospective study reported that 55 patients with VP shunt had bladder augmentation for neurogenic bladder, with shunt-related complications developing in 8 (15 %) during mean follow-up of 60 months (12–111): one extruded shunt tip through the former suprapubic tube site, five distal obstructions, and two exteriorized for bladder rupture. Of the five with obstructions, one had a pseudocyst diagnosed 14 months after augmentation, while the other four had simultaneous proximal shunt malfunction at 21–63 months after surgery. Patients underwent 1 day preoperative mechanical bowel preparation using GOLYTELY and oral plus intravenous antibiotics (not described) as well as intraoperative shunt isolation using antibiotic-soaked sponges (not described), with no acute shunt infections (Yerkes et al. 2001).

Bladder Rupture

Two series reported perforation of the augmentation in <10 % of patients during follow-up greater than 8 years.

One stated risk factors included sigmoid augment (versus ileum), and bladder neck procedures.

A retrospective review of 500 augmentations with minimum follow-up of 2 years and mean of 13 years reported that 43 (9 %) patients ruptured. A total of 54 perforations occurred (two in nine patients and three in one patient), one-third within 2 years of surgery and another third >6 years postoperatively. One patient death resulted from sepsis. There was no difference in rupture based on diagnosis (7/42 [17 %] bladder exstrophy, 31/336 [9 %] spinal dysraphism, $p = 0.167$), but sigmoid augments had a 3.5-fold increased risk (95 % CI [1.63–7.30]) versus ilium. Bladder neck surgery also increased risk (29/105 [28 %] with versus 13/304 [4 %] without, $p < 0.05$; no information in 91) (Metcalfe et al. 2006b).

Four of 86 (5 %) children followed a mean of 8.6 years had perforation occurring up to 11 years postoperatively, in one secondary to blunt abdominal trauma (Kispal et al. 2011).

Malignancy

A prospective assessment at median follow-up 27 years after enterocystoplasty found smoking and immunosuppression (after renal transplantation), but not augmentation, associated with increased malignancy risk.

A matched cohort study also found augmentation did not increase malignancy.

Markov modeling raised doubts that annual screening for malignancy using cystoscopy and cytology would be cost-effective.

Prospective data were maintained on 153 patients after enterocystoplasty for neurogenic bladder (97), exstrophy (38), and posterior urethral valves (18), with minimum follow-up 10 years and median follow-up, 27 (10–53). Seven (5 %) developed malignancy at a median time of 32 years (22–52); two smokers had transitional cell carcinoma, two with renal transplant and immunosuppressive medications had adenocarcinomas of the bowel segment, and three with bladder exstrophy had multifocal adenocarcinoma within the bladder, which was considered a disease-specific risk rather than risk secondary to augmentation (Husmann and Rathbun 2008).

In a subsequent study, this population was compared to a matched 1:1 cohort using intermittent catheterization for similar etiologies of bladder dysfunction, reporting that augmentation did not increase cancer risk (7 [5 %] augmented versus 4 [3 %] controls, $p=0.54$), while renal transplantation and immunosuppressive medications did (3/20 [15 %] on immunosuppressives versus 8/286 [3 %], $p=0.03$) (Higuchi et al. 2010).

Four of 119 (3 %) gastrocystoplasty patients developed adenocarcinoma (3) or poorly differentiated transitional cell carcinoma 11–14 years postoperatively in a retrospective report combining outcomes from two institutions. Three had spina bifida, and one had posterior urethral valves. None smoked. One used imminuosuppressives after renal transplantation. Two had cystoscopy 1 year before tumor diagnosis, showing "severe wall inflammation without mass" in one. Diagnosis was made during evaluation for new hydronephrosis or gross hematuria (Castellan et al. 2007).

Markov modeling compared two screening strategies, including annual cystoscopy and cytology, for patients with myelodysplasia following augmentation. Despite using higher than expected risks of malignancy and "highly optimistic" estimates of efficacy of screening, the models found annual screening unlikely to be cost-effective at willingness to pay thresholds (Kokorowski et al. 2011).

Ureterocystoplasty

One study reported ureterocystoplasty was not successful when only a distal ureteral segment was used for augmentation, when a non-refluxing megaureter was <1.5 cm in distal diameter, or when there was compliance <20 cm H_2O preoperatively with a refluxing megaureter.

A retrospective study combined all patients from five institutions undergoing ureterocystoplasty over a 15-year period, comprising 64 children with neurogenic bladder (46) or posterior urethral valves (18). When a refluxing ($n=8$) or non-refluxing ($n=16$) distal megaureter segment (5–8 cm) was used, there was minimal change, with a median capacity gain of 0.14-fold and median compliance loss of −0.11-fold. Twenty-three of 24 were considered to need re-augmentation. In the remaining 40 children, the entire ureter was used. Six of 9 non-refluxing megaureters with preoperative distal ureteral diameter on ultrasound >1.5 cm had median sixfold capacity increase and 50-fold compliance increase, versus 3/9<1.5 cm with 0.6 and 0.7-fold changes in capacity and compliance that led to re-augmentation in all three. Of 31 cases of refluxing megaureters, ureterocystoplasty was successful in those whose preoperative UD had compliance >20 mL/cm H_2O, but 21/26 with <20 mL/cm H_2O compliance had re-augmentation. Fifteen of 64 had progressive upper tract deterioration associated with decreased bladder compliance, and ureterocystoplasty was unsuccessful in each (Husmann et al. 2004).

Mitrofanoff Procedures

Appendix Versus Monti

Retrospective case series report the need for additional procedures in >20 % of Mitrofanoff channels from either appendix or reconfigured intestine (Monti).

The most common complications are stomal stenosis and incontinence, with Monti segments also elongating/angulating or forming diverticulum.

Bladder stones occur in approximately 10–25 % of patients after augmentation with Mitrofanoff procedures, as discussed above.

A retrospective review of 169 children followed a mean of 5.8 years (8 months to 15 years) with Mitrofanoff procedures for a variety of indications (neurogenic bladder in 36 %) reported that 67 (39 %) had at least one surgical revision: 18 % stoma revision at skin level, 4 % revision for mucosa prolapse, 8 % revision beneath the fascia, and injection for incontinence in 8 %. Event-to-time analysis showed no significant differences for complications related to appendix versus Monti channel, or umbilical versus lower quadrant stoma, with ≥65 % of skin stenoses and incontinence diagnosed within 3 years (Leslie et al. 2011).

Another retrospective review comprised Mitrofanoff procedures in 92 patients from 1994 to 1999 for several conditions, including neurogenic bladder in 21 (23 %). Appendix was used in 69 and small bowel Monti in 25 (8 single-segment and 17 double-segment joined end-to-end), with all stomas except one placed in the right or left lower quadrants. With mean follow-up of 37 months (6.7–65) after appendicovesicostomy and 25 months (6–66) after Monti, problems with catheterization occurred in 18 (26 %) appendix channels versus 15 (60 %) with reconfigured small bowel, $p<0.001$. However, comparison of surgical revision rates found no significant differences (10/69 versus 5/25, $p=0.7$) (Narayanaswamy et al. 2001).

A review of 56 Mitrofanoff procedures (48 appendix, 2 Monti, 6 ureter) performed in association with 86 bladder augmentations (53 [62 %] for neurogenic bladder), reported 16 (29 %) required surgical revision at a mean time of 6.6 years (1 month to 16 years) postoperatively. Complications included stoma stenosis ($n=4$), incontinence ($n=4$), difficulty with CIC ($n=6$), and mucosa prolapse ($n=2$), all following appendicovesicostomy (Kispal et al. 2011).

A retrospective evaluation of 199 Monti channels mostly done in children with neurogenic bladder (88 %), reported complications requiring surgical revision during a mean 28 months follow-up. Stoma revisions were done in 16 (8 %), mostly for stenosis or mucosa prolapse. These stomas had been placed at either the umbilicus (105, 53 %) or in lower abdominal quadrants. Channel or bladder-level problems developed in 17 (8.5 %) for elongated and angulated channels or deficient tunnel length (Cain et al. 2008).

Mitrofanoff into Bladder Versus Bowel

No randomized trial or cohort study reports outcomes of Mitrofanoff channels reimplanted into bladder versus bowel. Retrospective case series suggest similar outcomes with either technique.

A retrospective review concerned Mitrofanoff channels (20 appendix and 12 Monti) implanted into bowel (colon in 26 and ilium in 6) rather than the bladder, reporting follow-up a mean of 26 months. Revision was needed in 6/32 (18 %). Incontinence occurred in four (12.5 %), due to short Monti tunnel length in three undergoing reoperation; three others had stoma stenosis (Franc-Guimond and Gonzalez 2006).

Another retrospective study included 35 Mitrofanoff procedures done using appendix in 21 and ileal Monti in 14. These channels were implanted into bladder in 24 and intestinal augment in 11 patients (appendix versus Monti not stated). With mean follow-up 2.8 years (6 months to 6 years), reoperation was done for difficult catheterization ($n=2$), urinary leakage ($n=3$), or mucosal prolapse ($n=2$), with no difference in outcomes based on implantation in bladder or bowel (Boemers et al. 2005).

Health-Related Quality of Life

Two surveys found bladder reconstructive surgery did not change reported overall health quality of life in patients.

Parents in one small survey reported their children to have improved health-related quality of life after surgery.

One survey found little difference in self-reported health-related quality of life in sling patients with and without augmentation.

The Parkin disease-specific health-related quality of life score was obtained preoperatively and postoperatively in 31 consecutive children and adolescents undergoing lower tract reconstructions for urinary incontinence secondary to myelodysplasia. Despite improved continence, overall scores did not significantly change, although there were significant improvements in independence and emotional domains. The authors concluded that a single system change in a multisystem disability might be insufficient to change overall scores, and that improved continence might only improve caregiver quality of life (MacNeily et al. 2009).

In a prospective evaluation of ten children aged 2–18 years (mean 10) with spina bifida undergoing reconstructive surgery, health-related quality of life of patients and their parents was separately assessed using the PedsQL 4.0 validated health-related quality of life questionnaire both preoperatively and postoperatively. At baseline, children had similar summary scores reported by healthy children except for physical health and social functioning, which were lower. Compared to children with chronic illness, their summary scores were similar except for physical functioning, which was lower in patients with spina bifida. At baseline, parents reported significantly lower mean physical and psychosocial health and emotional, social, and school functioning in their children than did parents of the general population. They also reported lower emotional, social, and school functioning scores versus parents of children with chronic illnesses. Postoperatively, children had no significant differences in summary scores; however, parents reported significant improvement in social and school functioning, and psychological social health in their children. No demographic or clinical factors were predictors of health quality of life in this small sample (Parekh et al. 2006).

Another study noted that no validated instrument existed to evaluate functional and health status changes after bladder reconstructive surgery and so developed a satisfaction questionnaire related to continence, urinary system management, and participation in daily activities. Then consecutive patients returning for follow-up after sling with ($n=18$) and without ($n=23$) augment were analyzed. There were no differences based on age, gender, ambulatory status, or perceived continence between the two groups. AC use was significantly greater in the non-augmented patients. Median survey scores were the same between groups except for one question, which asked if patients had "achieved more independence with self-directed care." For that question, augmented patients scored 5 (2–5) versus 4 (1–5), $p=0.02$ (Snodgrass et al. 2009).

Antegrade Continence Enema

ACE Versus Retrograde Enema

Our review found only three studies comparing ACE to other bowel managements, including retrograde enemas. None reported added benefit to ACE to achieve fecal continence.

Two report greater independence with ACE versus retrograde enemas in children.

One reported significantly greater volume of tap water for ACE.

A multicenter European study retrospectively reviewed bowel management in 423 children >10 years old (mean 22, 10–47). Three hundred eighty-two were medically treated with a variety of methods (digital stimulation, oral laxatives, retrograde enemas), while 47 had ACE and were assessed a mean of 3 years postoperatively. Combining "rare" and "never" outcomes for soiling, fecal continence was achieved in 245/382 (64 %) with medical treatment versus 26/47 (55 %) by ACE, $p=0.3$ (Lemelle et al. 2006).

Retrospective analysis was done in 80 children with myelodysplasia 5–18 years (mean 13) following a treatment algorithm beginning with osmotic laxatives, then retrograde water enemas (self-administered after age 10 years), then ACE, if unsuccessful. Fecal continence was no soiling, achieved in 8 with no treatment, 5/13 (38 %) using laxatives without enemas, 21/26 (81 %) with retrograde enemas, and 16/20 (80 %) with ACE. Only 12 % using retrograde enemas were independent, versus 50 % following ACE, $p=0.001$ (Vande Velde et al. 2007).

Another retrospective review was done in 25 children with spina bifida, 13 using retrograde enemas (mean age 8 years, 4–15) and 12 following ACE (mean age 14 years, 4–23). Those receiving ACE did not first have retrograde enemas, but represented patients undergoing other reconstructive surgery. Warmed tap water was used for irrigation, recommended every 2 days but adjusted by families according to perceived need (no difference between groups). With mean follow-up at 28 months, fecal continence (no soiling) was 76 % in both groups. Time to perform enemas was also the same at mean 37 min (20–60). Water volume was significantly greater for ACE (800 cc [400–1,500] versus 550 cc [300–1,500], $p=0.03$). Both had similar abdominal pain during the procedure, 38.5 % retrograde versus 50 % ACE, $p=0.8$. Independence performing enemas was greater with ACE, 67 % versus 23 %, $p=0.047$, in patients who were significantly older (Matsuno et al. 2010).

ACE Versus LACE

Systematic literature review found no difference in fecal continence (approximately 68 %), but significantly smaller volume and less toilet time (30 versus 50 min) with LACE versus ACE.

Systematic literature review pooled results from publications between 2002 and 2007 concerning ACE or LACE:

- LACE, 9 publications reported a total of 93 patients at mean age 10 years, 70 % having neuropathic bowel. Mean enema volume was 400 mL (250–600), and mean toilet time was 30 min (5–60). Mean follow-up was 15 months (1–17) with complete fecal continence in 72 % achieved at a mean time of 4 months.
- ACE, 16 publications reported 583 patients at mean age 10 years, 66 % with neuropathic bowel. Mean enema volume was 600 mL (180–3,000), and mean toilet time was 50 min (5–60). During follow-up a mean of 29 months (6–64), complete continence was achieved by 81 %; time to continence was not stated.
- Enema volume and toilet time were significantly less with LACE, with no difference in continence (Sinha et al. 2008).

Imbricated Versus Non-imbricated ACE

Two retrospective studies reported that cecal imbrication of the appendix during ACE significantly reduced stoma leakage, while another found significantly greater leakage with imbrication.

A retrospective review included 75 patients, median age 8 years at surgery, 85 % with spina bifida, assessed at a mean of 3.5 years (6 months to 11 years). Appendicovesicostomy was non-imbricated in 67 (51 done laparoscopically) and imbricated in 12 (reasons for different technique during open surgery not stated). Four not originally imbricated were subsequently (three for leakage) and were reported in both categories. Zero of 12 imbricated had leakage, versus non-imbricated with no leakage (46, 69 %) or slight leakage ≤1 episode/month (13, 19 %), $p<0.001$ (Henrichon et al. 2012).

Another retrospective study compared imbricated ($n=34$) versus non-imbricated ($n=10$) ACE in 44 children mostly having anorectal malformations; reasons for different surgical management were not explained. In 21 months' mean follow-up, stomal leakage occurred in 4 (9 %), $p=0.002$ (Lawal et al. 2011).

A third retrospective study with 44 consecutive patients having mostly neurogenic bladder compared ACE with ($n=25$) and without ($n=19$) cecal "wrap." Stomal leakage occurred in six with and zero without at a median 4 months postoperatively, $p=0.03$ (Koivusalo et al. 2006).

Bowel Versus Button ACE

One study found complications requiring reoperation were greater after ACE, but nonoperative complications were more likely with a button.

Button complications include dislodgement, granulation tissue, stool leakage, and infection.

MIC-KEY gastrostomy button was used in 12 children and ACE in another 37 with non-Hirshsprung functional constipation at mean age 10 years. At mean of 18 months, follow-up requiring further surgery only occurred in the ACE group, in 24 %, with stoma stenosis the most frequent problem occurring in 11 %. Complications not needing surgery were significantly more common in the button group (92 % versus 19 %), including stool leakage around the device in 42 %, granuloma in 33 %, and pain at the entry site in 17 % (Cascio et al. 2004).

Button cecostomies (Chait) were performed on 69 children at mean age 11 years, 62 % having neuropathic bowel during a 10-year period ending in 2007. Tubes were changed annually. A standardized questionnaire was used before and after insertion. With mean follow-up at 4 years, complications developed in 28 (41 %), including tube dislodgement in 9 (13 %), granulation tissue in 11 (16 %) or infection at entry site in 3 (4 %), and pressure sores from the tube in 5 (7 %). No mention was made of leakage around the tube, nor of patient satisfaction with a tube except to note that overall satisfaction reported by parents/patients on the questionnaire was 2.7 out of possible 3 (Wong et al. 2008).

Twenty-nine Chait cecostomies were performed in children mean age 8 years (3–21), mostly having neurogenic bowel or anorectal malformation. At review all were at least 1 month postoperative, but actual follow-up duration was not stated. Two removed the device at 1 and 2.5 years when it was no longer needed for stool continence, leaving 22 with follow-up. Three had hypertrophic granulation tissue around the entry site, 12 (55 %) had leakage around the tube, and 7(32 %) found the button "not very esthetic" (Becmeur et al. 2008).

Results of 31 left colon buttons were assessed by telephone questionnaire done in 28 at a median time of 92 months (66–145). Thirteen (46 %) no longer used the device, 7 due to resolution of constipation and 6 due to failure. At least 5 had been removed, leaving 23 tubes in place. Complications included granulation tissue in six (26 %), leakage in three (13 %), entry site infection in one (4 %), and bleeding in one (4 %) (Blackburn et al. 2012).

Enema Fluid and Volume

Tap water, saline, and GoLYTELY solutions have similar results.

A retrospective review reported outcomes of a treatment algorithm used in 236 children with neurogenic bowel following ACE. Tap water was instilled beginning with 50 mL nightly, increasing by 50 mL every 3 days until continence. Eighty-three percent achieved fecal continence (no soiling) using a mean of 650 mL (100–1,000) (Bani-Hani et al. 2008b).

Another retrospective analysis stated that patients were begun on normal saline irrigation and changed to GoLYTELY if not successful. Of 87 patients using their ACE a median of 61 months later, 61 % use GoLYTELY and 31 % saline (others used tap water). Infusion volume was a mean 850 mL. Success was reported in 66 (76 %) (based on this analysis, but 69 % overall as discussed below) (Siddiqui et al. 2011).

Long-Term Follow-up

Three series with follow-up >5 years reported that 10–45 % of patients no longer use the ACE. Fecal continence ranged from 33 to 70 %.

Consecutive patients who had ACE between 1993 and 1999 were contacted for long-term follow-up >5 years, with data available in 61 at mean age 22 years (15–35) of which 44 % had spina bifida. Mean follow-up was 11 years (8–14), and 25 (41 %) reported they no longer used their ACE, 14 (23 %) because it was ineffective and 5 (8 %) from complications, including stoma stenosis or leakage. Of the 36 still using the ACE, 19 (53 %) reported abdominal pain, with 12 (33 %) rating the pain >5 on a visual analog scale of 1–10(very painful). Ease of use was scored 1–5 (very difficult), with users rating a median 2. Thirty-two responded with information about soiling, with 11 (34 %) reporting total fecal continence, but of those still using the ACE, satisfaction scored 1–5 (very) was 4.1 (overall satisfaction including all 61 patients was not reported) (YardLey et al. 2009).

Retrospective chart review was done in 117 patients with ACE, 45 % neuropathic bowel, and median follow-up in 105 of 61 months (mean 68, 7–178). Seventy-two (69 %) had "success," defined as ≤1 soiling episode/weekly, while 12 (11 %) no longer used the ACE. Ninety-three percent had initial success, with late failures occurring a mean of 88 months later (99 months in spina bifida patients), with reasons for late failure not stated. Mean toilet time was 50 min (10–180) (Siddiqui et al. 2011).

The review by Blackburn et al. (2012) described above included 31 children, 19 % with spina bifida, who had left-sided ACE buttons at median age 7 years (2–17). At median follow-up of 92 months (66–145), 28 were reached for telephone questionnaire. Thirteen (46 %) no longer used the device, 7 due to resolution of constipation and 6 due to failure. Of 15 continuing use, median toilet time was 25 min and 10 (67 %) reported no soiling.

Complications

The most common anatomic complications are stoma stenosis (15–50 %) and stoma leakage (3–35 %).

Stoma infection was reported in one series occurring in 25 % of patients at a mean of 14 months.

Pain during irrigation has been reported in several series, occurring in from 17 % to over 50 %, but not mentioned by others. Severity has been described as mild to severe. Pain was reported in patients using phosphate, saline, or tap water enemas.

Retrospective review included 236 patients with neurogenic bowel and ≥6-month follow-up (median 50). Appendix was used in 86 %, with cecal imbrications, and the stoma was umbilical in 46 % or lower quadrant in 54 %. Other technical details, including means of stoma creation, were not described. Apparently all were ACE. Of these, 39 (17 %) had revisions for stomal stenosis (32, 14 %), stoma leakage (7, 3 %), and channel fibrosis (7, 3 %). Channel obliteration occurred significantly more often in patients with colon flaps or cecal lengthening procedures (Bani-Hani et al. 2008a).

Another retrospective study with 117 patients (45 % neuropathic bowel) stated that 63 % had complications during median follow-up of 61 months. Appendix was used in 83 %. Stoma stenosis developed in 44 (38 %) at a mean of 8 months, stoma leakage in 41 (35 %) at a mean of 19 months, and stoma infection in 29 (25 %) at mean of 14 months (Siddiqui et al. 2011).

Forty-two patients, mean age 12 years, with spina bifida had ACE procedures, 93 % using appendix, and had follow-up to a mean of 2.5 years (2 months to 6 years). Complications occurred in seven (17 %), including stoma stenosis in six, and abscess in one (Webb et al. 1998).

Malone reviewed his results in 31 children, 37 % with neuropathic bowel, operated at a mean age of 8 years (1–18) and with mean follow-up of 3 years (1–6). Appendix was used in 84 %. Complications included stoma stenosis in 17 (55 %), channel fibrosis in 2 (6 %), and pain during irrigation in 18 (58 %). In addition, there were three (10 %) who developed phosphate toxicity from its instillation (Curry et al. 1998).

Patients reported by YardLey et al. (2009) described above with follow-up over 5 years reported that abdominal pain with irrigation (fluid not stated, an earlier publication indicated phosphate enemas) persisted and was rated five out of a possible ten on a visual analog scale.

Review of 29 patients with spina bifida who underwent ACE at mean age 9 years and were followed a mean of 4 years (4 months to 7 years) reported abdominal pain with irrigation in 21 (72 %), described as "severe" in 6 (23 %). "Standard saline and phosphate enemas" were used (Kim et al. 2009).

The retrospective comparison between retrograde enemas and ACE by Matsuno et al. (2010) mentioned above, in which tap water was used for irrigations, found that at 28 months mean follow-up 44 % noted abdominal pain, with no difference between groups. Severity of pain was not described.

Another review included 18 patients operated at mean age 13 years, 94 % having neuropathic bowel. All have LACE, and used either saline or tap water irrigations. At mean follow-up of 2 years, three (17 %) noted "mild cramping pain or nausea" during instillation (Churchill et al. 2003).

Health-Related Quality of Life

Quality of life surveys following ACE procedures generally report improved self-esteem and independence.

The FICQOL (fecal continence and constipation quality of life) instrument was used to evaluate

23 patients with spina bifida, 23 before and 18 following ACE (5 did not respond). Median age at surgery was 11 years, and post-surgical survey was done at ≥6 months. Soiling decreased from 4 to 0.3 episodes per week, but total time for bowel care remained a constant 45 min. Both patient and caretaker anxiety regarding soiling significantly reduced (Ok and Kurzrock 2011).

Psychosocial functioning and mental health were assessed preoperatively and at 6 and 16 months following ACE in 20 children mean age 11 years with spina bifida, using a structured clinical interview and three validated questionnaires. Responses were compared to a control group of 20 children median age 14 years of age chosen at random from an epidemiologic study of mental health. Mean toilet time was 50 min. Nineteen reported improved self-reliance, and 16 (80 %) reported fecal continence or rare soiling. There were significant differences in patients versus controls, with parents of patients reporting more behavioral and emotional problems and patients lower self-esteem. Postoperative patient scores indicated significantly improved self-esteem and close friend ratings that were similar to controls (Aksnes et al. 2002).

Twenty-five patients who had ACE at mean age 11 years (6–17), 66 % neuropathic bowel, were queried by telephone using a quality-of-life instrument 6 months to 9 years later (mean not stated). Seven (28 %) were no longer using the ACE due to stomal complications or perforations in five and two who "did not like the idea of it." Sixteen (64 %) reported fecal continence. Mean toilet time was 45 min, maximum was 90 min, with 8 (32 %) stating the procedure required more than 1 h. Quality of life was significantly improved from preoperative scoring, mean 6 (2–9) versus 11.5 (5–14) on a maximum 14-point scale, $p<0.001$ (Tiryaki et al. 2010).

Urologic Outcomes of Surgery for Tethered Cord

Primary Tethered Cord

Several retrospective series indicate that normal preoperative UD can become abnormal after detethering, and that abnormal preoperative UD can improve.

One report stated detrusor overactivity potentially resolved after detethering, while decreased compliance did not improve.

The retrospective review by Macejko et al. (2007) described above analyzed all cases of tethered cord release during a 7-year period to identify infants and children <3 years of age with a primary tethered cord. UD was obtained in 69/79 patients before neurosurgery was done at mean age 10 months, and was considered normal in 30 (55 %), with varying findings in the remainder (overactivity, "hypotonia," DSD, poor compliance, high voiding pressures). Mean follow-up after tethered cord release was 5 years (6 months to 11 years), with 49 (62 %) described as having no urologic problems, 6/43 (14 %) having "delayed toilet training," and 6/79 (8 %) children requiring CIC. Normal preoperative UD remained normal in 18/28 (64 %) and became abnormal in 10 (36 %) patients having both studies. Abnormal preoperative UD became normal in 8/22 (36 %) and remained abnormal in 14 (63 %) having both studies. In total, abnormal postoperative UDs were found in 24/50 (48 %) studies (Macejko et al. 2007).

Nogueira et al. (2004) reported outcomes from tethered cord release in 19 patients at mean age 8 years (8 months to 14 years) diagnosed because of orthopedic anomalies, of which 7 had postoperative UD showing resolution of preoperative detrusor overactivity in 2 of 3 and new onset of overactivity in 1. Of 16 patients diagnosed at an earlier age because of cutaneous lesions (mean 1 year, 1 month to 11 years), postoperative UD in 9 indicated that all 4 with preoperative detrusor overactivity had resolution.

A third retrospective review included 24 patients diagnosed with tethered cord, presenting at median age 6 years (1 month to 12 years) and undergoing preoperative and postoperative UD (at mean of 6 months). Seven of 14 toilet-trained were incontinent. Preoperative UD was abnormal in 21(91 %): 17 with detrusor overactivity, and 4 with decreased compliance. Postoperative UD showed detrusor overactivity resolved in 10/17; those with decreased compliance did not improve. Two of 3 with normal preoperative UD had adverse changes postoperatively, one with detrusor overactivity and the other with decreased compliance. Of all 24 patients, postoperative UD was abnormal in 14. Of the seven with preoperative incontinence, six became continent, and no patient had new incontinence (Guerra et al. 2006).

Secondary Tethered Cord

One study reported that uncorrected secondary tethering resulted in progressive urologic symptoms.

One retrospective study identified 45 patients with symptomatic tethered cord (flexion contractures, urinary incontinence, UTI) after myelomeningocele repair, representing 2.8 % of 1,435 myelodysplastic patients followed. Tethered cord release was not done, and during mean follow-up of 12 years (1–41) progressive orthopedic and urologic symptoms occurred in 40 (89 %). Age of patients at diagnosis of tethered cord was not stated (Phuong et al. 2002).

Another study reported 20/120 (17 %) myelodysplastic children developed symptomatic tethered cord (motor symptoms in 13, progressive scoliosis in 6, and incontinence in 1) at median age 8 years (2–13). UD was considered abnormal in all, and after tethered cord release were considered improved in 35 %, worse in 5 %, and unchanged in the remainder (Abrahamsson et al. 2007).

References

Abrahamsson K, Olsson I, Sillen U. Urodynamic findings in children with myelomeningocele after untethering of the spinal cord. J Urol. 2007;177(1):331–4. discussion 4.

Abrams P, Cardozo L, Fall M, Griffiths D, Rosier P, Ulmsten U, et al. The standardisation of terminology of lower urinary tract function: report from the Standardisation Sub-committee of the International Continence Society. Neurourol Urodyn. 2002;21(2): 167–78.

Adams RC, Vachha B, Samuelson ML, Keefover-Hicks A, Snodgrass WT. Incidence of new onset metabolic acidosis following enteroplasty for myelomeningocele. J Urol. 2010;183(1):302–5.

Aksnes G, Diseth TH, Helseth A, Edwin B, Stange M, Aafos G, et al. Appendicostomy for antegrade enema: effects on somatic and psychosocial functioning in children with myelomeningocele. Pediatrics. 2002; 109(3):484–9.

Austin PF, Westney OL, Leng WW, McGuire EJ, Ritchey ML. Advantages of rectus fascial slings for urinary incontinence in children with neuropathic bladders. J Urol. 2001;165(6 Pt 2):2369–71. discussion 71–2.

Bani-Hani AH, Cain MP, Kaefer M, Meldrum KK, King S, Johnson CS, et al. The Malone antegrade continence enema: single institutional review. J Urol. 2008a;180(3): 1106–10.

Bani-Hani AH, Cain MP, King S, Rink RC. Tap water irrigation and additives to optimize success with the Malone antegrade continence enema: the Indiana University algorithm. J Urol. 2008b;180(4 Suppl): 1757–60. discussion 60.

Barroso U, Jednak R, Fleming P, Barthold JS, Gonzalez R. Bladder calculi in children who perform clean intermittent catheterization. BJU Int. 2000;85(7): 879–84.

Barthold JS, Rodriguez E, Freedman AL, Fleming PA, Gonzalez R. Results of the rectus fascial sling and wrap procedures for the treatment of neurogenic sphincteric incontinence. J Urol. 1999;161(1):272–4.

Becmeur F, Demarche M, Lacreuse I, Molinaro F, Kauffmann I, Moog R, et al. Cecostomy button for antegrade enemas: survey of 29 patients. J Pediatr Surg. 2008;43(10):1853–7.

Bergman J, Lerman SE, Kristo B, Chen A, Boechat MI, Churchill BM. Outcomes of bladder neck closure for intractable urinary incontinence in patients with neurogenic bladders. J Pediatr Urol. 2006;2(6):528–33.

Blackburn SC, Parkar S, Prime M, Healiss L, Desai D, Mustaq I, et al. Ileal bladder augmentation and vitamin B12: levels decrease with time after surgery. J Pediatr Urol. 2010;8(1):47–50.

Blackburn SC, Fishman JR, Geoghegan N, Dave K, Madden N, Haddad M. The first 5-year follow-up of distal antegrade continence enema stomas. J Pediatr Urol. 2012;8(1):17–9.

Boemers TM, van Gool JD, de Jong TP, Bax KM. Urodynamic evaluation of children with the caudal regression syndrome (caudal dysplasia sequence). J Urol. 1994;151(4):1038–40.

Boemers TM, Beek FJ, van Gool JD, de Jong TP, Bax KM. Urologic problems in anorectal malformations. Part 1: urodynamic findings and significance of sacral anomalies. J Pediatr Surg. 1996;31(3):407–10.

Boemers T, Schimke C, Ardelean M, Ludwikowski B. Evaluation of urinary and faecal continent stomas. J Pediatr Urol. 2005;1(2):85–8.

Bolduc S, Moore K, Lebel S, Lamontagne P, Hamel M. Double anticholinergic therapy for refractory overactive bladder. J Urol. 2009;182(4 Suppl):2033–8.

Brough RJ, O'Flynn KJ, Fishwick J, Gough DC. Bladder washout and stone formation in paediatric enterocystoplasty. Eur Urol. 2009;33(5):500–2.

Cain MP, Dussinger AM, Gitlin J, Casale AJ, Kaefer M, Meldrum K, et al. Updated experience with the Monti catheterizable channel. Urology. 2008;72(4): 782–5.

Cascio S, Flett ME, De la Hunt M, Barrett AM, Jaffray B. MACE or caecostomy button for idiopathic constipation in children: a comparison of complications and outcomes. Pediatr Surg Int. 2004;20(7):484–7.

Castellan M, Gosalbez R, Labbie A, Ibrahim E, Disandro M. Bladder neck sling for treatment of neurogenic incontinence in children with augmentation cystoplasty: long-term followup. J Urol. 2005;173(6):2128–31. discussion 31.

Castellan M, Gosalbez R, Perez-Brayfield M, Healey P, McDonald R, Labbie A, et al. Tumor in bladder reservoir after gastrocystoplasty. J Urol. 2007;178 (4 Pt 2):1771–4. discussion 4.

Chin-Peuckert L, KomLos M, Rennick JE, Jednak R, Capolicchio JP, Salle JL. What is the variability between 2 consecutive cystometries in the same child? J Urol. 2003;170(4 Pt 2):1614–7.

Chin-Peuckert L, Rennick JE, Jednak R, Capolicchio JP, Salle JL. Should warm infusion solution be used for urodynamic studies in children? A prospective randomized study. J Urol. 2004;172(4 Pt 2):1657–61. discussion 61.

Chrzan R, Dik P, Klijn AJ, de Jong TP. Sling suspension of the bladder neck for pediatric urinary incontinence. J Pediatr Urol. 2009;5(2):82–6.

Churchill BM, Gilmour RF, Khoury AE, McLorie GA. Biological response of bladders rendered continent by insertion of artificial sphincter. J Urol. 1987;138(4 Pt 2):1116–9.

Churchill BM, De Ugarte DA, Atkinson JB. Left-colon antegrade continence enema (LACE) procedure for fecal incontinence. J Pediatr Surg. 2003;38(12):1778–80.

Cohen RA, Rushton HG, Belman AB, Kass EJ, Majd M, Shaer C. Renal scarring and vesicoureteral reflux in children with myelodysplasia. J Urol. 1990;144(2 Pt 2):541–4. discussion 5.

Curry JI, Osborne A, Malone PS. How to achieve a successful Malone antegrade continence enema. J Pediatr Surg. 1998;33(1):138–41.

Dajusta D, Gargollo P, Snodgrass W. Dextranomer/hyaluronic acid bladder neck injection for persistent outlet incompetency after sling procedures in children with neurogenic urinary incontinence. J Pediatr Urol. 2012 (in press). doi:10.1016/j.jpurol.2012.03.013.

De Vocht TF, Chrzan R, Dik P, Klijn AJ, De Jong TP. Long-term results of bulking agent injection for persistent incontinence in cases of neurogenic bladder dysfunction. J Urol. 2010;183(2):719–23.

Decter RM, Bauer SB, Khoshbin S, Dyearo FM, Krarup C, Colodny AH, et al. Urodynamic assessment of children with cerebral palsy. J Urol. 1987;138(4 Pt 2): 1110–2.

Decter RM, Harpster L. Pitfalls in determination of leak point pressure. J Urol. 1992;148(2 Pt 2):588–91.

DeFoor W, Minevich E, Reddy P, Sekhon D, Polsky E, Wacksman J, et al. Bladder calculi after augmentation cystoplasty: risk factors and prevention strategies. J Urol. 2004;172(5 Pt 1):1964–6.

Dik P, Klijn AJ, van Gool JD, de Jong-de Vos van Steenwijk CC, de Jong TP. Early start to therapy preserves kidney function in spina bifida patients. Eur Urol. 2006;49(5):908–13.

Dushi G, Frey P, Ramseyer P, Vernet O, Meyearat BJ. Urodynamic score in children with lipomyelomeningocele: a prospective study. J Urol. 2011;186(2): 655–9.

Franc-Guimond J, Gonzalez R. Effectiveness of implanting catheterizable channels into intestinal segments. J Pediatr Urol. 2006;2(1):31–3.

Game X, Mouracade P, Chartier-Kastler E, Viehweger E, Moog R, Amarenco G, et al. Botulinum toxin-A (Botox) intradetrusor injections in children with neurogenic detrusor overactivity/neurogenic overactive bladder: a systematic literature review. J Pediatr Urol. 2009;5(3):156–64.

Granberg C, Cost N, Gargollo P, Snodgrass W. Urodynamic parameters to determine management of infants with myelomeningocele: early intervention versus continued observation. AAP (American Academy of Pediatrics) National Conference and Exhibition, Boston, MA, 2011.

Guerra LA, Pike J, Milks J, Barrowman N, Leonard M. Outcome in patients who underwent tethered cord release for occult spinal dysraphism. J Urol. 2006;176(4 Pt 2):1729–32.

Guerra LA, Moher D, Sampson M, Barrowman N, Pike J, Leonard M. Intravesical oxybutynin for children with poorly compliant neurogenic bladder: a systematic review. J Urol. 2008;180(3):1091–7.

Guys JM, Fakhro A, Louis-Borrione C, Prost J, Hautier A. Endoscopic treatment of urinary incontinence: long-term evaluation of the results. J Urol. 2001;165(6 Pt 2):2389–91.

Hafez AT, McLorie G, Bagli D, Khoury A. A single-centre long-term outcome analysis of artificial urinary sphincter placement in children. BJU Int. 2002; 89(1):82–5.

Henrichon S, Hu B, Kurzrock EA. Detailed assessment of stomal incontinence after Malone antegrade continence enema: development of a new grading scale. J Urol. 2012;187(2):652–5.

Herndon CD, Rink RC, Shaw MB, Simmons GR, Cain MP, Kaefer M, et al. The Indiana experience with artificial urinary sphincters in children and young adults. J Urol. 2003;169(2):650–4. discussion 4.

Higuchi TT, Granberg CF, Fox JA, Husmann DA. Augmentation cystoplasty and risk of neoplasia: fact, fiction and controversy. J Urol. 2010;184(6):2492–6.

Hoebeke P, De Kuyper P, Goeminne H, Van Laecke E, Everaert K. Bladder neck closure for treating pediatric incontinence. Eur Urol. 2000;38(4):453–6.

Hopps CV, Kropp KA. Preservation of renal function in children with myelomeningocele managed with basic newborn evaluation and close followup. J Urol. 2003;169(1):305–8.

Husmann DA, Rathbun SR. Long-term follow-up of enteric bladder augmentations: the risk for malignancy. J Pediatr Urol. 2008;4(5):381–5. discussion 6.

Husmann DA, Snodgrass WT, Koyle MA, Furness 3rd PD, Kropp BP, Cheng EY, et al. Ureterocystoplasty: indications for a successful augmentation. J Urol. 2004;171(1):376–80.

Jawaheer G, Rangecroft L. The Pippi Salle procedure for neurogenic urinary incontinence in childhood: a three-year experience. Eur J Pediatr Surg. 1999;9 Suppl 1Suppl 1:9–11.

Joseph DB. The effect of medium-fill and slow-fill saline cystometry on detrusor pressure in infants and children with myelodysplasia. J Urol. 1992;147(2): 444–6.

Kaefer M, Pabby A, Kelly M, Darbey M, Bauer SB. Improved bladder function after prophylactic treatment of the high risk neurogenic bladder in newborns with myelomentingocele. J Urol. 1999;162(3 Pt 2):1068–71.

Karaman MI, Kaya C, Caskurlu T, Guney S, Ergenekon E. Urodynamic findings in children with cerebral palsy. Int J Urol. 2005;12(8):717–20.

Kim HY, Jung SE, Lee SC, Park KW, Kim WK. Is the outcome of the left colon antegrade continence enema better than that of the right colon antegrade continence enema? J Pediatr Surg. 2009;44(4):783–7.

Kispal Z, Balogh D, Erdei O, Kehl D, Juhasz Z, Vastyan AM, et al. Complications after bladder augmentation or substitution in children: a prospective study of 86 patients. BJU Int. 2011;108(2):282–9.

Koivusalo A, Pakarinen MP, Rintala RJ. Treatment of a leaking ACE conduit with Deflux injections. Pediatr Surg Int. 2006;22(12):1003–6.

Kokorowski PJ, Routh JC, Borer JG, Estrada CR, Bauer SB, Nelson CP. Screening for malignancy after augmentation cystoplasty in children with spina bifida: a decision analysis. J Urol. 2011;186(4):1437–43.

Lawal TA, Rangel SJ, Bischoff A, Pena A, Levitt MA. Laparoscopic-assisted Malone appendicostomy in the management of fecal incontinence in children. J Laparoendosc Adv Surg Tech A. 2011;21(5):455–9.

Lemelle JL, Guillemin F, Aubert D, Guys JM, Lottmann H, Lortat-Jacob S, et al. A multicentre study of the management of disorders of defecation in patients with spina bifida. Neurogastroenterol Motil. 2006;18(2):123–8.

Leonardo CR, Filgueiras MF, Vasconcelos MM, Vasconcelos R, Marino VP, Pires C, et al. Risk factors for renal scarring in children and adolescents with lower urinary tract dysfunction. Pediatr Nephrol. 2007;22(11):1891–6.

Leslie B, Lorenzo AJ, Moore K, Farhat WA, Bagli DJ, Pippi Salle JL. Long-term followup and time to event outcome analysis of continent catheterizable channels. J Urol. 2011;185(6):2298–302.

Liard A, Seguier-Lipszyc E, Mathiot A, Mitrofanoff P. The Mitrofanoff procedure: 20 years later. J Urol. 2001;165(6 Pt 2):2394–8.

Lopez Pereira P, Somoza Ariba I, Martinez Urrutia MJ, Lobato Romero R, Jaureguizar ME. Artificial urinary sphincter: 11-year experience in adolescents with congenital neuropathic bladder. Eur Urol. 2006;50(5):1096–101. discussion 101.

Lopez Pereira P, Moreno Valle JA, Espinosa L, Alonso Dorrego JM, Martinez Urrutia MJ, Lobato Romera R, et al. Are urodynamic studies really needed during bladder augmentation follow-up? J Pediatr Urol. 2009;5(1):30–3.

Lorenzo AJ, Wallis MC, Cook A, Buffett-Fairen A, Bozic D, Bagli DJ, et al. What is the variability in urodynamic parameters with position change in children? Analysis of a prospectively enrolled cohort. J Urol. 2007;178(6):2567–70.

Lottmann HB, Margaryan M, Lortat-Jacob S, Bernuy M, Lackgren G. Long-term effects of dextranomer endoscopic injections for the treatment of urinary incontinence: an update of a prospective study of 61 patients. J Urol. 2006;176(4 Pt 2):1762–6.

Macejko AM, Cheng EY, Yerkes EB, Meyer T, Bowman RM, Kaplan WE. Clinical urological outcomes following primary tethered cord release in children younger than 3 years. J Urol. 2007;178(4 Pt 2):1738–42. discussion 42–3.

MacNeily AE, Jafari S, Scott H, Dalgetty A, Afshar K. Health related quality of life in patients with spina bifida: a prospective assessment before and after lower urinary tract reconstruction. J Urol. 2009;182(4 Suppl):1984–91.

Maerzheuser S, Jenetzky E, Zwink N, Reutter H, Bartels E, Grasshoff-Derr S, et al. German network for congenital uro-rectal malformations: first evaluation and interpretation of postoperative urological complications in anorectal malformations. Pediatr Surg Int. 2011;27(10):1085–9.

Matsuno D, Yamazaki Y, Shiroyanagi Y, Ueda N, Suzuki M, Nishi M, et al. The role of the retrograde colonic enema in children with spina bifida: is it inferior to the antegrade continence enema? Pediatr Surg Int. 2010;26(5):529–33.

Matthews GJ, Churchill BA, McLorie GA, Khoury AE. Ventriculoperitoneal shunt infection after augmentation cystoplasty. J Urol. 1996;155(2):686–8.

McGuire EJ, Woodside JR, Borden TA, Weiss RM. Prognostic value of urodynamic testing in myelodysplastic patients. J Urol. 1981;126(2):205–9.

Metcalfe PD, Casale AJ, Kaefer MA, Misseri R, Dussinger AM, Meldrum KK, et al. Spontaneous bladder perforations: a report of 500 augmentations in children and analysis of risk. J Urol. 2006a;175(4):1466–70. discussion 70–1.

Metcalfe PD, Cain MP, Kaefer M, Gilley DA, Meldrum KK, Misseri R, et al. What is the need for additional bladder surgery after bladder augmentation in childhood? J Urol. 2006b;176(4 Pt 2):1801–5. discussion 5.

Moore KN, Fader M, Getliffe K. Long-term bladder management by intermittent catheterisation in adults and children. Cochrane Database Syst Rev (Online). 2007(4):CD006008.

Mosiello G, Capitanucci ML, Gatti C, Adorisio O, Lucchetti MC, Silveri M, et al. How to investigate neurovesical dysfunction in children with anorectal malformations. J Urol. 2003;170(4 Pt 2):1610–3.

Narayanaswamy B, Wilcox DT, Cuckow PM, Duffy PG, Ransley PG. The Yang-Monti ileovesicostomy: a problematic channel? BJU Int. 2001;87(9):861–5.

Neveus T, von Gontard A, Hoebeke P, Hjalmas K, Bauer S, Bower W, et al. The standardization of terminology of lower urinary tract function in children and adolescents: report from the Standardisation Committee of the International Children's Continence Society. J Urol. 2006;176(1):314–24.

Nogueira M, Greenfield SP, Wan J, Santana A, Li V. Tethered cord in children: a clinical classification with urodynamic correlation. J Urol. 2004;172(4 Pt 2):1677–80. discussion 80.

Ok JH, Kurzrock EA. Objective measurement of quality of life changes after ACE Malone using the FICQOL survey. J Pediatr Urol. 2011;7(3):389–93.

Palmer LS, Richards I, Kaplan WE. Age related bladder capacity and bladder capacity growth in children with myelomeningocele. J Urol. 1997;158(3 Pt 2):1261–4.

Parekh AD, Trusler LA, Pietsch JB, Byearne DW, DeMarco RT, Pope JC, et al. Prospective, longitudinal evaluation of health related quality of life in the pediatric spina bifida population undergoing reconstructive urological surgery. J Urol. 2006;176(4 Pt 2):1878–82.

Perez LM, Smith EA, Broecker BH, Massad CA, Parrott TS, Woodard JR. Outcome of sling cystourethropexy in the pediatric population: a critical review. J Urol. 1996;156(2 Pt 2):642–6.

Phuong LK, Schoeberl KA, Raffel C. Natural history of tethered cord in patients with meningomyelocele. Neurosurgery. 2002;50(5):989–93. discussion 93–5.

Richardson I, Palmer LS. Clinical and urodynamic spectrum of bladder function in cerebral palsy. J Urol. 2009;182(4 Suppl):1945–8.

Rosenbaum DH, Cain MP, Kaefer M, Meldrum KK, King SJ, Misseri R, et al. Ileal enterocystoplasty and B12 deficiency in pediatric patients. J Urol. 2008;179(4): 1544–7. discussion 7–8.

Salle JL, McLorie GA, Bagli DJ, Khoury AE. Urethral lengthening with anterior bladder wall flap (Pippi Salle procedure): modifications and extended indications of the technique. J Urol. 1997;158(2):585–90.

Shiroyanagi Y, Suzuki M, Matsuno D, Yamazaki Y. The significance of 99mtechnetium dimercapto-succinic acid renal scan in children with spina bifida during long-term followup. J Urol. 2009;181(5):2262–6. discussion 6.

Siddiqui AA, Fishman SJ, Bauer SB, Nurko S. Long-term follow-up of patients after antegrade continence enema procedure. J Pediatr Gastroenterol Nutr. 2011;52(5):574–80.

Sidi AA, Dykstra DD, Gonzalez R. The value of urodynamic testing in the management of neonates with myelodysplasia: a prospective study. J Urol. 1986;135(1):90–3.

Sillen U, Hansson E, Hermansson G, Hjalmas K, Jacobsson B, Jodal U. Development of the urodynamic pattern in infants with myelomeningocele. Br J Urol. 1996;78(4):596–601.

Sinha CK, Butler C, Haddad M. Left Antegrade Continent Enema (LACE): review of the literature. Eur J Pediatr Surg. 2008;18(4):215–8.

Snodgrass WT, Elmore J, Adams R. Bladder neck sling and appendicovesicostomy without augmentation for neurogenic incontinence in children. J Urol. 2007;177(4):1510–4. discussion 5.

Snodgrass W, Keefover-Hicks A, Prieto J, Bush N, Adams R. Comparing outcomes of slings with versus without enterocystoplasty for neurogenic urinary incontinence. J Urol. 2009;181(6):2709–14. discussion 14–6.

Snodgrass W, Barber T, Cost N. Detrusor compliance changes after bladder neck sling without augmentation in children with neurogenic urinary incontinence. J Urol. 2010;183(6):2361–6.

Spiess PE, Capolicchio JP, Kiruluta G, Salle JP, Berardinucci G, Corcos J. Is an artificial sphincter the best choice for incontinent boys with Spina Bifida? Review of our long term experience with the AS-800 artificial sphincter. Can J Urol. 2002;9(2):1486–91.

Tarcan T, Bauer S, Olmedo E, Khoshbin S, Kelly M, Darbey M. Long-term followup of newborns with myelodysplasia and normal urodynamic findings: is followup necessary? J Urol. 2001;165(2):564–7.

Tiryaki S, Ergun O, Celik A, Ulman I, Avanoglu A. Success of Malone's antegrade continence enema (MACE) from the patients' perspective. Eur J Pediatr Surg. 2010;20(6):405–7.

Torre M, Guida E, Bisio G, Scarsi P, Piatelli G, Cama A, et al. Risk factors for renal function impairment in a series of 502 patients born with spinal dysraphisms. J Pediatr Urol. 2011;7(1):39–43.

Vande Velde S, Van Biervliet S, Van Renterghem K, Van Laecke E, Hoebeke P, Van Winckel M. Achieving fecal continence in patients with spina bifida: a descriptive cohort study. J Urol. 2007;178(6):2640–4. discussion 4.

Vanderbrink BA, Cain MP, King S, Meldrum K, Kaefer M, Misseri R, et al. Is oral vitamin B(12) therapy effective for vitamin B(12) deficiency in patients with prior ileocystoplasty? J Urol. 2010;184(4 Suppl): 1781–5.

Webb HW, Barraza MA, Stevens PS, Crump JM, Erhard M. Bowel dysfunction in spina bifida—an American experience with the ACE procedure. Eur J Pediatr Surg. 1998;8(1):37–8.

Wilmshurst JM, Kelly R, Borzyskowski M. Presentation and outcome of sacral agenesis: 20 years' experience. Dev Med Child Neurol. 1999;41(12):806–12.

Wong AL, Kravarusic D, Wong SL. Impact of cecostomy and antegrade colonic enemas on management of fecal incontinence and constipation: ten years of experience in pediatric population. J Pediatr Surg. 2008;43(8): 1445–51.

Wu HY, Baskin LS, Kogan BA. Neurogenic bladder dysfunction due to myelomeningocele: neonatal versus childhood treatment. J Urol. 1997;157(6): 2295–7.

YardLey IE, Pauniaho SL, Baillie CT, Turnock RR, Coldicutt P, Lamont GL, et al. After the honeymoon comes divorce: long-term use of the antegrade continence enema procedure. J Pediatr Surg. 2009;44(6):1274–6. discussion 6–7.

Yerkes EB, Rink RC, Cain MP, Luerssen TG, Casale AJ. Shunt infection and malfunction after augmentation cystoplasty. J Urol. 2001;165(6 Pt 2):2262–4.

Urolithiasis

17

Linda A. Baker and Nicol C. Bush

The initial aim in stone management is relief of symptoms.

Secondary aims:

1. **Achieve stone-free status.**
2. **Reduce or prevent stone recurrence.**

Summary of evidence for these aims:

- **The most common presenting complaint is abdominal pain. Our review found no study evaluating medical therapy to control acute renal colic in children.**
- **Although studies in adults conclude that alpha-blockers promote spontaneous stone passage, evidence in children is not conclusive.**
- **Two studies reported spontaneous stone passage in 34 and 47 % of children.**
- **Reported stone-free rates for renal stones <1 cm were 63–86 % for shock wave lithotripsy (SWL) and 50–90 % for ureteroscopy. Efficiency quotients (EQ) were only reported for SWL, with approximately 25 % needing additional procedures. However, at least a third of patients undergoing ureteroscopy needed a period of stenting to dilate the ureter before the stone could be accessed, and most had postoperative stents, meaning some had as many as three procedures to achieve stone-free status.**
- **Unlike adults, lower pole stones in children are as effectively treated by SWL as those in other renal locations.**
- **One trial compared monotherapy percutaneous nephrolithotomy (PCNL) to SWL for renal stones 1–2 cm, finding stone-free rates greater with PCNL, 95 % versus 85 %.**
- **One trial found no difference in stone recurrence in those stone-free versus having fragments <5 mm after SWL.**
- **Recurrence after stone-free status occurred in ≤10–33 % of patients. One study reported significantly fewer recurrences with potassium citrate therapy.**
- **Low-sodium high-potassium diet resolved hypercalciuria in 50 % of children, but was difficult to maintain.**
- **Indications and duration of medical therapy with potassium citrate or thiazides are not defined for children.**
- **Our review found no study evaluating stone recurrence rates in children with versus without 24-h urine stone-risk profile determinations in first-time pediatric stone formers.**

Medical Evaluation

Clinical Presentation

Four retrospective studies reported that pain was the most common chief complaint. Hematuria and UTI were other common presenting complaints of pediatric stones.

L.A. Baker, M.D. (✉) • N.C. Bush, M.D., M.S.C.S.
Department of Pediatric Urology, University of Texas Southwestern Medical Center and Children's Medical Center Dallas, 1935 Medical District Drive, MS F4.04, Dallas, TX 75235, USA
e-mail: linda.baker@childrens.com

W.T. Snodgrass (ed.), *Pediatric Urology: Evidence for Optimal Patient Management*,
DOI 10.1007/978-1-4614-6910-0_17, © Springer Science+Business Media New York 2013

Two studies found younger children more likely to have renal stones versus ureteral stones in older patients.

Two studies reported spontaneous stone passage in 34 % (renal and ureteral) and 47 %.

Most stones analyzed in children were calcium oxalate or phosphate.

One hundred and twenty-six consecutive children referred to a Turkish urology department with urinary stones were divided into two cohorts based on age at presentation, 48 (58 % male) aged 0–5 years and 78 (63 % male) aged 6–15 years. At presentation, kidney/ureteral stone percentages were 65 %/35 % in younger and 38 %/62 % in older patients, $p=0.006$ (Koyuncu et al. 2011).

A retrospective review identified 80 US children (46 % males) evaluated with stones during a 7-year period ending in 2007, 39 <10 years and 41 >10 years of age at presentation. There was no age difference in the chief complaint, which was pain in 62.5 %, hematuria in 10 %, and UTI in 12.5 %. Stone location was renal in 57 % versus 31 % of younger versus older children, $p=0.02$. Mean renal stone size was 7 mm (1–22) in both groups. Spontaneous passage of these renal stones occurred in 32 % and 0 % of younger and older children. Ureteral stones were more common in those >10 years old, with no differences by age in stone size, 7 mm versus 5 mm (1–17), or spontaneous passage rate of 42 %. Overall spontaneous passage rate (renal and ureteral stones) was 34 %. During follow-up a mean of 36 months (2–17), new stones occurred in 16 %, with no age difference. There were no differences in stone composition between 17/39 (44 %) and 16/41 (39 %) analyzed in the two age groups, with 85 % calcium oxalate and 48 % containing calcium phosphate. There were no differences in metabolic assessments done in 59 % and 46 % of younger versus older children, with hypercalciuria in 33 % and hypocitraturia in 62 % (Kalorin et al. 2009).

Retrospective review found 72 children (56 % males), mean age 11 years, who presented with first known stone disease to a tertiary children's hospital in Canada over a 5-year period ending in 2004. Family history was positive for stones in 25 %. Chief complaint was flank pain in 63 %, with 49 % having nausea/vomiting, 18 % gross hematuria, 10 % lower tract symptoms, and 4 % UTI. The diagnosis was "incidental" in 21 %. UPJO was found in four (6 %). Spontaneous passage occurred in 47 %, with stones a mean diameter of 4 mm; 35 % had surgical intervention, and 18 % continued with their stone. Of 42 stones analyzed, 93 % were calcium oxalate or phosphate. During follow-up at a mean of 1.5 years, stones recurred in 21 % of 70 patients (excluding two with cystinuria) (Kit et al. 2008).

Clinical symptoms were described for 197 children (54 % males), mean age 9±4 years, evaluated in a pediatric nephrology unit lacking emergency services. Recurrent abdominal pain was the most common chief complaint in 17 %, acute abdominal pain in 6 %, dysuria in 6 %, microscopic hematuria in 6 %, and gross hematuria in 4 %; the remainder had various combinations of these (Polito et al. 2012).

Prevalence of Metabolic Abnormalities

Stone Formers

Two prospective studies evaluating consecutive children with stones reported widely divergent results of urine stone risk profiles: one found metabolic abnormalities in 43 % of stone formers, mostly hypocitraturia, while the other found 81 % had abnormalities, mostly hypercalciuria.

Prospective data were collected in the 126 consecutive Turkish children with urinary stones reported by Koyuncu et al. (2011) mentioned above, including two to three 24-h urine stone risk profiles. Children were divided into two cohorts based on age at presentation, 48 (58 % male) aged 0–5 years and 78 (63 % male) aged 6–15 years. Metabolic evaluation of calcium, citrate, and oxalate reported no significant differences in abnormalities based on age group, 50 % versus 38 %, for a total of 43 %, but other risk factors, such as low urine volume, cystine, and magnesium, were not reported. These comprised

10 % hypercalciuria, 12 % hyperoxaluria, 24 % hypocitraturia (Koyuncu et al. 2011).

Prospective 24-h urine stone risk profile data were recorded in 197 children (54 % males), mean age 9 ± 4 years, evaluated in an Italian pediatric nephrology unit by Polito et al. (2012) reported above. Of these, 38 (19 %) had normal profiles. There was a positive family history in 77 %. Three 24-h urine collections were performed at home, and highest values were used to classify defects in the 81 % with abnormalities:

- 48 % Hypercalciuria
- 7 % Hyperoxaluria
- 4 % Hypocitraturia
- 19 % Hyperuricosuria
- 4 % Cystinuria

Another study evaluated 112 children (54 % males), mean age 4 years (1 month–18 years), with stones referred to a Turkish pediatric nephrology department. Positive family history was reported in 55 %. Stones were located in the kidney in 94 %, ureter in 2 %, and both in 4 %, with 23 % having multiple stones bilaterally. Metabolic evaluation reported abnormalities in 92 %:

- 38 % Hypercalciuria
- 42 % Hyperoxaluria
- 49 % Hypocitraturia
- 18 % Hyperuricosuria
- 4 % Cystinuria

More than one risk factor was seen in 22 (20 %) (Gurgoze and Sari 2011).

Retrospective review was done in 104 children (53 % males) presenting to a pediatric nephrology clinic with stones in Turkey. Metabolic factors were analyzed by either two 24-h urine collections or spot urine sampling (percentages of each not provided). Fifty percent had a positive family history. Reported urine abnormalities were found in 87 %, and included:

- 31 % Hypercalciuria
- 30 % Hyperoxaluria
- 38 % Hypocitraturia
- 24 % Hyperuricosuria
- 6 % Citraturia (Alpay et al. 2009)

Retrospective review of 221 consecutive children (108 males, mean 11 years) referred to the Mayo clinic for stone evaluation demonstrated metabolic abnormalities in 42 %; however, 24-h metabolic evaluation was variable, as reflected below. Presenting symptoms were pain (47 %), hematuria (33 %), and infection (11 %). Infection-related stones were diagnosed in 41 (19 %), including 6 patients with bladder stones after exstrophy repair. Ten patients had urinary diversion. Thirty-seven percent of children had a positive family history for stones.

- 49/145 (34 %) Hypercalciuria
- 25/124 (20 %) Hyperoxaluria
- 11/32 (34 %) Cystinuria
- 8/96 (8 %) Hyperuricosuria
- 5/54 (9 %) Hypocitraturia (Milliner and Murphy 1993)

Stone Formers Versus Controls

One study showed higher urine calcium and super saturation indices in pediatric stone formers compared to their non-stone-forming siblings and healthy controls, with no difference in other parameters. Two studies comparing stone formers to controls reported patients had significantly increased urinary calcium and oxalate and significantly lower urinary citrate. A third study found calcium excretion similar but oxalate higher and citrate lower in patients.

A study of 129 stone formers (6–17 years) versus 105 non-stone-forming siblings and 183 healthy children without family history of stones was performed. The stone formers had higher urine calcium excretion (calcium >200 mg versus 170 mg versus 140 mg/1.73 m^2 in stone formers, siblings, and controls). They also had higher calcium super-saturation indices, but similar levels of hyperoxaluria, hypocitraturia, low urine volume, and abnormal pH (Bergsland et al. 2012).

A cross-sectional study compared 24-h urine stone risk profiles in 142 children (46 % males), median age 14 years (3–18), with newly diagnosed stones to 210 children, median age 15 years (3–18), without stones (source of controls not described). Stone formers had significantly increased calcium and oxalate and significantly lower citrate than controls (Spivacow et al. 2008).

A 24-h urine metabolic evaluation was done in 78 stone formers and 24 controls (source not described) with similar gender and a mean age of 7 years. Of patients, 42 % had multiple stones, 19 % bilateral stones, and 5 % staghorn stones; 57 (73 %) were evaluated after a first stone, and the others had recurrent stones (frequency not stated). Median citrate was lower and median oxalate higher in stone formers versus controls, while calcium excretion was similar. Multivariable analysis found only hypocitraturia an independent risk factor for stones (Tekin et al. 2000).

A tertiary Scottish referral clinic recruited 24 stone-formers (62 % males), median age 10 years (1–17), and 32 controls (41 % males), median age 7 years (1–15), for analysis of random urine samples tested for creatinine, calcium, oxalate, urate, citrate, and glycosaminoglycans (GAGs). There was no difference in ages between stone patients and controls. Compared to controls, stone formers had significantly lower citrate and significantly higher calcium excretion, as well as higher promoter–inhibitor ratios (calcium × oxalate/citrate × GAGs). Control males and females showed no differences in parameters. Controls showed significant inverse correlations between age and all urinary constituents tested expressed as ratios to calcium (MacDougall et al. 2010).

Solitary Versus Recurrent Stone Formers

One study found children with hypocitraturia, hyperoxaluria, and/or hypercalciuria were more likely to have stone recurrence versus children without these risk factors.

One study reported patients with multiple or recurrent stones had significantly greater prevalence of hypercalciuria and hypocitraturia than those with a single stone and no recurrence.

Another found no difference in urine risk factors between first-time stone formers and those with recurrent stones.

The prospective study by Koyuncu et al. (2011) described above demonstrated a higher recurrence rate in children with versus those without metabolic abnormalities (50 % versus 14 %, $p<0.0001$) with average follow-up of 43 months.

A retrospective study analyzed two cohorts, children with a single stone at presentation and no recurrence ($n=88$) and those with either multiple stones at presentation and/or recurrent stone ($n=51$). Mean age (13 years) and gender were similar, as was follow-up a mean of approximately 3 years. The 24-h urine stone risk profiles demonstrated significantly greater prevalence of hypercalciuria (73 % versus 57 %, $p=0.02$) and hypocitraturia (30 % versus 13 %, $p=0.003$) in multiple/recurrent stone patients (DeFoor et al. 2010).

The study by Tekin et al. (2000) described above included 78 children categorized as first-time stone formers ($n=57$, 73 %) or recurrent stone formers (frequency not defined). In contrast to DeFoor et al. (2010) above, patients with multiple stones at presentation were not classified as recurrent. Multivariable analysis did not find any difference in metabolic defects.

Pediatric Versus Adult Stone Formers

One study comparing children mean age 9 years to adults mean age 42 years found most stones in both age groups were calcium oxalate, but children were more likely to have hypocitraturia versus adults who more likely had hypercalciuria.

The 24-h urine stone risk profiles were analyzed in 71 children (59 % male), mean age 9 years (1–14), and 285 adult (59 % male) stone formers, mean age 42 years (14–71). Mean stone frequency was 2 (1–4) in children versus 3 (2–8) in adults; stones analyzed in 63 and 44 % of patients were calcium oxalate in 84 % of children and 75 % of adults. Metabolic factor analysis was abnormal in 90 % of patients in both groups, but with hypocitraturia significantly more often in children (58 % versus 45 %, $p=0.046$), and hypercalciuria significantly more often in adults (51 % versus 27 %, $p<0.01$) and no differences in hyperoxaluria or hyperuricosuria (Karabacak et al. 2010).

Risk for Urolithiasis in Children with Hypercalciuria

Three studies reported onset of urolithiasis in children diagnosed with hypercalciuria because of abdominal pain, hematuria, dysuria, or voiding dysfunctions. During 3–7 years of follow-up, stones were diagnosed in 4–16 %.

One study included 104 children without known urolithiasis who were diagnosed with hypercalciuria on the basis of abdominal pain, gross or microscopic hematuria, or various voiding symptoms as discussed below (Tabel and Mir 2006). Patients were treated with a diet that included sodium restriction, which most did not comply with, and followed for a mean of 4 years (6 months to 16 years). Systematic renal imaging was not described. A total of seven stones developed in 103 (7 %) treated with diet changes.

Another searched a database to identify 94 children diagnosed with hypercalciuria without urolithiasis, of which 50 were randomly selected for follow-up assessment; 33 (42 % males) with mean age 12 years (8–17) agreed to the follow-up. This secondary evaluation was done a mean of 7 years (4–11) after initial diagnosis, which was made secondary to dysuria/frequency (55 %), incontinence/enuresis (18 %), abdominal/flank pain (15 %), and hematuria (48 %). Calcium–creatinine ratio was mean 0.32 (0.22–0.45) with 24-h excretion measured in 22 (67 %) between 4.5 and 9 mg/kg/day. Initially, renal US showed only two with "minimal" renal calcifications; no imaging was done in seven (21 %). Therapy included increased fluids, salt restriction, RDA of calcium and protein; eight (24 %) were also prescribed thiazides. At follow-up at 7 years, 21 % still had symptoms considered minor. None continued on medication, and 63 % ate an unrestricted diet; the others followed a "somewhat" salt-reduced and/or low calcium diet. Only three (9 %) continued high fluid intake. Repeated urine samples showed 48 % to be hypercalciuric and 51 % normocalciuric. US was done in 23 (70 %), finding only one (4 %) "small" renal calcification. None had symptomatic urolithiasis (Alon and Berenbom 2000).

A third study of children with hematuria found 58 (71 % male), mean age 8 years, with hypercalciuria. Seventy-four percent of these had a positive family history for stones. Hypercalciuria was categorized as renal leak in 33 %, absorptive in 41 %, and uncertain in 26 %. All had US at diagnosis and annually. During follow-up at a mean of 3 years (1–6), 16 % developed a stone, not associated with subtype of hypercalciuria (Garcia et al. 1991).

Hypercalciuria and Bone Density

Two studies found decreased bone mineral density (BMD) in 32–47 % of children with hypercalciuria ± stones.

A retrospective chart review was done to indentify 98 children with hypercalciuria ± urolithiasis (61 without and 37 with stones). BMD was obtained in all cases, finding a *Z* score <–1 in 47 %, and <–2 in 25 %, numbers representing bone density that is >1 and >2 SD below healthy age, gender, and race-matched controls, respectively. Mean BMD for children with normal scores was 0.4 ± 1.3 versus –2.3 ± 1 for those with low bone density. There were no significant differences between those with normal versus low BMD in patient age (mean 9 ± 3 years), gender, or calcium excretion. Stone patients had significantly lower bone density scores and a higher percentage of *Z* scores <–2 (Schwaderer et al. 2008).

BMD was determined in 88 children (57 % male), median age 9 years (2–18), with hypercalciuria (three samples with >4 mg/kg/day) versus 29 normal controls (siblings of the patients but without hypercalciuria). Hypercalciuric patients included 49 (56 %) stone formers. There were no differences in the groups by gender, age, BMI, or bone age, but BMD *Z* scores were significantly less in hypercalciuric patients (–0.7, –2.2 to 1.7 versus 0.0, –0.9 to 1.7), $p < 0.001$. Thirty-two percent of patients had osteopenia (*Z* score <–2) at diagnosis of hypercalciuria (Penido et al. 2003).

Hypercalciuria and UTI

One study reported hypercalciuria in 43 % of children mean age 8 years with recurrent UTI.

A prospective study was designed to evaluate the possible relationship between recurrent UTI and hypercalciuria in 75 children >5 years of age (mean 8 years). The mean of ≥3 random morning urine calcium–creatinine ratios was used to define hypercalciuria; UTI was $>10^5$ CFU/cm^3 in midstream urine and recurrent UTI was two or more infections with an intervening sterile culture and symptom-free interval. Febrile versus non-febrile infection was not stated. All had renal US and DMSA for renal scar, with VCUG if either upper tract test was abnormal. All had recurrent UTI, and 83 % of patients were female. Hypercalciuria (mean calcium–creatinine ratio 0.5 ± 0.2 mg/mL, mean 24-h calcium excretion 6.5 mg/kg/day) was found in 32 (43 %). There were no differences in voiding dysfunction (73 %, means to diagnose not described) or in anatomic anomalies (27 %) between hypercalciuric and normocalciuric children (Biyikli et al. 2005).

Urine Stone Risk Profiles in Tube-Fed Children with Stones

One retrospective evaluation comparing tube-fed patients to otherwise healthy stone-forming controls reported similar rates of hypercalciuria and hypocitraturia but significantly higher urine pH and more calcium phosphate stones in those who were tube-fed.

A retrospective review was done comparing 16 stone patients with gastrostomy feeding to 32 age-matched controls who formed stones but were considered otherwise healthy. Ninety-four percent of gastrostomy patients were immobile, and duration of tube feeding prior to stone onset was mean of 35 months (4–96), with no apparent differences between enteral formulas used. A 24-h urine collection was done in 10/16 patients and 28/32 stone-forming controls, finding similar rates of hypercalciuria (29 %), hypocitraturia (13 %) and low urine volume (65 %, <40 cm^3/kg/day). However, urine pH was significantly higher (mean 6.9 versus 6.2) in gastrostomy patients, and stone composition was significantly more likely calcium phosphate stones in gastrostomy patients versus calcium oxalate in controls (Smith et al. 2011).

Medical Management

Stone Expulsion Therapy

Although alpha-blocker therapy in adults significantly improves spontaneous stone passage, one trial in children comparing doxazosin to controls reported no difference in either rate of spontaneous passage or time to passage of distal ureteral stones.

Another pediatric trial compared tamsulosin to placebo, reporting increased spontaneous stone passage and decreased time to passage, but 45 % of treated patients had residual fragments after SWL or PCNL, while all those on placebo presented with ureteral stones.

Systematic literature review of alpha-antagonist (16 studies) and calcium channel blocker therapy (9 studies) reported that these agents significantly improve spontaneous stone passage in adults >18 years of age:

- Alpha-antagonists RR 1.6 (95 % CI 1.4–1.7), number need to treat three
- Calcium channel blockers RR 1.5 (95 % CI 1.3–1.7), number needed to treat four

Side effects from alpha-blockers were noted in 4 % (Singh et al. 2007).

One trial in children 2–14 years old with distal ureteral stones <10 mm randomized patients to 20 controls receiving ibuprofen versus 19 receiving doxazosin 0.03 mg/kg/day. Mean follow-up was 19 days. There was no difference in spontaneous stone passage rates, 70 % versus 84 %, or in time to passage, 6 days in both groups. No gender differences were noted in response either. The authors stated that there were fewer pain episodes with alpha-blocker therapy, but added that this was not objectively assessed. There were no reported complications from alpha-blocker treatment (Aydogdu et al. 2009).

Another trial randomized 61 children (59 % males), mean age 8 ± 7 years, with distal ureteral stones to either tamsulosin (0.2 mg daily if <4 years; 0.4 mg if >4 years of age) or placebo. Patient groups were similar for gender, age, and stone size. However, 45 % of tamsulosin patients had ureteral fragments after SWL or PCNL, with none of these randomized to the placebo group. Tamsulosin treatment resulted in increased spontaneous passage, 88 % versus 64 %, and decreased time to passage, 8 days versus 14.5 days, $p<0.001$. Patients receiving tamsulosin reported significantly fewer pain episodes (1.4 ± 1.2 versus 2.2 ± 1.4); 25 % also reported "mild" somnolence and nasal congestion (Mokhless et al. 2012).

Hypercalciuria

Two studies found diet changes (decreased sodium, increased potassium) resolved hypercalciuria in 33–50 %; one reported that hypercalciuria recurred in half of responders due to difficulties maintaining a low-sodium diet.

Most non-responders treated with either thiazides or potassium citrate became normocalciuric.

Optimal duration of medication therapy is unknown.

Hypercalciuria diagnosed on the basis of calcium–creatinine ratio >0.21 in three consecutive morning urinalyses or urinary calcium >4 mg/kg/day on 24-h collections (percentages of each not stated), in children evaluated in a pediatric nephrology clinic for abdominal pain (60 %), hematuria (56 %), or urination disturbance including UTI (24 %), dysuria (45 %) or enuresis (14 %). There was a total of 131 children (53 % male), mean age 3 years (1–15). Fifty-five percent of patients had a family history of urolithiasis. Stones were diagnosed in 27 (20 %) at presentation. All were recommended a diet with liberal fluids (>1,500 mL/m^2/day), decreased sodium (1–2 mg/kg/day) and increased potassium ("according to RDA") and followed by calcium–creatinine and sodium–potassium (Na–K) rates in spot urines monthly for 3 months and then every 3 months. Hydrochlorothiazide (1–2 mg/kg for a mean of 8 months, 3–18) was prescribed for 20 children (19 with stones) subcategorized with renal leak hypercalciuria unresponsive to dietary treatment after 1 year. Mean follow-up was 4 years (6 months to 16 years):

- Only 27 % had normal calcium–creatinine and Na–K ratios on the first spot urine after beginning dietary management.
- Hypercalciuria resolved with diet in 65 (50 %), but then recurred in 30 (time to recurrence, dietary habits at recurrence not stated).
- Hypercalciuria persisted in 50 (38 %), all with high Na–K ratios.
- Nineteen (95 %) thiazide-treated patients resolved hypercalciuria, but four discontinued therapy for symptoms, and hypercalciuria recurred in a total of ten (apparently when medication stopped).
- Eight of 104 (8 %) without stones at presentation developed stones, including 1 treated with thiazide.

The authors stated that most patients did not comply with sodium restriction (Tabel and Mir 2006).

A pediatric nephrology unit identified 33 children (from a group of 44, 55 % male, mean age 10 years) with known urolithiasis diagnosed with hypercalciuria by 24-h urine collection or spot urine calcium–creatinine ratios if not toilet-trained. Treatment included high fluid intake (not defined), and a low-sodium, high-potassium, and RDA protein diet. Those with persistent hypercalciuria were then treated with thiazide (15–25 mg/kg/day) and/or potassium citrate (1–1.5 mEq/kg/day). Of the 33 patients:

- Thirteen had diet changes alone; two had persistent "mild" hypercalciuria (not defined).
- Fifteen used potassium citrate.
- Four started thiazide, but one added and two changed to potassium citrate.

Thirty-one (94 %) became normocalciuric. No new stones developed on therapy. Three ending or stopping medication had recurrent hypercalciuria and new stones. Recommended duration of medication treatment was not stated (Alon et al. 2004).

Hypocitraturia

One study reported that potassium citrate significantly increased urine pH and citrate and decreased urinary calcium.

A retrospective chart review reported potassium citrate treatment (1 mEq/kg/day) for hypocitraturia (< 320 mg/1.73 m^2/day) in 64 consecutive children (65 % males), median age 7 years (1–15), with stones. With mean follow-up of 22 months (3–67), no adverse drug reactions were recorded. Therapy resulted in significant median changes from baseline at both 3 months and at last visit, including pH (5.3 ± 0.3 to 6.3 ± 0.5), citrate (197 ± 72 to 621 ± 173), and calcium (3.5 ± 2.7 to 2.7 ± 2.4). Of the children, 20 (31 %) had recurrent stones at entry; during follow-up, 93 % had no new stones or stone growth, while 3 with prior history of recurrent stones had additional recurrence. Recommended duration of therapy was not discussed (Tekin et al. 2002).

Surgical Therapy

Renal Stones

Shock Wave Lithotripsy

Several retrospective analyses reported SWL achieved stone-free status after one treatment in 50–80 % of kidneys.

Stone-free rates were consistently found to be significantly greater with stones <1 cm versus >2 cm, 63–86 % versus 25–62.5 %.

One study contrasted results in children younger than 6 versus those 7–15 years of age, and found that younger patients had significantly higher stone-free rates after one treatment.

Two studies reported both stone-free rates and EQ (taking into account additional post-operative procedures). Both indicated that secondary procedures were needed in approximately 25 % for stones <1 cm.

One study reported that Houndsfield Units determined from the stone center predicted SWL success, with significantly greater clearance for those <1,000 HU.

Only one reviewed study reported the frequency with which US, KUB, and CT were used to determine stone-free status.

Steinstrasse occurred in from 0.6 to 11 % of patients.

A retrospective study considered SWL efficacy for varying stone burdens in 260 children mean age 7 years (3 months to 16 years) and 279 renal units treated with the Lithostar Modularis. Mean stone burden was 1 cm^2, mean number of sessions was 1.4 (1–3), and mean shock waves per session was 2,260 (500–3,500). IVP or non-contrast CT were done in all patients (numbers of each not stated) 3 months after the last treatment. Stone-free rate was 77 % with SWL. Additional postoperative procedures (double-J stent, PCNL, or ureteroscopy) were included in an EQ calculation. Overall success was 87.5 %, with EQ of 0.62. There was a significant decrease in stone-free rates and EQ as stone burden increased: <1 cm^2 87 %, 0.71; 1–2 cm^2 74 %, 0.61; >2 cm^2 33 %, 0.29. There were no procedure-related complications. Steinstrasse occurred in 28 (11 %) patients, 4 treated with a second SWL and the others “conservatively” managed (Turunc et al. 2010a).

Another review included 149 children, mean age 14 years (3–17), with mean total stone diameter of 1.4 cm (0.2–9) who had SWL using Medirex Tripter X1 or Medstone STS. No single stone was >2 cm diameter. Mean time to imaging after SWL was 21 days (13–93), but imaging modalities used were not stated. One-session stone-free status was 71 %, with 8 % undergoing a second session; EQ was 0.63. Multivariable analysis showed stone diameter related to success, but not age, gender, BMI, or stone location (lower pole versus others). Stone-free rates and EQ were 80 %, 0.74 for stones <1 cm; 59 %, 0.5 for stones 1–2 cm; and 45 %, 0.35 for those >2 cm (McAdams et al. 2010a).

A third retrospective study reported SWL using the HM3 machine in 157 children mean age 6 years (10 months to 12 years) with mean stone diameter 1.5 cm and maximum 5.5 cm. Stent or nephrostomy was placed before treatment in 42 % of patients for stones >2 cm, staghorn stones, or high-grade obstruction. Stone-free rates were determined 3 months after SWL, but imaging was not described. Overall 80 % were stone-free apparently after one session, with others having one to two additional SWL sessions. Stone-free rates after one session for those <1 cm were 86 % versus 62.5 % if >2 cm, $p=0.03$. One un-stented patient developed steinstrasse, leading to nephrostomy tube and spontaneous stone passage (Landau et al. 2009).

SWL using the Compact Delta was reported in 101 children, mean age 10.5 years (10 months to 19 years), with mean stone diameter of 8 mm and a solitary stone in 76 %. Of these, one session was done in 78 % (mean size not stated) and mean shock waves per session was 2,250. Outcome assessment was done at a mean of 5 months, using US in 92 % of cases. Stone-free rate after one session was 50 %, and 59 % overall, more likely with stones <1 cm (63 % versus 25 %, $p=0.01$). Hospital admission was needed in 3 % of sessions—for febrile UTI (fUT) in three and ureteral obstruction in two (Nelson et al. 2008).

Retrospective analysis was done in 164 children, mean age 46 months (4–178), treated with SWL monotherapy using the PeizoLith 3000 lithotripter for solitary renal calcium stones <2.5 cm in length. Patients were divided into two cohorts by age <6 years (mean 28 months) versus those 7–15 years (mean 119 months). Follow-up included KUB, renal US, and/or CT (relative use within the two cohorts not stated). There were no differences in stone location, mean stone size (10 mm, 5–25), mean shock waves per session (2,233 versus 2,147), or mean energy applied (0.6 mJ/mm^2 versus 0.7 mJ/mm^2):

- The number of sessions was significantly less in the younger children, mean 1.6 (1–5) versus 2.9 (1–6).
- Stone-free rate after one session was 68 % versus 39 % for younger versus older children, $p=0.04$.
- Stone-free rates between younger and older patients were similar for all locations except the lower pole calyx, where one session was effective in 36 % versus 78 %, $p=0.2$.
- Overall stone-free rate was the same—93 % for the entire group (Goktas et al. 2012).

Preoperative stone attenuation was studied in 53 children, mean age 10 years (1–18), undergoing SWL for stones a mean of 1 cm (4 mm–4 cm) in diameter. Attenuation was determined in HU from the center of the stone. Stone-free rates were reported based on US, KUB, or CT (relative use not described) from 2 weeks to 3 months. While univariate analysis showed both stone size and attenuation to predict stone-free rates, multivariable analysis showed that only attenuation was an independent factor. For successful versus failed cases, mean attenuation was 710 ± 294 HU versus 994 ± 379 HU, $p=0.007$. Stone-free rate was 77 % for stones <1,000 HU versus 33 % for >1,000 HU (McAdams et al. 2010b).

Percutaneous Nephrolithotomy

Three reviewed retrospective studies reported stone-free rates after PCNL ranging from 61 to 86 % of kidneys.

None reported EQ to take into account additional procedures, including second looks.

Complications included postoperative fever, renal pelvis perforation, and blood loss requiring transfusion (4–15 %).

PCNL was reported for 169 children (188 kidneys) ranging in age from 1 to16 years with mean stone burden ranging from 19 to 33 mm. Single access was used in 94 %, with a 17-Fr scope in 71 % and a 26-Fr scope in the others. Postoperative imaging was not described. Sixty-one percent were stone-free using only PCNL; second looks were not described, and SWL was used for additional therapy. Postoperative fever lasting ≤48 h occurred in 49 % of patients, and seven (4 %) had transfusion (Samad et al. 2006).

Results of PCNL were reviewed in 45 children, mean age 6 ± 4 years, with 51 treated kidneys. Procedures were all done using a 20-Fr access sheath and 170-Fr nephroscope, with one access in 43 (84 %) kidneys. Indications were SWL-resistant stones and those >2 cm^2, and were single in 27, multiple in 12, and staghorn in 12 kidneys. Postoperative imaging included KUB and renal US at ≤4 weeks, 6 months, and annually with mean follow-up of 16 ± 12 months. Forty-four (86 %) kidneys were stone-free. Analysis in 43 patients showed calcium oxalate stones in 79 % and struvite in 21 %. Complications included blood loss requiring transfusion in three (7 %), colon perforation "treated conservatively" in one, and "prolonged" urine leak in one, as well as fever in six (13 %, duration not stated) (Dogan et al. 2011b).

Another retrospective series included 26 children, median age 3 years (6 months to 6 years), treated by PCNL using 14-Fr access sheaths for stone burden ranging from 100 to 1,380 mm^2. Three (12 %) patients needed two to three access sites. Twenty-four of 28 (86 %) kidneys were stone-free after one session. Complications included need for transfusion in four (15 %) and leakage from insertion site requiring double-J stent in one (Bilen et al. 2010).

SWL Versus PCNL

One review compared treatments in renal stones 1–2 cm, finding higher stone-free rates for PCNL, with one patient needing transfusion after PCNL versus one steinstrasse after SWL.

One retrospective study evaluated 166 children undergoing either SWL or PCNL for renal stones 1–2 cm in size according to surgeon preference, with SWL done in 91 (93 kidneys, 53 %) and PCNL in 75 (82 kidneys). SWL was done using electromagnetic Lithotriptor S, and a maximum of three sessions was used with maximum 2,000 shock waves each. PCNL used 22-Fr access sheaths and ultrasonic lithotripsy or 30-Fr access with intact extraction (in "older" children, age not stated). Mean age was similar at 6 years, as was mean stone diameter of 14 mm (11–20) and location (pelvis, calyces, both). Stone-free rates were reported using US (and CT, number not stated) at 3 months. One-session stone-free rates were 87 % for PCNL and 45 % for SWL. PCNL monotherapy stone-free rate was 95 % versus 85 % for SWL, $p=0.05$. Complications included bleeding needing transfusion and renal pelvic perforation requiring 4 days nephrostomy diversion in two patients after PCNL versus one steinstrasse treated with ureteroscopy after SWL. Postoperative fever developed in two (3 %) PCNL and zero SWL patients. During follow-up a mean of 31 months (6–84), recurrence in prior stone-free patients was similar (10 %) (Shokeir et al. 2006).

Ureteroscopy

Three studies reported ureteroscopy for renal stones, all with mean size ≤1 cm.

Stone-free rates ranged from 50 to 97 %.

Each reported inability to access the upper tract initially in from 30 to 43 % of patients, in some despite active dilation of the distal ureter, managed by double-J stent placement.

Two reported postoperative double-J stenting in all cases.

None reported EQ to take into account unsuccessful initial access or need for an additional anesthetic to retrieve a stent.

Prospectively entered data were analyzed in 167 children (89 boys) mean age 5 years (3 months to 18 years) who had a mean stone burden of 6 mm (3–24) and underwent flexible ureteroscopy. Of these, 101 stones were above the UPJ. Access was not possible at initial attempt in 57 % of patients, who then had a ureteral stent placed for passive dilation for 1–2 weeks; active dilation was not done. All were stented after ureteroscopy, with approximately 50 % having a retrieval string. Stone-free rate for renal stones was 97 % with one intervention. Mean follow-up was 20 months (6–39); no complications were reported, but postoperative imaging was not discussed (Kim et al. 2008).

A retrospective study found 80 children (69 males), mean age 9.5 years (6–12), who had ureteroscopy for upper ureteral or UPJ stones with a mean stone burden of 10 mm (7–16). Retrograde access included active dilation using cone-tipped metal dilators followed by flexible ureteroscopy (scope size not stated) in 65 %, while another 31 % had pretreatment double-J stenting for passive dilation (when unable to dilate or pass the ureteroscope). The number with stents after ureteroscopy was not reported. Postoperative imaging was at the discretion of the operating surgeon. Single-session stone-free rate was reported as 90 %, with no perforations or other major complications noted (Nerli et al. 2011).

A retrospective review was reported in 50 children (52 kidneys), mean age 8 years (1–14), after ureteroscopy using a 7.5-Fr flexible scope, with holmium:YAG lithotripsy done in 54 %. Ureteroscopy was initial therapy in 90 %, with 54 % having stones in the renal pelvis and 25 % in the lower pole. Mean stone size was 8 mm (1–16). In 33 % of cases, a 4.8-Fr or 6-Fr stent was placed solely to passively dilate the ureter before intervention a mean of 21 days (7–40) later. Ureteral dilation was done in 35 %, and an access sheath used in 48 %. Stents were left in all but one ureter, with retrieval strings in 57 %, while a second anesthetic solely to remove the stent was needed in five (10 %). Postoperative imaging was by US in 24 (46 %), CT in 14 (27 %), and KUB in 4 (10 had no imaging because of second look or were lost to follow-up). Stone-free status was 25 (50 %) patients with a single session. Patient age, gender, or stone location did not predict need for additional intervention, but 50 % of stones >6 mm had additional treatment versus none <6 mm. There were no complications (Tanaka et al. 2008).

Another series evaluated ureteral access for renal/proximal ureteral stones in 30 children. All had active dilation using an 8/10-Fr coaxial dilator. Ureteroscopy was then possible in 18 (60 %); no differences were seen in mean age (10 years) between those that were successful and those that were not. Failure was due to a small ureteral orifice ($n=3$), difficulty passing the iliac vessels ($n=4$), a narrow UPJ ($n=3$), and various other problems, such as reimplanted ureter or duplication anomaly ($n=2$). A 3.7-Fr or 4.8-Fr stent was left for 1–2 weeks for passive dilation in those with failed access, apparently with subsequent ability to reach the kidney. Early complications included two ureteral perforations, one requiring percutaneous urinoma drainage. At mean follow-up of 8 months with imaging by US (44 %), CT (23 %), or KUB (31 %), no obstruction was noted (Corcoran et al. 2008).

Staghorn Stones

One study reported SWL monotherapy to be successful after one session in 61 %, and overall in 83 % of staghorn stones.

Three studies using PCNL reported one-session success in 58–74 %. Complications included urinoma, urine leak requiring stenting, hydro-pneumothorax, hyponatremia with seizure, and transfusions.

SWL monotherapy was reported for 23 children ranging from 5 months to 12 years of age with complete ($n=6$) or partial staghorn stones with two or more caliceal branches. Stone burden was >2 cm in 91 %. Treatment used either a Sonolith 3000 or Nova machine and a maximum of 3,000 shocks per session, with no difference in results. Double-J stent was used in five (22 %) children, all >6 years of age. One-session stone-free rate was 14/23 (61 %), and overall stone-free rate with SWL monotherapy was 19 (83 %). There were no steinstrasse (Lottmann et al. 2001).

PCNL was used in 12 children mean age 12 years (4–16) for "branched stones occupying more than 1 portion of the collecting system" (AUA guideline definition for staghorn) that ranged in size from 300 to 1,150 mm^2. The 24-Fr sheaths were placed, and a pneumatic lithoclast was used. Flexible renoscopy was not done. KUB ± renal US or CT was obtained on postoperative day 1, with second-look procedures only done for known fragments. Seven patients (58 %) were considered stone-free after one session using one access. Additional procedures included three second looks (two with additional access), one SWL, and one ureteroscopy to become stone-free in 11 (92 %). Complications included one abdominal urinoma; mean hemoglobin loss was 1 mg % (apparently none transfused). Stone composition was only reported in six, with five calcium oxalate monohydrate and one struvite. Follow-up after treatment was not described (Kumar et al. 2011).

A retrospective review was done in patients with PCNL, identifying 51 children with 53 complex stones (staghorn, or stones >300 mm^2, involving more than one calyx, upper ureteral or in an anomalous kidney). Tract dilation was done to 20–30-Fr, and fragmentation used ultrasonic and pneumatic lithotripters. A single tract was sufficient in 60 % of renal units. Antegrade nephrostograms were obtained 48 h after the procedures. One treatment session was successful in 39 (74 %) renal units. Complications included 17 % transfusions, 6 % urine leaks (after nephrostomy tube removal, required double-J stenting), and 2 % hydro-pneumothorax (Ozden et al. 2008).

One other retrospective review included 38 children (69 % male), mean age 8 years (1–13), with 45 renal units having a mean stone burden of 3 cm who underwent PCNL. A complete staghorn stone was present in 12. "Stone-free" was defined as absent fragments or fragments <4 mm on KUB or renal US 2 weeks post-procedure. Single 26–30-Fr access sheaths were used to place pneumatic or ultrasonic lithotripters. Simultaneous transurethral lithotripsy was done in nine (24 %) but not further described. Based on their definition of success, 67 % were considered stone-free after one treatment. Complications included transfusion in one, hyponatremia with seizure in one (sterile water was used for irrigation in all cases), and fever for 1–7 days in eight (Etemadian et al. 2012).

Lower Pole Stones

In contrast to adults, lower pole stones in children are just as effectively treated by SWL as stones in the renal pelvis or other calyces.

One study compared SWL for lower pole stones ($n=50$) versus those in other locations for 131 children (157 kidneys) mean age 8 years (1–16). Median stone burden was 0.6 cm^2 in the lower pole. A Lithostar machine was used for one to three sessions with a mean of 1,500 shock waves per session. Outcomes were assessed at 12 weeks using US or IVP. Single-session stone-free rate for lower pole stones was 42 %, which was not different from those in other locations. Total stone-free rate and EQ was 71.5 and 43 % for the lower pole, which was also not different from stones elsewhere. One patient with a lower pole stone developed a steinstrasse (Demirkesen et al. 2006).

SWL specifically for lower calyceal stones <2.5 cm was compared between adults ($n=282$, mean age 48 ± 13 years) and children ($n=54$, mean age 48±42 months) in a retrospective review. Mean stone size was 8 mm (5–25), apparently not different between groups. The PiezoLith 3000 was used; post-treatment imaging included KUB and renal US ± CT (relative use in the two cohorts not described), with final assessment for stone-free status at 3 months. Sixty-seven percent versus 28 % of children versus adults were stone-free after one session, $p=0.001$ (Goktas et al. 2011).

Ureteroscopy for lower pole stones was reviewed in 21 children, mean age 15 years (1–20), having mean stone burden of 12 mm. In 11 (52 %), the procedure was secondary to prior SWL, ureteroscopy, or PCNL. Preoperative stenting was done in 38 % (reasons, decision-making not described). Active dilation with balloons or dilators was used in 81 and 43 % when the scope would not pass. Postoperative stenting was done in 71 %. Time for analysis to determine stone-free status was not stated; overall follow-up was mean 11 ± 14 months. Stone-free status apparently was achieved in 13 (62 %) after one treatment and overall in 76 %. Total number of procedures, including that to place and retrieve stents, was not stated. No "major" complications occurred (Cannon et al. 2007).

Anomalous Kidneys

One report indicated that PCNL could be effectively and safely performed in children with horseshoe, malrotated or cross-fused kidneys.

PCNL was described for six children, mean age 7 years (5–12), with anomalous kidneys, including three horseshoe, two malrotated, and one cross-fused. Indications were failed SWL in two and large stone burden in the others, mean surface area of 3 cm^2. All procedures were done prone in one session, including access and lithotripsy, with mean operating time of 43 min (25–70). One treatment achieved stone-free status in five, while a second look was needed in one. No child needed transfusion, and one had puncture of the renal pelvis treated with 5 days nephrostomy diversion (Abdeldaeim et al. 2011).

Treatment Effects on Renal Function

Three studies reported pre- and post-SWL renal function and scarring using nuclear renography. None reported new renal scar. Two reported no decrease in ipsilateral function, while another reported transient decrease in 2 % and decrease without recovery in 1 %.

One retrospective review reported 6 % of patients had ≥10 % ipsilateral renal function decrease after PCNL, but did not describe access sheath size or number of access sites.

A prospective study included 100 children mean age 8 years (3–14) who had DMSA and DTPA pre- and 6 months post-SWL (for those stone-free). Mean number of sessions was 1.5 (1–3), with a mean of 2,000 (800–2,600) shocks per session. Average stone size was 1 cm (8 mm–2.7 cm). Eighty-eight percent were stone-free, and none demonstrated new renal cortical scar on DMSA. Ipsilateral GFR was measured by DTPA and also unchanged in all patients (Fayad et al. 2010).

SWL was used in 182 children mean age 5 years (5 months to 20 years) over a 20-year period, for which there was pre- and ≥6 month posttreatment DMSA in 94 (52 %), who were all stone-free at follow-up imaging. Of these, three (3 %) had >5 % decrease in function, which recovered in two from a transient 8 % decrease. None developed new cortical scars. The number of treatment sessions for the entire group was one to four (mean not stated) with median 3,000 shocks per session (IQR 2,600–3,005), but data specific to those with DMSA were not provided (Griffin et al. 2010).

SWL was used for 23 complete or partial staghorn stones by Lottmann et al. (2001) described above, in 21 children ranging from 5 months to 12 years of age with complete ($n=6$) or partial staghorn stones with ≥2 caliceal branches. Stone burden was >2 cm in 91 %. Treatment used either a Sonolith 3000 or Nova machine and a maximum of 3,000 shocks per session. Total sessions used were one ($n=12$, 52 %), two ($n=8$, 35 %), 3 ($n=1$), and four ($n=2$). DMSA was obtained pre-SWL and at 6 months after treatment, with no scars of "significant changes in renal function attributable to SWL."

PCNL effects on renal function were studied in 65 children (72 kidneys), mean age 6 years (9 months to 16 years). Sizes of access sheaths were not described, nor were number of sites per kidney. Lithotripsy was done in 57 %, while the remainder had stones removed intact. DMSA scans were obtained only postoperatively, sometime during follow-up between 6 and 72 months, and were described as showing "no significant gross cortical scarring." DTPA scans apparently were done both preoperatively and postoperatively, with four (6 %) demonstrating a ≥10 % function loss (data not shown) (Dawaba et al. 2004).

Stone Fragments After SWL

One trial reported no difference in new stone formation in patients with versus those without fragments after SWL. Both groups had significantly fewer recurrences on potassium citrate therapy (6 %) than observation alone (33 %).

Ninety-six children (60 % males) had SWL, with 52 becoming stone-free and 44 having persistent stone fragments <5 mm by 4 weeks post-treatment. These patients were then randomized into two groups, one receiving potassium citrate 1 mEq/kg/day for 1 year ($n=48$, mean age 9 years), or another receiving no medication or other preventative measures ($n=48$, mean age 7 years). Stone growth was not defined other than as "enlargement" during follow-up. All radiologic assessment was by US and KUB. Duration of follow-up was mean 24 months (12–36):

- In stone-free children, recurrence was reported in 8 % on therapy versus 35 % observed, $p=0.04$.
- In residual fragment patients, recurrence was found in 5 % on therapy versus 32 % observed, $p=0.04$.
- There was no difference in new stone formation in patients who were stone-free versus those with residual fragments after SWL.

Although 24-h urine stone risk profiles were done in each patient, results were only provided for those with residual fragments, with none having hypercalciuria, 81 % having hypocitraturia, and 31 % hyperoxaluria. It was not stated if randomization resulted in equal balance of patients with metabolic abnormities into the two groups (Sarica et al. 2006).

A retrospective review had 25 children, mean age 9 years (3–14), and 26 renal units with residual fragments ≤5 mm after SWL ± additional procedures. Metabolic evaluation was done in 20, reporting hypercalciuria in 7 and cystinuria in 3 (12 %). History of stone activity before SWL was not reported. Follow-up was a mean of 48 months, with stone growth determined using US or KUB and considered an increase in diameter of ≥50 %. Nine stones met this criteria, but seven were in patients with metabolic conditions. Excluding these, 4/17 (24 %) had renal colic, and 3 had gross hematuria. Eight stones were stable, and four passed (Afshar et al. 2004).

Ureteral Stones

SWL Versus Ureteroscopy

One trial randomized children with distal ureteral stones, mean burden 36 mm², to either ureteroscopy or SWL, reporting that stone-free rates from one treatment were significantly better with ureteroscopy (82 % versus 62 %).

One patient needed reimplant following perforation during ureteroscopy.

EQ for the two procedures was not reported.

A RCT allocated 100 consecutive children with distal ureteral stones to either SWL using the Compact Delta II (mean 1,530 shock waves per session) or ureteroscopy using a 6-Fr (48 cases) or 8.5-Fr semirigid scope with holmium laser or pneumatic lithotripsy. Post-treatment imaging included US at 2 weeks and IVP at 3 months, with success defined as no stones. There were no differences in age (mean 6 years), gender (56 males), or stone burden (mean 36 mm²). Stone-free rates at 3 months were significantly greater after one treatment by ureteroscopy versus SWL, 82 % versus 62 %, $p=0.001$. In contrast to series described above and in the following section, the authors state that they did not encounter difficulties with access for ureteroscopy. In addition, they did not report postoperative ureteral stenting. Ureteral perforation occurred in two patients, one managed with a double-J stent and the other by reimplantation. Steinstrasse occurred in three following SWL but was not described, and management was not mentioned (Basiri et al. 2010).

Ureteroscopy

Three retrospective studies discussed ureteroscopy for ureteral stones in children. Two reported stone-free success greater for distal than proximal stones.

One study described passive ureteral dilation with a double-J stent in 54 %, while active orifice dilation was done in 8 and 31 % in the other two.

Two reported 1 and 4 % distal ureteral injuries with ureterovesical junction obstruction.

A retrospective multicenter analysis was done in Turkey for 642 children mean age 90±51 months managed with semi-rigid ureteroscopy and having 72 % distal, 11 % middle, and 14 % proximal ureteral stones. Mean stone burden was 9 mm (3–32). Instrument size was <8-Fr in 42 % of cases. Preoperative stenting was not described for these patients, although orifice dilation was done in 31 %. Lithotripsy was pneumatic in 55 %, holmium:YAG in 21 %, and basketing in 24 %. Mean operative time was 46 min (10–180). Mean postoperative stenting used in 62 % was 28±29 days. Stone-free status was determined by KUB±US at ≤4 weeks. At mean follow-up of 13 months (1–120), 93 % were stone-free, with significantly greater success for distal versus proximal stones, 96 % versus 82.5 % $p<0.01$. EQ was reported to be 0.93 versus 0.85 in distal versus proximal stones, but reconciliation of that calculation with procedures involving stents was not discussed. Complications occurred in 8 % of patients, including inability to access the stone (1 %), ureteral perforation (1 %), and UVJO (1 %) (Dogan et al. 2011a).

Another retrospective review included 61 consecutive patients mean age 8 years (6 months to 16 years) with ureteral stones a mean of 8 mm (4–20) that were in the distal ureter in 75 %, middle in 14 %, and upper in 11 %. An 8-Fr rigid ureteroscope was used, with balloon dilation to 15-Fr done in five (8 %). Pretreatment stenting, if done, was not described; post-treatment stenting was done in 55 %, with subsequent removal under anesthesia in 1–2 weeks. Stone-free rates were determined 1 day after surgery using KUB, reported as 90 % for distal, 67 % for middle, and 71.5 % for upper ureteral stones (significantly better for distal stones). No complications were reported (Turunc et al. 2010b).

Ureteroscopy was reviewed in 100 children, mean age 13 years (58 % female), who had stones in the kidney in 33 % and upper, middle, and distal ureter in 19 %, 11 %, and 37 %, respectively. Passive dilation with a stent was used in 54 %, and active dilation was done in 66 %. Overall stone-free rate was 91 % (not reported for various locations), with seven patients having more than one procedure. Follow-up was a mean of 10 months; complications included five perforations and four ureterovesical junction strictures needing reimplantation (Smaldone et al. 2007).

References

Abdeldaeim HM, Hamdy SA, Mokhless IA. Percutaneous nephrolithotomy for the management of stones in anomalous kidneys in children. J Pediatr Urol. 2011;7(3):239–43.

Afshar K, McLorie G, Papanikolaou F, Malek R, Harvey E, Pippi-Salle JL, et al. Outcome of small residual stone fragments following shock wave lithotripsy in children. J Urol. 2004;172(4 Pt 2):1600–3.

Alon US, Berenbom A. Idiopathic hypercalciuria of childhood: 4- to 11-year outcome. Pediatr Nephrol. 2000;14(10–11):1011–5.

Alon US, Zimmerman H, Alon M. Evaluation and treatment of pediatric idiopathic urolithiasis—revisited. Pediatr Nephrol. 2004;19(5):516–20.

Alpay H, Ozen A, Gokce I, Biyikli N. Clinical and metabolic features of urolithiasis and microlithiasis in children. Pediatr Nephrol. 2009;24(11):2203–9.

Aydogdu O, Burgu B, Gucuk A, Suer E, Soygur T. Effectiveness of doxazosin in treatment of distal ureteral stones in children. J Urol. 2009;182(6):2880–4.

Basiri A, Zare S, Tabibi A, Sharifiaghdas F, Aminsharifi A, Mousavi-Bahar SH, et al. A multicenter, randomized, controlled trial of transureteral and shock wave lithotripsy—which is the best minimally invasive modality to treat distal ureteral calculi in children? J Urol. 2010;184(3):1106–9.

Bergsland KJ, Coe FL, White MD, Erhard MJ, DeFoor WR, Mahan JD, et al. Urine risk factors in children with calcium kidney stones and their siblings. Kidney Int. 2012;81(11):1140–8.

Bilen CY, Gunay M, Ozden E, Inci K, Sarikaya S, Tekgul S. Tubeless mini percutaneous nephrolithotomy in infants and preschool children: a preliminary report. J Urol. 2010;184(6):2498–502.

Biyikli NK, Alpay H, Guran T. Hypercalciuria and recurrent urinary tract infections: incidence and symptoms in children over 5 years of age. Pediatr Nephrol. 2005;20(10):1435–8.

Cannon GM, Smaldone MC, Wu HY, Bassett JC, Bellinger MF, Docimo SG, et al. Ureteroscopic management of lower-pole stones in a pediatric population. J Endourol. 2007;21(10):1179–82.

Corcoran AT, Smaldone MC, Mally D, Ost MC, Bellinger MF, Schneck FX, et al. When is prior ureteral stent placement necessary to access the upper urinary tract in prepubertal children? J Urol. 2008;180(4 Suppl):1861–3. discussion 3–4.

Dawaba MS, Shokeir AA, Hafez AT, Shoma AM, El-Sherbiny MT, Mokhtar A, et al. Percutaneous nephrolithotomy in children: early and late anatomical and functional results. J Urol. 2004;172(3): 1078–81.

DeFoor WR, Jackson E, Minevich E, Caillat A, Reddy P, Sheldon C, et al. The risk of recurrent urolithiasis in children is dependent on urinary calcium and citrate. Urology. 2010;76(1):242–5.

Demirkesen O, Onal B, Tansu N, Altintas R, Yalcin V, Oner A. Efficacy of extracorporeal shock wave lithotripsy for isolated lower caliceal stones in children compared with stones in other renal locations. Urology. 2006;67(1):170–4. discussion 4–5.

Dogan HS, Onal B, Satar N, Aygun C, Piskin M, Tanriverdi O, et al. Factors affecting complication rates of ureteroscopic lithotripsy in children: results of multi-institutional retrospective analysis by Pediatric Stone Disease Study Group of Turkish Pediatric Urology Society. J Urol. 2011a;186(3):1035–40.

Dogan HS, Kilicarslan H, Kordan Y, Celen S, Oktay B. Percutaneous nephrolithotomy in children: does age matter? World J Urol. 2011b;29(6):725–9.

Etemadian M, Maghsoudi R, Shadpour P, Mokhtari MR, Rezaeimehr B, Shati M. Pediatric percutaneous nephrolithotomy using adult sized instruments: our experience. Urol J. 2012;9(2):465–71.

Fayad A, El-Sheikh MG, Abdelmohsen M, Abdelraouf H. Evaluation of renal function in children undergoing extracorporeal shock wave lithotripsy. J Urol. 2010;184(3):1111–4.

Garcia CD, Miller LA, Stapleton FB. Natural history of hematuria associated with hypercalciuria in children. Am J Dis Child. 1991;145(10):1204–7.

Goktas C, Akca O, Horuz R, Gokhan O, Albayrak S, Sarica K. SWL in lower calyceal calculi: evaluation of the treatment results in children and adults. Urology. 2011;78(6):1402–6.

Goktas C, Akca O, Horuz R, Gokhan O, Albayrak S, Sarica K. Does child's age affect interval to stone-free status after SWL? A critical analysis. Urology. 2012;79(5):1138–42.

Griffin SJ, Margaryan M, Archambaud F, Sergent-Alaoui A, Lottmann HB. Safety of shock wave lithotripsy for treatment of pediatric urolithiasis: 20-year experience. J Urol. 2010;183(6):2332–6.

Gurgoze MK, Sari MY. Results of medical treatment and metabolic risk factors in children with urolithiasis. Pediatr Nephrol. 2011;26(6):933–7.

Kalorin CM, Zabinski A, Okpareke I, White M, Kogan BA. Pediatric urinary stone disease—does age matter? J Urol. 2009;181(5):2267–71. discussion 71.

Karabacak OR, Ipek B, Ozturk U, Demirel F, Saltas H, Altug U. Metabolic evaluation in stone disease metabolic differences between the pediatric and adult patients with stone disease. Urology. 2010;76(1):238–41.
Kim SS, Kolon TF, Canter D, White M, Casale P. Pediatric flexible ureteroscopic lithotripsy: the Children's Hospital of Philadelphia experience. J Urol. 2008;180(6):2616–9. discussion 9.
Kit LC, Filler G, Pike J, Leonard MP. Pediatric urolithiasis: experience at a tertiary care pediatric hospital. Can Urol Assoc J. 2008;2(4):381–6.
Koyuncu H, Yencilek F, Erturhan S, Eryildirim B, Sarica K. Clinical course of pediatric urolithiasis: follow-up data in a long-term basis. Int Urol Nephrol. 2011; 43(1):7–13.
Kumar R, Anand A, Saxena V, Seth A, Dogra PN, Gupta NP. Safety and efficacy of PCNL for management of staghorn calculi in pediatric patients. J Pediatr Urol. 2011;7(3):248–51.
Landau EH, Shenfeld OZ, Pode D, Shapiro A, Meretyk S, Katz G, et al. Extracorporeal shock wave lithotripsy in prepubertal children: 22-year experience at a single institution with a single lithotriptor. J Urol. 2009;182(4 Suppl):1835–9.
Lottmann HB, Traxer O, Archambaud F, Mercier-Pageyral B. Monotherapy extracorporeal shock wave lithotripsy for the treatment of staghorn calculi in children. J Urol. 2001;165(6 Pt 2):2324–7.
MacDougall L, Taheri S, Crofton P. Biochemical risk factors for stone formation in a Scottish paediatric hospital population. Ann Clin Biochem. 2010;47(Pt 2):125–30.
McAdams S, Kim N, Ravish IR, Monga M, Ugarte R, Nerli R, et al. Stone size is only independent predictor of shock wave lithotripsy success in children: a community experience. J Urol. 2010a;184(2):659–64.
McAdams S, Kim N, Dajusta D, Monga M, Ravish IR, Nerli R, et al. Preoperative stone attenuation value predicts success after shock wave lithotripsy in children. J Urol. 2010b;184(4 Suppl):1804–9.
Milliner DS, Murphy ME. Urolithiasis in pediatric patients. Mayo Clin Proc. 1993;68(3):241–8.
Mokhless I, Zahran AR, Youssif M, Fahmy A. Tamsulosin for the management of distal ureteral stones in children: a prospective randomized study. J Pediatr Urol. 2012;8(5):544–8.
Nelson CP, Diamond DA, Cendron M, Peters CA, Cilento BG. Extracorporeal shock wave lithotripsy in pediatric patients using a late generation portable lithotriptor: experience at Children's Hospital Boston. J Urol. 2008;180(4 Suppl):1865–8.
Nerli RB, Patil SM, Guntaka AK, Hiremath MB. Flexible ureteroscopy for upper ureteral calculi in children. J Endourol. 2011;25(4):579–82.
Ozden E, Sahin A, Tan B, Dogan HS, Eren MT, Tekgul S. Percutaneous renal surgery in children with complex stones. J Pediatr Urol. 2008;4(4):295–8.
Penido MG, Lima EM, Marino VS, Tupinamba AL, Franca A, Souto MF. Bone alterations in children with idiopathic hypercalciuria at the time of diagnosis. Pediatr Nephrol. 2003;18(2):133–9.
Polito C, Apicella A, Marte A, Signoriello G, La Manna A. Clinical presentation and metabolic features of overt and occult urolithiasis. Pediatr Nephrol. 2012;27(1):101–7.
Samad L, Aquil S, Zaidi Z. Paediatric percutaneous nephrolithotomy: setting new frontiers. BJU Int. 2006;97(2):359–63.
Sarica K, Erturhan S, Yurtseven C, Yagci F. Effect of potassium citrate therapy on stone recurrence and regrowth after extracorporeal shockwave lithotripsy in children. J Endourol. 2006;20(11):875–9.
Schwaderer AL, Cronin R, Mahan JD, Bates CM. Low bone density in children with hypercalciuria and/or nephrolithiasis. Pediatr Nephrol. 2008;23(12): 2209–14.
Shokeir AA, Sheir KZ, El-Nahas AR, El-Assmy AM, Eassa W, El-Kappany HA. Treatment of renal stones in children: a comparison between percutaneous nephrolithotomy and shock wave lithotripsy. J Urol. 2006;176(2):706–10.
Singh A, Alter HJ, Littlepage A. A systematic review of medical therapy to facilitate passage of ureteral calculi. Ann Emerg Med. 2007;50(5):552–63.
Smaldone MC, Cannon Jr GM, Wu HY, Bassett J, Polsky EG, Bellinger MF, et al. Is ureteroscopy first line treatment for pediatric stone disease? J Urol. 2007;178(5):2128–31. discussion 31.
Smith PJ, Basravi S, Schlomer BJ, Bush NC, Brown BJ, Gingrich A, et al. Comparative analysis of nephrolithiasis in otherwise healthy versus medically complex gastrostomy fed children. J Pediatr Urol. 2011;7(3):244–7.
Spivacow FR, Negri AL, del Valle EE, Calvino I, Fradinger E, Zanchetta JR. Metabolic risk factors in children with kidney stone disease. Pediatr Nephrol. (Berlin, Germany). 2008;23(7):1129–33.
Tabel Y, Mir S. The long-term outcomes of idiopathic hypercalciuria in children. J Pediatr Urol. 2006;2(5): 453–8.
Tanaka ST, Makari JH, Pope IV JC, Adams MC, Brock III JW, Thomas JC. Pediatric ureteroscopic management of intrarenal calculi. J Urol. 2008;180(5):2150–3. discussion 3–4.
Tekin A, Tekgul S, Atsu N, Sahin A, Ozen H, Bakkaloglu M. A study of the etiology of idiopathic calcium urolithiasis in children: hypocitruria is the most important risk factor. J Urol. 2000;164(1):162–5.
Tekin A, Tekgul S, Atsu N, Bakkaloglu M, Kendi S. Oral potassium citrate treatment for idiopathic hypocitruria in children with calcium urolithiasis. J Urol. 2002;168(6):2572–4.
Turunc T, Gonen M, Kuzgunbay B, Bilgilisoy UT, Dirim A, Tekin MI, et al. The effects of hydronephrosis and stone burden on success rates of shockwave lithotripsy in pediatric population. J Endourol. 2010a;24(6): 1037–41.
Turunc T, Kuzgunbay B, Gul U, Kayis AA, Bilgilisoy UT, Aygun C, et al. Factors affecting the success of ureteroscopy in management of ureteral stone diseases in children. J Endourol. 2010b;24(8):1273–7.

Index

W.T. Snodgrass (ed.), *Pediatric Urology: Evidence for Optimal Patient Management*,
DOI 10.1007/978-1-4614-6910-0, © Springer Science+Business Media New York 2013